D1707627

Evaluating Drug Literature

Evaluating Drug Literature
A Statistical Approach

Richard L. Slaughter, M.Sc., FCCP
Professor and Chair
Department of Pharmacy Practice
College of Pharmacy and Allied
    Health Professions
Wayne State University
DETROIT, MICHIGAN

David J. Edwards, Pharm.D.
Professor
Department of Pharmacy Practice
College of Pharmacy and Allied
    Health Professions
Wayne State University
DETROIT, MICHIGAN

McGraw-Hill
Medical Publishing Division

*New York   Chicago   San Francisco   Lisbon   London   Madrid   Mexico City
Milan   New Delhi   San Juan   Seoul   Singapore   Sydney   Toronto*

McGraw-Hill

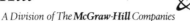

A Division of The **McGraw·Hill** Companies

Evaluating Drug Literature: A Statistical Approach

1 2 3 4 5 6 7 8 9 0 DOC/DOC 0 9 8 7 6 5 4 3 2 1

ISBN 0-07-134729-1

This book was set in Horley Oldstyle by North Market Street Graphics.
Project management was provided by North Market Street Graphics.
The production manager was Clare B. Stanley.
The cover designer was Aimee Nordin.
The index was prepared by North Market Street Graphics.
R.R. Donnelley & Sons was printer and binder.

This book is printed on acid-free paper.

Library of Congress Cataloging-in-Publication Data

Slaughter, Richard L.
    Evaluating drug literature : a statistical approach / Richard L. Slaughter,
David J. Edwards.
        p. cm.
    Includes bibliographical references.
    ISBN 0-07-134729-1
        1. Pharmacy—Research.   2. Statistics.   3. Pharmacy—Statistical methods.
I. Edwards, David J., Pharm.D.   II. Title.
RS122.S58 2001
615'.1'0727—dc21
                                                                        00-045206

CONTENTS

Contributors   vii

Preface   ix

Chapter 1
Introduction to Drug Literature   1
Richard L. Slaughter

Chapter 2
Searching Drug Literature   17
Richard L. Slaughter and Ellen Marks

Chapter 3
The Publication Process   39
David J. Edwards

Chapter 4
Classification of Study Design: Observational Research   63
David J. Edwards

Chapter 5
Study Design: Experimental Research   83
David J. Edwards

Chapter 6
Data Measurement, Description, and Presentation   105
David J. Edwards

Chapter 7
Concepts in Inferential Statistics: Distributions,
Confidence Intervals, and Hypothesis Testing   127
David J. Edwards

Chapter 8
Evaluating Statistical Results: Parametric Tests   153
Richard L. Slaughter

Chapter 9
Evaluating Statistical Results: Nonparametric Tests   179
Richard L. Slaughter

Chapter 10
Evaluating Statistical Results: Correlation, Regression,
Survival Life Analysis   201
Richard L. Slaughter

Chapter 11
Critical Appraisal of Meta-analysis   229
John Devlin

Chapter 12
Evaluating Pharmacoeconomic Literature   249
James G. Stevenson and Daniel R. Touchette

Chapter 13
Managing Uncertainty in Decision Analysis
with Sensitivity Analysis   269
James G. Stevenson, Daniel R. Touchette,
Muhammad M. Mamdani, and R. Michael Massanari

Chapter 14
Ethical Concerns in Drug Research and Literature Evaluation   295
David J. Edwards

Chapter 15
The Future of Drug Information and the Internet   313
Richard L. Slaughter

Answer Key   333
Appendix A. *z*-Score for a Normal Distribution   347
Appendix B. The *t* Distribution   349
Appendix C. The χ^2 Distribution   351
Appendix D. *F*-Table for $p < 0.05$ and $p < 0.01$ 352
Appendix E. Health Care–Related Web Sites   354
Glossary   357
Index   361

CONTRIBUTORS

John Devlin, Pharm.D., BCPS
Clinical Pharmacy Specialist, Surgery/Critical Care
Detroit Receiving Hospital and University Health Center
Adjunct Assistant Professor of Pharmacy Practice
College of Pharmacy and Allied Health Professions
Wayne State University
DETROIT, MICHIGAN

David J. Edwards, Pharm.D.
Professor
Department of Pharmacy Practice
College of Pharmacy and Allied Health Professions
Wayne State University
DETROIT, MICHIGAN

Muhammad M. Mamdani, Pharm.D., M.A., M.P.H.
University of Toronto
Institute for Clinical Evaluative Sciences
NORTH YORK, ONTARIO, CANADA

Ellen Marks, M.S. in L.S.
Director, Shiffman Medical Library
Wayne State University
DETROIT, MICHIGAN

R. Michael Massanari, M.D., M.S.
Director, Center for Healthcare Effectiveness Research
Professor of Medicine and Community Medicine
Wayne State University School of Medicine
DETROIT, MICHIGAN

Richard L. Slaughter, M.Sc., FCCP
Professor and Chair
Department of Pharmacy Practice
College of Pharmacy and Allied Health Professions
Wayne State University
DETROIT, MICHIGAN

James G. Stevenson, Pharm.D.
Director of Pharmacy Services
University of Michigan Health System
Professor and Associate Dean for Clinical Services
College of Pharmacy
University of Michigan Hospitals
ANN ARBOR, MICHIGAN

Daniel R. Touchette, Pharm.D.
Assistant Professor of Pharmacy Practice
Pharmacoeconomics and Outcomes Research
Colleges of Pharmacy
Oregon State University
PORTLAND, OREGON

PREFACE

Accessing, evaluating, and disseminating information are integral parts of the profession of pharmacy. As one of the most trusted and accessible professionals, pharmacists have to respond routinely to questions concerning drug therapy from patients and health care professionals. Easy access of information through the Internet, increased media exposure concerning pharmaceuticals, and direct-to-consumer advertising by pharmaceutical companies are just some of the reasons consumers are more educated and involved in their health care. Patients are savvier and bring many more questions about the treatment of their disease to pharmacists. A pharmacist is utilized as much as a resource of drug information as a provider of medications. These efforts have coincided with professional changes that are shifting the role of the pharmacist toward greater responsibility for the overall care of the pharmacy needs of patients. This is recognized by the accrediting guidelines established by the American Council on Pharmaceutical Education. Standard No. 10, "Professional Competencies and Outcome," states that students who are in pharmacy programs should be able to retrieve, evaluate, and manage professional information and literature. Further drug information and literature evaluation are required core components of the pharmacy curriculum. The importance of information and education in the practice of pharmacy is reinforced by the following goal of the American Pharmaceutical Association, which was adopted in January 2000:

> Goal 2: Equip pharmacists and others allied to the profession with information and education resources to support provision of patient care.

The ability of the pharmacists to retrieve and interpret information is an integral component of everyday practice. The primary purpose of this textbook, *Evaluating Drug Literature: A Statistical Approach,* is to focus not only on the retrieval of information but also on how drug information is presented, accessed, and evaluated by the end user. How journals are using the Internet and how the Internet is used to deliver drug information are discussed.

The chapters on statistics will introduce the reader to statistical procedures. They are designed such that prior exposure to basic statistical concepts is beneficial. While an introduction to confidence intervals is given, the chapters focus heavily on hypothesis testing that evaluates the probability that a null hypothesis statement occurs by chance alone. Basic parametric and nonparametric tests are covered with a focus on understanding the factors that are important in evaluating the statistical results. Some exposure is given to the mathematics of statistics; however, the relationships that are derived from equations are emphasized. Application to specific literature examples is provided throughout these chapters.

We have used several techniques to enhance reader understanding of what at times can be a complex topic. Throughout the text, we have used Key Concept boxes to highlight key elements being discussed. These allow the reader to focus on those areas that are critical for understanding these important concepts. These are also used to help simplify and demystify some of the statistical components addressed. Examples are broadly used throughout the text. Each chapter includes examples, or case studies, taken from recent drug literature to illustrate how to apply principles to actual examples of published literature. These are designed to illustrate and reinforce in a practical manner specific issues discussed. At the end of each chapter is a set of study questions (with an answer key preceding the appendixes). These are primarily based on recent literature examples that reinforce the understanding of the principal concepts that were reviewed. Finally, a listing of health- and drug-related Web addresses is provided in Appendix E at the end of the book. These should serve as an easy source of sites from which to build personal bookmarks that will facilitate searching for information on the World Wide Web.

This book is not a drug information textbook and it is not a statistics text. Rather, it is a book on how to retrieve and interpret information found. This text is designed for use in courses that focus on drug literature evaluation. A strong focus is given on study design and statistics, as these are the cornerstones of interpreting primary drug literature. Some chapters have been included that go beyond basic statistics. These include a chapter on meta-analysis, which has become an increasingly important process that is used to make more definitive conclusions on therapeutic comparisons. Chapters are also included that introduce the reader to concepts important for the evaluation of pharmacoeconomic literature.

This book will assist pharmacy students and pharmacists in being able to retrieve drug literature. Their skill in evaluating and interpreting literature, including study design and statistical procedures, will be enhanced by this text. It is hoped that this will lead to informed decision making concerning drug therapy issues that relate to specific patients.

Chapter 1

Introduction to Drug Literature

Richard L. Slaughter

OUTLINE

Goals and Objectives

Importance of Drug Literature

Sources of Drug Literature

    Tertiary Drug Literature

    Secondary Drug Literature

    Primary Drug Literature

Online Drug Literature

Summary

Study Questions

References

KEY WORDS

Case reports
Internet
Online
Pharmacoeconomic studies
Primary
Research studies
Secondary
Tertiary

Goals and Objectives

The goal of this chapter is to introduce the reader to the different types and formats of drug literature. The objectives are as follows:

1. To explain the difference between primary, secondary, and tertiary literature
2. To review examples of tertiary drug literature

1

3. To provide examples of commonly used sources of secondary literature such as Medline, *Current Contents,* and Toxline

4. To provide examples of the different types of primary literature, including clinical studies, pharmacoeconomic studies, adverse drug reaction literature, and case reports

5. To introduce the Internet as a source of drug information

Importance of Drug Literature

The ability of a pharmacist to access and evaluate sources of drug literature is an important component of pharmacy practice. Pharmacists today are as much purveyors of information about drugs as they are dispensers of medications. The ability of pharmacists to provide up-to-date knowledge about drug products and their ability to counsel patients on the proper use of medications was identified as a major reason for the selection of a pharmacist by older patients.[1] Practicing pharmacists are inundated with information coming from a wide variety of sources. These typically include promotional materials provided by drug company representatives, peer-reviewed and non-peer-reviewed journal articles, textbook information, information available through public resources, and online information. The rate of growth of drug literature is expansive. Practicing pharmacists need to be able to read and evaluate this information and be capable of disseminating this information to the wide variety of clients they serve. As a result of recent technology developments and changes in drug advertising, patients have direct access to drug information prior to seeing their pharmacist or physician. The ready availability and use of the Internet for communications is further accelerating the growth of drug information at an unprecedented pace. Direct-to-consumer prescription drug advertising through broadcast media (TV and radio), Web sites, and printed advertisements increases awareness of prescription drugs by consumers. This translates into more questions to pharmacists to clarify issues raised by these types of advertisements. It has been estimated that as many as 12.1 million people have asked for and received a prescription as a result of this type of advertising. This results in enhanced need of the pharmacists to be able to retrieve and interpret drug information. A survey indicates that older patients (greater than 60 years of age) seek pharmacists who guide them on how to use prescribed medications. A major consideration on how older consumers decide which pharmacies to obtain their medications from is the level of information received by the pharmacy.

Drug literature serves pharmacists in many purposes. These include the following:

- Providing information in response to questions concerning drug products from patients and health care workers (physicians, nurses) who are involved in the prescribing of pharmaceuticals.
- Preparing documents (newsletters, presentations) on therapeutic issues.

• Preparing evaluations of drug products for inclusion in drug formularies.

• Updating knowledge about drug therapy issues for personal growth and education.

On a daily basis, every pharmacist is exposed to literature in some format concerning the use of drugs. The ability to retrieve and interpret literature for one's own consumption and for the delivery of services should be a part of every pharmacist's practice.

Sources of Drug Literature

Drug information can be obtained from a wide variety of sources, ranging from published clinical research studies, review articles in peer review journals, textbooks, compendia, and newsletters to information available through the World Wide Web. Drug literature sources can be divided into *primary, secondary,* and *tertiary* sources of information. Each type of source will be overviewed.

Tertiary Drug Literature

Tertiary literature contains information about a topic that has been compiled from primary reference sources. Examples of tertiary literature include textbooks, review articles, and compendia. Table 1-1 shows some examples of tertiary sources of drug information. An advantage of tertiary resources is that they provide information on a given topic that someone else has already compiled. Often the bibliographies can be used as an excellent source of secondary literature. This is particularly true for review articles, which often will have very exhaustive and complete bibliographies. The disadvantage of tertiary literature is that the information presented can be out of date because of the lag time associated with preparing and publishing the information. For published reviews this will typically be 12 to 18 months while for textbooks it will commonly exceed 2 years. The frequency with which new editions are published will provide an assessment of how current a given text may be. As an example, the following are commonly used textbooks with different time periods for new editions that will reflect how current the information is in each text. The *AHFS Drug Information* text published by the American Society of Health-System Pharmacists is a publication of drug monographs that is updated on annual basis. Further monographs are updated by fax throughout the year. This is an example of a textbook that remains as current as is feasible. Another example is the therapeutics textbook *Pharmacotherapy: A Pathophysiologic Approach,* published by Appleton & Lange. This is currently being updated every 2 years, so that information presented is dated by approximately 3 years (given the publication lag time). This text is reasonably current, although it will become dated toward the time for a new edition to appear. In contrast, the most recent edition of the pharmacology textbook *Pharmacological Basis of Therapeutics* [9th ed; JG Hardman, AG Gilman, LE Limbird (eds), McGraw-Hill, New York] is updated every 5 years. This textbook tends to be out of date after 3 years or so

TABLE 1-1. **Examples of Tertiary Literature**

Textbooks	*Applied Therapeutics*
	Pharmacotherapy: A Pathophysiologic Approach
	Textbook of Therapeutics
	Applied Biopharmaceutics and Pharmacokinetics
	Drug Interactions
	Goodman & Gilman's Pharmacological Basis of Therapeutics
	Handbook of Nonprescription Medications
Compendia	*American Society of Health-System Pharmacists Formulary Service*
	Drug Facts and Comparisons
	Physician's Desk Reference (PDR)
	Handbook of Injectable Drugs
Review articles	
Online sources	Mosby's GenRx: www.mosby.com/mosby/open/hfea_genr
	RxList: www.rxlist.com

into a given edition. Some instructors will supplement or replace this text with another pharmacology text when it is felt the information is too dated.

Often tertiary literature is the first source that pharmacists will use in answering questions. Common examples include the package insert material for a given drug, or texts that are common in pharmacies, such as *Drug Facts and Comparisons* or the *Physician's Desk Reference.* Unfortunately, tertiary resources are limited in their utility because they are not as current as primary drug information sources. Often the information needed to provide an answer to a question cannot be found in a tertiary source, requiring the use of primary literature. The other disadvantage is that the information presented represents the biases of the authors, as tertiary references are not subjected to the same peer review process that is applied to primary references.

KEY CONCEPT

Tertiary literature consists primarily of textbooks or review articles that have compiled information on a topic from primary literature sources.

Secondary Drug Literature

Secondary drug literature involves sources that are used to find information from other sources of drug information. These may include primary sources, as discussed in the next section, or tertiary sources (see preceding section) such as review articles, newsletters, and other sources of cited literature. Secondary literature is used to identify primary literature sources that can be used to answer a specific question. In the past these indexes have been primarily available in printed format. However, in recent years these have shifted to being available in electronic form, with many being easy to use from a desktop personal computer. Examples of index services that were available and frequently used in print format included *Index Medicus, Current Contents, International Pharmaceutical Abstracts,* and the *Iowa Drug Information System.* Table 1-2 provides a summary of sources of secondary literature.

Currently, numerous online databases are available free of charge. It is possible to perform literature searches using an online database that will provide an immediate listing of sources relating to a search. In addition, online abstracts are available. For a fee, actual reproductions of articles can be forwarded to a specified e-mail address. However, more and more frequently full-text articles are becoming available at no charge. Examples of online databases, with Web address and database descriptions, are provided in Table 1-3. Chapter 2 provides more detail on the application of online databases and reviews methods of searching Medline using the search tool PubMed.

TABLE 1-2. **Examples of Secondary Literature Sources**

Source	Description
Current Contents	Provides tables of contents of over 1000 publications; published weekly
Index Medicus	Index of over 3000 journals; published monthly
International Pharmaceutical Abstracts	Abstracting service for information relevant to pharmacy and pharmaceutical sciences; published semimonthly; includes information from over 750 pharmaceutical, medical, and health-related journals
Iowa Drug Information System	Index service that can retrieve complete articles; published monthly; provides access to information on drugs and human drug therapy found in the primary literature of over 190 medical and pharmaceutical journals
Medline	Database of biomedical literature containing about 370,000 references; available in CD-ROM or online
Science Citation Index	Index that provides citation frequency for authors' journal articles; updated weekly

TABLE 1-3. **Examples of Online Secondary Literature Sources**

Source	Web Address	Comments
PubMed	www.ncbi.nlm.nih.gov/PubMed	Free online Medline service
Current Contents	www.isinet.com	
Science Citation Index	www.isinet.com	
Biosis	www.biosis.org	Databases such as Toxline available through online vendors such as OVID
BIDS Embase	www.bids.ac.uk	Provides access to the *Excerpta Medica* database providing international coverage of drug-related research
Center Watch	www.centerwatch.com	Listing of clinical trials and new drug approvals
Medscape	www.medscape.com	Access to Medline, AIDSline, Toxline, and free full-text online articles

KEY CONCEPT

Secondary literature consists primarily of databases, such as Medline, that are used to identify primary sources of drug information.

Primary Drug Literature

The most direct source of drug information is primary literature, which consists of articles in journals that publish the results of research studies. These studies are typically published in journals that use both editorial and peer review to ascertain the quality and reputability of a study before presenting it to the journal's readership. The accuracy of information in primary literature is a function of the authors of the manuscript and the rigors of the peer review process used before publishing. Readers should always know whether the journals they are reading are peer reviewed. Those that are peer reviewed provide for detailed critiques of manuscripts by experts in the field of study prior to publication. This process provides for a higher-quality, more reliable product than that of journals that are not peer-reviewed.

Not all journals are peer reviewed, and peer-reviewed journals often have sections that are not reviewed. Some peer-reviewed journals will publish supplements on meetings or symposia that focus on a specific drug or disease state. Often these supplements are sponsored by pharmaceutical companies, and they may or may not be peer reviewed. For example, the journal *Pharmacotherapy* frequently publishes supplements, such as the supplement titled "Progress in the Treatment of Epilepsy" that appeared with the August 2000 issue. The editor notes on the inside cover that all of the manuscripts in the supplement underwent the normal peer review process. However, this supplement was based on the proceedings of a closed symposium supported by an educational grant from Novartis Pharmaceuticals Corporation. Although still peer reviewed, one of the main purposes of this supplement was to provide educational material on Novartis's new antiepileptic drug Trileptal (oxcarbazepine) in a format more scientifically acceptable than advertising. Other supplements may not undergo any peer review process and can be more easily influenced by the sponsoring company.

It should be realized, however, that even in non-peer-reviewed journals manuscripts are typically screened and edited by the editorial staff. Examples of non-peer-reviewed journals include *Drug Topics* and *US Pharmacist*. The subject of peer review is covered in detail in Chap. 3. Examples of pharmacy journals that publish peer-reviewed clinical studies are shown in Table 1-4. Journals that publish clinical pharmacology and clinical pharmacokinetic studies include *Clinical Pharmacology and Therapeutics* and the *Journal of Clinical Pharmacology*. Other commonly used journals that are good sources of primary drug literature include the *New England Journal of Medicine, Annals of Internal Medicine, Archives of Internal Medicine,* and the *Journal of the American Medical Association.* These journals provide information and studies with a general drug and health focus. Specialty journals publish clinical studies in areas related to that specialty. Examples include the *Journal of Infectious Diseases,* the *Journal of Allergy and Clinical Immunology, American Review of Respiratory Diseases, Cancer,* and the *American Heart Journal.* Primary literature can also be characterized as clinical studies, pharmacoeconomic studies, studies that focus on adverse drug reactions (ADRs), and case reports. This chapter briefly overviews the general types of studies commonly found in drug literature, while a more detailed analysis is presented in Chap. 4.

KEY CONCEPT

Primary literature describes the result of research studies or case reports.

Clinical Studies. Clinical studies involve the comparison of two or more drugs. The comparison may be between an active drug and a placebo, or between two or more drugs. The endpoint may be mortality (how many patients died); endpoints may also be clinical in nature, such as control of blood pressure, or they may be phar-

TABLE 1-4. **Examples of Peer-Reviewed Pharmacy Journals**

Journal Title	Organization
American Journal of Health-Systems Pharmacy	American Society of Health-Systems Pharmacists
American Journal of Pharmaceutical Education	American Association of Colleges of Pharmacy
American Pharmacy	American Pharmaceutical Association
Annals of Pharmacotherapy	
Consultant Pharmacist	American Society of Consultant Pharmacists
Journal of Managed Care Pharmacy	Academy of Managed Care Pharmacy
Journal of Pharmacy Teaching	
Pharmacotherapy	American College of Clinical Pharmacy

macokinetic [drug clearance, area under the serum concentration vs. time curve (AUC)]. The number of patients studied may vary from small numbers (6 to 8 per treatment group) to numbers that are very large (10,000 per treatment group). Patient numbers typically depend on the endpoint reached and the degree of difference expected between the treatment groups.

EXAMPLES

The following is an example of a clinical study published in the *New England Journal of Medicine.*

> Johnson DW, Jacobson S, Edney PC, Hadfield P, Mundy ME, Shuh S: A comparison of nebulized budesonide, intramuscular dexamethasone, and placebo for moderately severe croup. N Eng J Med 339:498–503, 1998.

This study compared 4 mg of nebulized budesonide, 0.6 mg/kg of intramuscular dexamethasone, and placebo in children with moderately severe croup. A total of 144 children were studied, with 49 in the placebo group, 48 in the budesonide group, and 47 in the dexamethasone group. The primary endpoint was hospitalization; secondary endpoints were the change in croup score and the number of additional raceepinephrine treatments. The results of this study can be used to determine if nebulized budesonide can be used to treat croup in children.

The following is an example of a clinical study performed in healthy volunteers with pharmacokinetic endpoints.

Kantola T, Kivisto KT, Neuvonen PJ: Erythromycin and verapamil considerably increase serum simvastatin and simvastatin acid concentrations. Clin Pharmacol Ther 64:177–182, 1998.

In this study 8 male and 4 female healthy volunteers (ages 20 to 29 years) received 500 mg erythromycin, 80 mg verapamil, or placebo orally three times a day for 2 days. On day 2 they received 40 mg simvastatin. The primary endpoints of this study were pharmacokinetic variables (C_{max}, t_{max}, AUC, and $t_{1/2}$) of simvastatin and simvastatin acid. The results of this study can be used to determine if the pharmacokinetics of simvastatin and simvastatin acid are influenced by erythromycin or verapamil.

Pharmacoeconomic Literature. Pharmacoeconomic literature assesses the economic implications of drug use. These studies will be similar in design to clinical studies; however, they will have a measure of drug costs or health care costs as a primary endpoint. There are various types of pharmacoeconomic studies, which other texts deal with in more detail [JL Bootman, RJ Townsend, WF McGhan (eds): *Principles of Pharmacoeconomics,* Harvey Whitney, 1991]. These studies can be classified as cost minimization, cost-effectiveness, cost-benefit, and cost-utility studies. A *cost minimization* study analyzes and compares two or more treatments of equal efficacy with the goal of showing cost differences between treatments. A *cost-effectiveness* study assesses differences in both cost and efficacy between two or more treatments. A *cost-benefit* analysis evaluates and assesses both the costs of treatment and the costs associated with the consequences of treatment. A *cost-utility* analysis studies the consequences of treatment in terms of quality of life and the willingness to pay for one treatment over another. See Chap. 12 for more information on pharmacoeconomic literature.

KEY CONCEPT

Pharmacoeconomic studies evaluate the effect of treatment on cost, disease outcomes, and quality of life.

EXAMPLES

Cost Minimization. This study is an example of a study that compares costs of antihypertensive therapy across five classes of drugs in patients with equivalent responses.

Hilleman DE, Mohiuddin SM, Lucas BD Jr., Stading JA, Stoysich AM, Ryschon K: Cost-minimization analysis of initial antihypertensive therapy in patients with mild-to-moderate essential diastolic hypertension. Clin Ther 16:88–102, 1994.

This was a retrospective study assessing total costs of therapy in patients with controlled mild to moderate hypertension who were treated with monotherapy. Mean total costs by drug class were reported as $895 for beta blockers, $1043 for diuretics, $1165 for centrally acting α_2 agonists, $1243 for angiotensin converting enzyme (ACE) inhibitors, and $1425 for calcium channel blockers. This study shows that with equal efficacy, beta blockers are the least expensive therapy and calcium channel blockers are the most expensive therapy for the management of mild to moderate hypertension.

Cost Effectiveness. The following is an example of a study that compares two treatments that differ in efficacy and cost between two treatment groups.

> Hempel AG, Wagner ML, Maaty MA, Sage JI: Pharmacoeconomic analysis of using Sinemet CR over standard Sinemet in parkinsonian patients with motor fluctuations. Ann Pharmacother 32:878–883, 1998.

This study was a retrospective study of the charts of patients who had been maintained on Sinemet therapy for at least 6 months and then switched to Sinemet CR for at least 6 months. Prior to conversion to Sinemet CR, the mean number of hours without chorea was 6.12 h, which increased to 8.32 h while on Sinemet CR. The total daily drug costs were higher on Sinemet CR ($10.03 vs. $8.26). However, the cost-effectiveness ratio (daily cost of therapy/daily hours without chorea) was calculated to be lower with Sinemet CR (3.70 vs. 6.55).

Cost Utility. The following study is an example that demonstrates equal efficacy between two treatment groups with a difference in the two groups in quality of life measurements.

> Testa A, Anderson RB, Nackley JF, Hollenberg NK, and the Quality of Life Hypertension Study Group: Quality of life and antihypertensive therapy in men. N Engl J Med 328:907–913, 1993.

This study compared the effects of enalapril, captopril, and placebo on blood pressure and quality of life. Changes in quality of life were compared to changes in life events, such as divorce or major personal illness. This study was performed in 379 men with mild to moderate hypertension; 192 were randomized to captopril treatment and 187 to enalapril. Blood pressure response was equivalent between the two groups, while captopril-treated patients had a more favorable quality of life than those treated with enalapril. The magnitude of differences between groups corresponded to life events such as major change in work responsibilities, in-law troubles, or mortgage foreclosure.

Adverse Drug Reaction (ADR) Literature. Adverse drug reaction literature assesses the incidence of ADRs and provides an indication for the overall importance that a specific ADR may have for a given drug. Some investigators have established algorithms or protocols to establish the probability that an adverse event is related to a given drug.[2,3,4] This literature can be used to determine the overall safety of a given drug. Decisions by either the Food and Drug Administration (FDA) or drug companies concerning the safe use of drugs are made from this literature.

EXAMPLE

In 1996 dexfenfluramine was approved by the FDA for the long-term treatment of obesity and was frequently used in combination with phentermine in a combination known as "fen-phen." After the occurrence of cardiac valvular insufficiency in 33 women who had taken the combination, the FDA issued a public health advisory in July 1997. Subsequent to these reports, the manufacturer discontinued marketing fenfluramine and dexfenfluramine. The following report definitely associates valvular dysfunction with the use of fenfluramine, dexfenfluramine, and their combination.

> Kjan MA, Herzog CA, St. Peter JV, Hartley GG, Madlon-Kay R, Dick CD, Asinger RW, Vessey JT: The prevalence of cardiac valvular insufficiency assessed by transthoracic echocardiography in obese patients treated with appetite-suppressant drugs. N Engl J Med 339:713–718, 1998.

In this study, the occurrence of valvular dysfunction assessed from echocardiography was compared in patients who participated in appetite suppressant studies ($n = 257$) to a group of matched controls ($n = 239$). The incidence of cardiac valve abnormalities was 1.3% in the control subjects, 12.8% in patients exposed only to dexfenfluramine, 22.6% in patients exposed to dexfenfluramine and phentermine, and 25.2% in patients given fenfluramine and phentermine. When compared to control subjects, the odds ratio of having cardiac valve abnormalities on fenfluramine and phentermine was 26.3 (95% confidence interval: 7.9–87.1). This study demonstrated the high risk of cardiac valvular disorders associated with long-term appetite suppressant therapy and provided further justification for the removal of these products from the market.

Case Reports. Case reports present interesting or unusual clinical findings in either a single patient or a small number of patients. They frequently are used to justify larger studies that identify the incidence and possible mechanism of the event or reaction identified in the case report. Several journals (e.g., *Annals of Pharmacotherapy, Pharmacotherapy, New England Journal of Medicine,* and *Annals of Internal Medicine*) have specific sections devoted to case reports.

EXAMPLE

The following is an example of a case report.

> Michalets EL, Smith LK, Van Tassel ED: Torsade de pointes resulting from the addition of droperidol to an existing cytochrome P450 drug interaction. Ann Pharmacother 1998; 32:761–765.

This report describes the occurrence of a serious ventricular tachyarrhythmia, torsade de pointes, in a patient who was receiving long-term fluoxetine and cyclobenzaprine therapy. Fluoxetine is a known inhibitor of the cytochrome P450 isozymes CYP2D6 and CYP3A4. The combination of fluoxetine and cyclobenzaprine resulted in prolongation of the QT interval in this patient. This woman experienced torsade de pointes, which progressed to ventricular fibrillation after the administration of droperidol, a butyrophenone derivative with class III antiarrythmic effects. A more detailed study evaluating this potentially serious drug interaction would be justified based on this case report.

Online Drug Literature

A growing amount of literature about pharmaceuticals is available online through the Internet. This includes information from sources ranging in credibility from pharmaceutical companies and colleges of pharmacy to private individuals who post whatever information they desire. Examples of online sources of information that may be relevant to drug therapy are provided in Table 1-5. These include sites for national organizations such as the National Institutes of Health, addresses for professional organizations such as the American Society of Health-System Pharmacists, journal sites, and listings for colleges of pharmacy and pharmaceutical companies. Colleges of pharmacies can be accessed through the Virtual Library Pharmacy, located at www.cpb.uokhsc.edu/pharmacy. A listing of pharmaceutical companies on the Web is provided at www.pharminfo.com/phrmlink.html#drugs _RandD by the Pharmaceutical Information Network.

A major difference between printed and online literature is that online literature may not be reviewed. This can result in a wide range in quality of information about a given topic. For example, a search using the search engine Infoseek (www.infoseek.com) for thrombolytic therapy and stroke resulted in 198 hits. As an example, one was very useful, the American Heart Association Guide to Heparin Therapy at www.amhrt.org/Scientific/statements/1994/039401.html. Another useful site was Grand Rounds at Froedtert Hospital, with a page entitled "Stroke," at www.grand-rounds.com/2no6.html. Also included in the search was a news-type article entitled "Angioplasty has Edge over 'Clot-Busting' Drugs Study Finds," published by Newstand@thrive. It was found at www.thriveonline.com/news-stand/todays/times3.06-05-97.html. This article provides a news summary of an article published in the *New England Journal of Medicine* comparing angioplasty to thrombolytic therapy in patients with heart attacks. More accurate information can be obtained by accessing the original article.

Online searches can provide very rapid response to questions. However, the lack of review of material requires that this information be reviewed and evaluated more critically than that of traditional printed media. The ready availability of this information to the public at large will increase the number of pharmacy- and drug therapy–related questions provided to health care providers.

TABLE 1-5. **Examples of Online Sources of Drug Information**

Description	Web Address
National organizations	
Food and Drug Administration	www.fda.gov
National Library of Medicine	www.nlm.nih.gov
Centers for Disease Control	www.cdc.gov
National Institutes of Health	www.nih.gov
Professional organizations	
American Society of Health-System Pharmacists	www.ashp.org
American Pharmaceutical Association	www.aphanet.org
American College of Clinical Pharmacy	www.accp.com
American Association of Colleges of Pharmacy	www.aacp.org
American Heart Association	www.amhrt.org
American Diabetes Association	www.diabetes.org
American Cancer Society	www.cancer.org
Journals	
Annals of Internal Medicine	www.acponline.org/journals/annals/annaltoc.htm
The Lancet	www.thelancet.com/newlancet
New England Journal of Medicine	www.nejm.com
Archives of Internal Medicine	www.ama-assn.org/public/journals/inte/intehome.htm
Journal of the American Medical Association (*JAMA*)	www.ama-assn.org/public/journals/jama/jamahome.htm
British Medical Journal	www.bmj.com
Colleges of pharmacy (listing of all colleges and schools)	www.pharmacy.org/schools.html
Pharmaceutical companies	
Listing of companies	www.pharminfo.com/phrmlink.html#drugs_RandD
Abbott	www.abbott.com
Bristol Myers Squibb	www.bms.com
Eli Lilly	www.lilly.com
Glaxo-Wellcome	www.glaxowellcome.co.uk
Merck	www.merck.com
Novartis	www.novartis.com
SmithKline Beecham	www.sb.com

KEY CONCEPT

Online sources of drug literature are readily accessible, but are not reviewed and may not be as reliable as printed information.

Summary

The reliance of consumers and health care professionals on pharmacists for rapid delivery of accurate drug information has created a need for pharmacy practitioners to have a good understanding of the types of drug literature that are available. Rapid dissemination and accessibility of information through news media and the Internet have increased the necessity for pharmacists to be knowledgeable regarding how to organize and retrieve information. While some information can be easily obtained from readily available tertiary sources of information, such as the package insert or the *Physician's Desk Reference,* much of this information may be out of date, and these references may not have any information related to the question at hand. Today drug literature, including primary literature, is readily accessible to the practicing pharmacist. Through the Internet, a secondary source of information such as Medline can be used to readily identify a primary source of information. This primary reference will supply the information required to provide sophisticated answers to questions that are asked by consumers or health care professionals. This accessibility allows for easy remote access of information from a computer, so that more detailed answers to increasingly complex questions can be found from a home- or work-based computer without requiring physical access to a university or health system library. This provides pharmacists with rapid and easy access to information. This will increase the reliance on and frequency of use of drug literature in daily practice.

Study Questions

1. The August 3, 2000, issue of the *New England Journal of Medicine* published a paper titled "Pravastatin Therapy and the Risk of Stroke." This paper describes a moderate effect of pravastatin in reducing the incidence of stroke in 4612 patients at as compared to a placebo group of 4502 patients. This is best categorized as what type of literature (primary, secondary, or tertiary)?

2. The July 15, 2000, issue of the *American Journal of Health-System Pharmacists* published a paper titled "Safety and Efficacy of Antiestrogens for Prevention of Breast Cancer." This article reviews issues concerning clinical trials of antiestrogen therapy for the prevention of breast cancer. This is best categorized as what type of literature (primary, secondary, or tertiary)?

3. The June 2000 issue of the *Annals of Pharmacotherapy* published a case report titled "Interaction Between Warfarin and Trazadone." This paper reported three cases of a change in INR of >1.0 in patients on warfarin after the initiation of discontinuation of trazadone. This is best categorized as what type of literature (primary, secondary, or tertiary)?

4. BIDS Embase is an example of what type of literature (primary, secondary, or tertiary)?

5. What are the positive and negative aspects of using the Internet to search for an answer to a drug information question?

References

1. Anon: Adults over 60 depend heavily on pharmacists for guidance in medication use. Am J Health-System Pharm 55:768–769, 1998.

2. Lanctot KL, and Naranjo CA: Comparison of the Bayesian approach and a simple algorithm for assessment of adverse drug events. Clin Pharmacol Ther 58:692–698, 1995.

3. Nanjo CA, Busto U, Sellers EM, et al: A method for estimating the probability of adverse drug reactions. Clin Pharmacol Ther 30:239–245, 1981.

4. Michel DJ, Knodel LC: Comparison of three algorithms used to evaluate adverse drug reactions. Am J Health-System Pharm 43:1709–1714, 1986.

Searching Drug Literature

Richard L. Slaughter
Ellen B. Marks

OUTLINE

Goals and Objectives

Introduction

Searchable Online Databases

    National Library of Medicine Databases

    Commercial Vendors

Performing a Search

    First Steps

    Boolean Operators

Case Examples: Searching for Drug Literature

    Citation Searching

Search Strategies

Summary

Study Questions

References

KEY WORDS

Boolean
Citation
Database
Free-text term
Indexed term
Medline
PubMed
Reference

KEY WEB SITES

Institute for Scientific Information   www.isinet.com
National Library of Medicine   www.nlm.nih.gov
   Gateway to all Databases   gateway.nlm.nih.gov/gw/Cmd
   Internet Grateful Med   igm.nlm.nih.gov
   PubMed   www.nlm.nih.gov/pubmed
   Toxnet   www.toxnet.nlm.nih.gov
OVID Technologies   www.ovid.com

Goals and Objectives

The goal of this chapter is to introduce the major drug and medical databases, including their basic searching principles with examples from Medline via PubMed. After reading this chapter, readers should:

1. Be able to identify databases that can be used to search for drug information

2. Be aware of government and commercial vendors that provide access to the drug and medical literature, including electronic journals

3. Understand the differences between standard and free-text search terms

4. Be able to use boolean operators while performing searches

5. Be able to access PubMed and perform an efficient search

6. Be able to perform searches using databases to answer specific drug information questions

Introduction

The drug and medical literatures are expansive. In the U.S. National Library of Medicine's (NLM) 40 databases alone, there are over 25 million records citing primary literature such as journal articles and, increasingly, linking to the full text of journals and other documents. With such a vast amount of literature to review, it is important to understand how to locate databases to search for and identify information or data that is helpful in answering questions. This chapter will review the major databases available and provide examples of how to perform a search in a commonly used database to answer a specific question.

When faced with a question, the type of question asked and the circumstances surrounding it will determine the source best used to find an appropriate answer. Some questions may be answered by looking in tertiary sources such as a drug's package insert or the material published in the *Physicians' Desk Reference* (PDR).[1] More detailed, evaluative answers may be found in compendia such as *Drug Facts & Comparisons*[2] or *AHFS Drug Information.*[3] Basic questions on pharmacology, such as a drug's mechanism of action, can be found in *Goodman & Gilman's Pharmacological Basis of Therapeutics.*[4] However, these secondary and tertiary sources may not provide the most current information or may fall short of addressing a specific question. In such cases, the pharmacist will need to access a database to identify primary sources of drug information to adequately answer a wide array of questions.

Methods of accessing and using databases have improved in recent years, significantly advancing the pharmacist's ability to find credible and timely information and data. One key advance is the availability of databases through the World Wide Web (Web). With a computer, communications mode (telephone, cable, network, or wireless), standard Web browser, and an Internet service provider (ISP), the highest-quality databases and related information resources are within easy reach of homes, pharmacies, laboratories, and offices. The Web has made it easier for database producers to introduce features that ease the search process for the user and features that interconnect a variety of different information resource types, including links among full text, related Web sites, and current awareness services. Another key advance is the recent elimination of charges for access to the medical, health, and toxicological databases by the NLM and other government agencies.

Searchable Online Databases

Major drug and medical databases available through the Web are produced by U.S. government agencies including NLM, the National Agriculture Library, and the National Cancer Institute. These databases (e.g., Medline, Agricola, or Cancerlit) are available at no cost to users connecting directly to an agency's Web site.* Moreover, there are many commercial database vendors that offer the same databases, along with numerous additional databases. Commercial vendors, such as OVID Technologies or the Institute for Scientific Information (ISI), offer their users the ability to search an array of databases using common search methods, as well as access to databases that are unavailable from other vendors. Commercial vendors charge for access in ways that can be transparent to users (when they are affiliated with a library or university, for example), or individual accounts may be established on a subscription or per-use basis.

> **KEY CONCEPT**
>
> Drug and medical databases are available through NLM, the National Agricultural Library, and the National Cancer Institute.

National Library of Medicine Databases

NLM's Medline (Medical Literature, Analysis, and Retrieval System Online) is the world's foremost database in the life sciences with a concentration on biomedicine. Medline indexes approximately 4500 international journals published in a number of languages and includes over 11 million records, composed mainly of bibliographic citations and English language abstracts. Medline is searchable through two different systems from NLM as well as through many other systems from commercial vendors or advertiser-supported Web sites. The two NLM

---

*Two systems for searching Medline may be found at the NLM at http://gateway.nlm.nih.gov/gw/cmd agricola, from the National Agriculture Library at www.nal.usda.gov, and from Cancerlit at http://cancernet.nci.gov as part of the most comprehensive system of cancer information through the National Cancer Institute.

systems, Internet Grateful Med (IGM) and PubMed, each have different attributes. Common elements of IGM and PubMed's delivery of Medline include searching by author name, title word, text word, journal name, phrase, or the medical subject heading (MeSH). MeSH is the thesaurus, or standardized vocabulary, used in Medline and a number of other NLM databases that can aid, in many circumstances, the development of effective search strategies.

KEY CONCEPT

NLM's Medline is the world's foremost biomedical literature database with over 11 million records. It is searchable through two NLM systems: IGM and PubMed.

Medline began in 1966 and is updated daily. When pharmacists are seeking biomedical literature published before 1966, consultation with a librarian is suggested to locate citations in Medline's predecessor, *Index Medicus,* other paper-based indexes, or the IGM database Oldmedline.

Although Medline's records have been traditionally composed of references to journal articles—requiring the user to note the source journal and seek the paper-based article through a library—new innovations are rapidly being introduced to eliminate obstacles to accessing the primary literature. Over 800 journals are linked from the PubMed record for direct access to an article's full text. Access to the electronic journal article in this way is typically available through the student or pharmacist's affiliated library as an institutional subscription, society membership, or by per-article charge. Some electronic journals are freely available. Generally, biomedical journals began publishing in electronic form around 1993 to 1995. Although there are exceptions, few biomedical electronic journals predate 1990.

Through Loansome Doc, a no-cost service available through Medline via IGM or PubMed, journal articles not available electronically can be ordered online and received via mail, e-mail, or fax. Charges may be associated with an article's delivery from a supplier library, but the cost per article ordered by health care providers through Loansome Doc tends to be lower than those purchased from commercial suppliers.

KEY CONCEPT

Over 800 journals are linked from PubMed to full-text online articles. At only a delivery charge, articles can be obtained by mail, e-mail, or fax through Loansome Doc.

. The NLM databases and an array of supporting resources are accessible from http://gateway.nlm.nih.gov/gw/Cmd. NLM has three systems for database access, all designed for user-cordial searching:

1. IGM, containing Medline and 14 other databases, is optimized with step-by-step guidance for developing a search strategy.

2. PubMed is the newer and more powerful means of searching Medline that includes integrated molecular biology databases (DNA and protein sequences, genome maps, and 3D structure data).

3. Toxnet (Toxicology Data Network) is a comprehensive system of computer data files, literature, and chemical information.

IGM. IGM is designed with a standard, easy method of searching databases ranging from bibliographic (citations and abstracts of journal articles—e.g., AIDSline, Bioethicsline, Medline, or Toxline), to Dirline (a database of health-related organizations and contact information), to databases containing complete files of data or full-text publications. For example, AIDStrials fully describes AIDS-related clinical trials of experimental treatments conducted under the Food and Drug Administration's investigational new drug regulations. AIDSdrugs describes the agents being tested in AIDS-related studies. Health Services Technology Assessment Texts (HSTAT) contains resources useful for health care decision making such as clinical practice guidelines, evidence reports, and consumer brochures.

Conducting a search through IGM is made easy by simple forms that guide the user to enter an author name, MeSH term, institution, text word, or other fields unique to a particular IGM database. Fields can easily be combined by using the form and can be limited in various ways including language of publication, publication type (e.g., review articles only), age of persons studied within an article, or year(s) of publication. IGM is notable for its online help embedded in each database. IGM is accessible at http://igm.nlm.nih.gov. The home page for IGM is shown in Fig. 2-1. More information about the databases searchable through IGM is shown in Table 2-1. A sample of the form used to search the database AIDSline is shown in Fig. 2-2, which shows how easy these databases are to use.

Toxnet. Toxnet contains databases on toxicology, hazardous chemicals, and broadly related areas. Factual information on toxicity and other hazards of chemi-

KEY CONCEPT

IGM provides access to numerous databases in addition to Medline. These include AIDSline, Bioethicsline, Toxline, ChemID, and Health-Star.

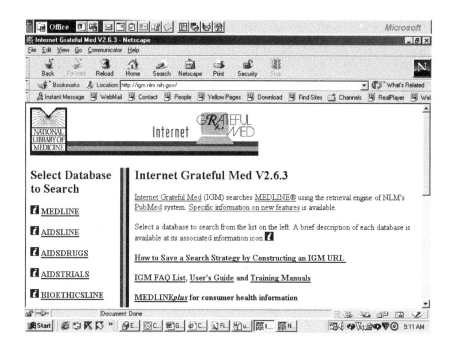

Figure 2-1 IGM home page.

cals is available through such databases as the Hazardous Substances Data Bank in the form of substantial monographs on human and animal toxicity, safety and handling, and environmental fate. The toxicology literature is referenced in Toxline, covering biochemical, pharmacological, physiological, and toxicological effects of drugs and chemicals in greater depth than Medline. Within Toxnet, the pharmacist can look up nomenclature, identification, and structure of chemicals, and have quick access via ChemID*plus* to chemical synonyms, structures, regulatory list information, and links to other databases containing information about chemicals. Table 2-2 summarizes the resources in Toxnet, which can be found at www.toxnet. nlm.nih.gov. Figure 2-3 shows the Toxnet home page.

Commercial Vendors

Access to online databases can be acquired through companies that hold licensing agreements to a large number of databases in a wide variety of fields. OVID Technologies (www.ovid.com) is one that specializes in bibliographic and full-text databases and electronic journals for health care and scientific research. Examples of databases available through OVID are given in Table 2-3.

Electronic journals with full text from 1993 to the present are available in one database of 500-plus titles as Journals@OVID. Just as costs are involved to access information from all commercial vendors, OVID charges for access to its databases

TABLE 2-1. Databases Searchable Through IGM*†

Database	Subject	Type	Size (No. of Records)	Frequency of Updates
AIDSline	AIDS	Bibliographic citations	>156,000	Weekly
Bioethicsline	Ethics and related public policy issues in health care and biomedical research	Bibliographic citations	>53,000	Bimonthly
Dirline	Directory of resources providing information services	Referral	>16,000	Quarterly
HealthStar	Clinical and nonclinical aspects of health care delivery	Bibliographic citations	>3.1 million	Weekly
HSRProj	Health services research, including health technology assessment and the development and use of clinical practice guidelines	Research project descriptions	>5,000	Quarterly
Medline	Biomedicine	Bibliographic citations	>9.2 million	Weekly
MeSH Vocabulary File	Thesaurus of biomedical-related terms	Factual	>96,000	Annually
Toxline	Toxicological, pharmacological, biochemical, and physiological effects of drugs and chemicals	Bibliographic citations	>2.4 million	Monthly

*Data current as of October 2000.
†IGM, Internet Grateful Med.

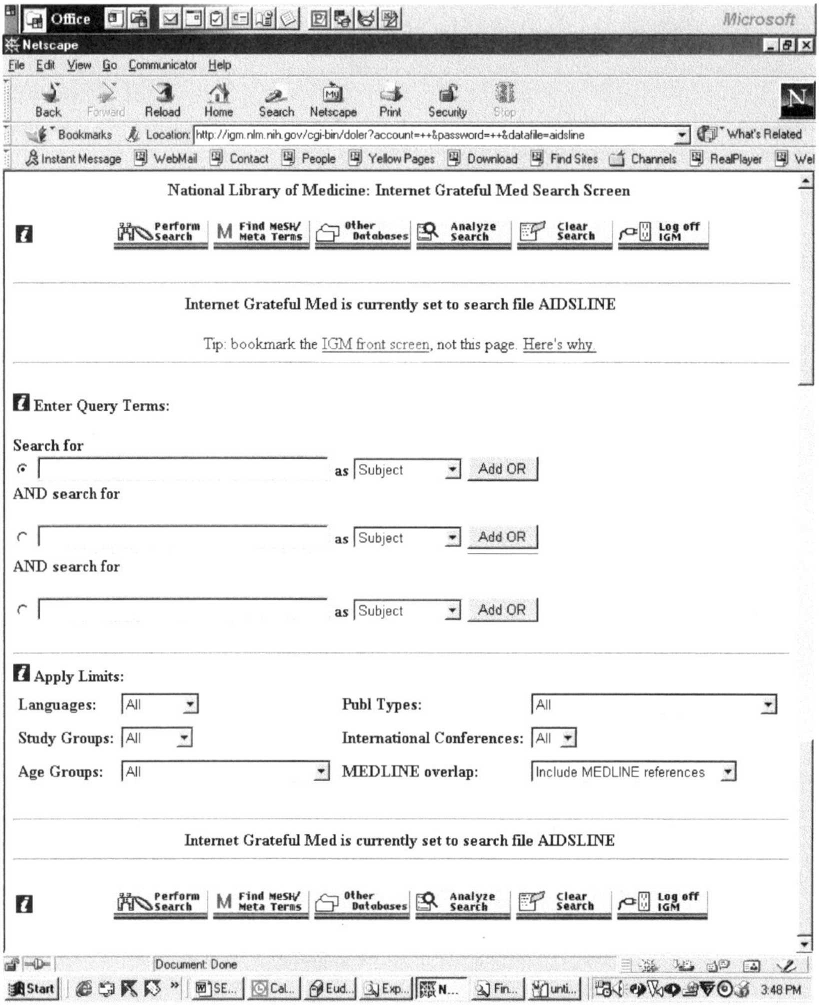

Figure 2-2 IGM search screen.

and electronic journals. A university may license online access on behalf of its students and faculty, but OVID also offers packages of databases and selected journals scaled to small organizations that may not otherwise have access to biomedical information resources. OVID journals include core clinical titles such as the *New England Medical Journal, Annals of Internal Medicine,* and the *British Medical Journal,* as well as specialized journals.

TABLE 2-2. **Searchable Databases Available Through Toxnet**

Database	Subject	Type	Size	Frequency of Updates
CCRIS[a]	Data provided by the National Cancer Institute	Bibliographic citations	8,000	
DART/ETIC[b]	Teratology, development, and reproductive toxicology	Bibliographic citations	>28,000	Yearly
Gene-Tox	Peer-reviewed mutagenicity test data from the EPA[c]	Factual	≈2,900	As needed
HSDB[d]	Hazardous chemicals, toxic effects, environmental fate, safety, and handling	Factual	>4,500	Continuous
IRIS[e]	Provided by the EPA in support of human health risk assessment	Factual	≈500	Continuous
TRI[f]	Annual estimated releases of toxic chemicals to the environment, amounts transferred to waste sites and sources reduction, and recycling data	Numeric	Up to >87,000	New file added annually

[a]CCRIS, Chemical Carcinogenesis Research Information System.
[b]DART/ETIC, Developmental and Reproductive Toxicology and Environmental Teratology Information Center.
[c]EPA, Environmental Protection Agency.
[d]HSDB, Hazardous Substances Data Bank.
[e]IRIS, Integrated Risk Information System.
[f]TRI, Toxics Release Inventory.

The ISI (www.isinet.com) has created citation databases that enable searches for biomedical or pharmaceutical literature in ways differing from standard bibliographic databases such as Medline. Web of Science, through which the *Science Citation Index** is accessible by license, is based on links among the citations found at the end of most scholarly publications. This unique method of seeking information is discussed later in this chapter.

*Databases searchable through Web of Science may also include *Social Science Citation Index* or *Arts and Humanities Citation Index,* depending on the license purchased by the library or organization. The citation indexes continue to be available as paper indexes subscribed to mainly by libraries.

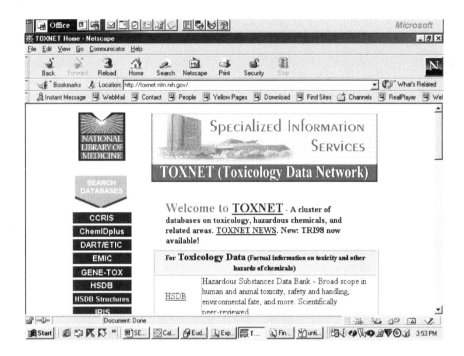

Figure 2-3 Toxnet home page.

Performing a Search

When faced with a drug information question, the type of question asked should guide the pharmacist's choice of databases. The databases selected should be those most likely to produce a set of good references that will lead, in turn, to publications containing the answer. As well, full-text databases to support drug and medical subjects may directly contain the answers.

First Steps

For many topics, Medline is a good first choice. Other more specialized databases may also be appropriate, but a preliminary search in Medline may provide useful

TABLE 2-3. **Databases Available Through OVID Technologies**

Database	Description	Availability
Drug Information Full Text	Complete text of evaluation monographs from AHFS Drug Information and the *Handbook of Injectable Drugs;* produced by the American Society of Health-System Pharmacists	Online pay-as-you-go Online fixed fee
Embase Drugs and Pharmacology	Contains the most important citations and abstracts to worldwide drug literature; published by Elsevier Science	Online pay-as-you-go Online fixed fee Local CD-ROM Network CD-ROM Magnetic network
Evidence-Based Medicine Reviews	Designed for use by clinicians and researchers, reflecting current practices in the medical field; available through OVID Technologies	Accessed via OVID online
International Pharmaceutical Abstracts	Provides worldwide coverage of pharmaceutical science and health-related literature; produced by the American Society of Health-System Pharmacists	Online pay-as-you-go Online fixed fee Local CD-ROM Network CD-ROM Magnetic network
Iowa Drug Information Service	Contains bibliographic records on human drug therapy	Pay-as-you-go

terminology with definitions, chemical registry numbers, or author names. A question on AIDS is most likely answered using AIDSline or AIDSdrugs. HealthStar would be used to find literature related to health services administration or research. Questions about a nondomestic drug might be addressed in *International Pharmaceutical Abstracts (IPA)*.

Clearly identifying the question at hand and breaking it down into parts—or its separate concepts—is the best way to begin the information searching process. The database user can enter these concepts into a database by using terms selected from a standardized list or thesaurus created by indexers to represent the central and peripheral content of an article. Or, words used to search for a concept may be those that the user predicts are likely to have been used by an article's author. These words—the everyday words of biomedicine or science—are called variously *free text, text words,* or *keywords.* For example, the word *automobile* might be the term selected for a hypothetical database's standardized word list. The database's indexers add *automobile* to every record concerned with that concept. When database users enter *automobile* into a database, they can be assured that the resulting set of records will include those that may use words such as *cars, autos, automobiles,* and so on. This results in a comprehensive set of records by automatically incorporating all synonyms, abbreviations, and other language variations.

Just as often, it may be important to find a specific word or phrase that is not on the standardized list, for example, *Dodge Viper.* Using this phrase will yield a highly precise set with records that have *Dodge Viper* written within them. Cutting-edge concepts, clinical jargon, or acronyms can be easily retrieved by using keywords or text words.

Boolean Operators

The operators *AND, OR,* and *NOT* are used in every major database to combine more than one term or text word. As well, terms or words can be combined with the names of authors, journal names, or other fields using boolean operators.

By using *AND* to connect two words, the resulting set of records (set) are those that have both words in common—the intersection. For example, enter *dogs AND greyhound* and the set will contain both words in every record. Using *OR* produces the union of two sets. Enter *greyhounds OR terriers* and the results obtained will have records that contain *both* greyhounds and terriers as well as records that contain *only* greyhounds or *only* terriers. *Greyhounds NOT buses* will exclude all instances of buses from a set.

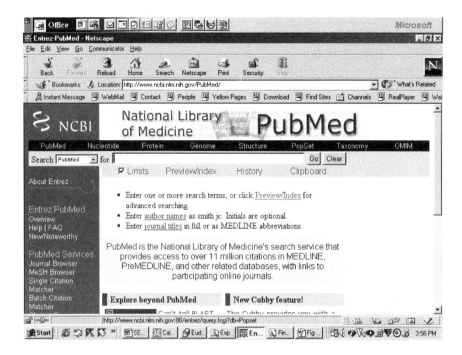

Figure 2-4 Example of the PubMed query box
(appears as accessed on October 18, 2000).

Case Examples: Searching for Drug Literature

The following examples apply basic search principles to the PubMed version of Medline. Testing these examples at www.ncbi.nlm.nih.gov/pubmed can be useful. PubMed makes it easy to perform quick searches. A word, phrase, or combinations of them can be entered directly into the PubMed query box (Fig. 2-4) and results retrieved. Many times, the results will be voluminous, requiring time-consuming browsing for one or two good records. One efficient way of starting a search is through the MeSH browser, located on the left side of the main PubMed screen.

Suppose the searcher's interest is in the use of protease inhibitors in the disease AIDS. These concepts can be entered into the query box as *aids AND protease inhibitors,* resulting in 901 records.* The word *aids,* however, can mean many things, and a number of irrelevant records may be retrieved.

Instead, click on the MeSH browser and enter the word *aids.* The response readily explains that the MeSH term is *acquired immunodeficiency syndrome.* This standard term can be immediately added to the search or further refined by click-

---

*Sample searches performed on October 7, 2000.

ing on Detailed Display. This display offers a selection of subheadings, such as Drug Therapy or Diagnosis, that can be added to create a specifically focused set. Likewise, entering the phrase *protease inhibitors* into the MeSH browser produces a hierarchical listing or tree of broader terms (e.g., *enzyme inhibitors*), narrower terms (e.g., *HIV protease inhibitors*), and terms that are narrower still (e.g., *Indinavir*). The term that the searcher would like to use or the term and one or more subheadings can be selected and incorporated into the search.

A search of *acquired immunodeficiency syndrome AND HIV protease inhibitors* results in 291 records. The set eliminates all irrelevant records but is time-consuming to review. By clicking on Limit, immediately below the query box, an array of ways to make the results more precise is available (Fig. 2-5). These include limiting by date of publication or type of publication, including clinical trials, practice guidelines, or review articles. Other options include eliminating animal studies or selecting one gender or age group, or limiting the search to a specified language such as English. Note that once the limits are "turned on," they will be applied to all subsequent searches unless the limit box is deliberately cleared.

Suppose a colleague has seen a good article on pharmacists' salaries but can't remember whether it was seen in the journal *Pharmacotherapy* or the *Annals of*

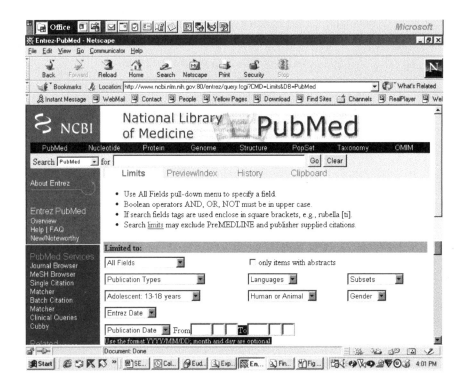

Figure 2-5. Example of use of limits in a PubMed search (appears as accessed on October 18, 2000).

Pharmacotherapy. The MeSH browser suggests the use of *salaries and fringe benefits.* The following example will demonstrate the use of PubMed's Preview/Index as the best way of constructing searches consisting of more than one concept:

- Click on Preview/Index located directly under the PubMed query box.

- Enter the standard MeSH phrase *salaries and fringe benefits* into the query box.

- Click on Preview to the right of the query box. (This step will create the first set and provide the total number of records retrieved.)

- Clear the query box using the button on the right.

- Enter the name *Annals of Pharmacotherapy* and click Preview, creating set #2.

- Entering the name *Pharmacotherapy* will result in over 800,000 records because it is a word commonly found in Medline records. Instead, note the Add Terms to Query Box near the bottom of the screen in the Preview/Index area. From its pull-down menu, select Journal Name as the field, enter *Pharmacotherapy,* and click Preview, resulting in set #3.

- These sets can be combined by typing their numbers into the PubMed query box as *#1 AND (#2 OR #3)* and clicking on Go. This search will retrieve records indexed with *salaries and fringe benefits* published in either the *Annals of Pharmacotherapy* or *Pharmacotherapy.* A summary of this search process is shown in Table 2-4, and the output of this search is shown in Fig. 2-6.

By clicking on the titles of each record retrieved, the full Display opens. This default view displays the bibliographic citation, abstract and links to related records, occasionally book chapters, and increasingly full-text links. The searcher can change the Display to *citation* from the default to examine all MeSH terms applied to the record. Taking note of these terms from one or two good records is an efficient way of reformulating a search to create a better one.

PubMed offers a variety of methods to create, refine, and save searches. The History feature keeps track of all search sets in a session; the Cubby is used to save

---

TABLE 2-4. **Summary of Example Search for Salary and Fringe Benefits**

Search Term	Comments	Number of Citations
1. Salary and fringe benefits	MeSH search terms	13,963
2. *Annals of Pharmacotherapy*	No limitations used	2,497
3. *Pharmacotherapy*	Limited to journal name	1,888
#1 AND (#2 OR #3)	Search criteria	5

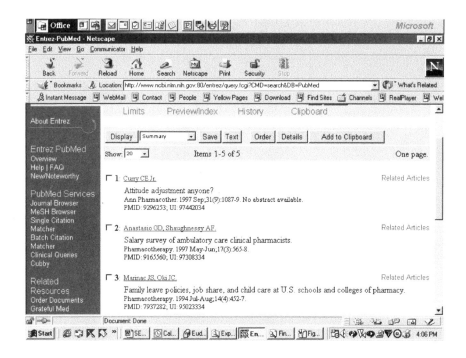

Figure 2-6 Example of an Output Form in a PubMed Search.

search strategies for use at a later time; and the downloading function is a step-by-step way of saving results on diskettes or importing results into bibliographic file management software such as EndNote. New capabilities are being introduced within PubMed at a rapid pace; checking on its development regularly will be worthwhile.

KEY CONCEPT

Databases such as PubMed are constantly changing in format and functions. At the time this chapter is read, the data and information shown in examples will have changed. Be aware of the how searchable databases change.

Citation Searching

The ISI is a commercial vendor of paper-based citation indexes such as *Science Citation Index,* typically available in academic libraries. The Web of Science (www.webofscience.com) is the Web interface to an expanded version of the *Index.*

Web of Science indexes an even greater number of journals than Medline and in a broader array of sciences. This database can be searched by author, by journal, by institution, or by topic as a general search. There is no standardized thesaurus, so subject searches use words that may be in the title, abstract, or supplied by the authors. After useful records are found, the searcher may click on the Related Records button to get lists of additional relevant records.

The most powerful advantage of using Web of Science, however, is citation searching. Every reference cited by an article's authors is included. This method enables the searcher to find, for one example, all articles that have cited a given article—providing a trail of meaningful references from the time of an article's publication to the present. The Cited Reference search can be used to find all articles citing a publication or all publications citing a particular author. A specific author, for example, Buxton AE, can be entered into the Cited Reference box. Over 187 references, in all likelihood referring to this one author, are returned. Figure 2-7 shows the most recent 10 references. The hits shown indicate that some of his publications have been cited over 40 times; he has an earlier publication (not shown) that has been cited 115 times, suggesting that he may be an expert in his field.

KEY CONCEPT

The Web of Science (www.webofscience.com) indexes more journals than Medline. This database can be searched by author, journal, institution, or topic as a general search. The major use of this database is to perform citation searches.

The sample record in Fig. 2-8 demonstrates the ease with which searches can be performed once a useful citation has been identified. For example, a search for the use of protease inhibitors in the treatment of HIV infection identified the article by Kakuda et al.[5] The references, or bibliography, of this article consist of approximately 125 articles' citations, all of which can be viewed by clicking Cited References. In addition, authors of at least 24 articles published after this article's 1998 publication have cited it, finding it important enough to reference. Clicking on Times Cited will produce a list of every article that has cited this one since 1998. Citing an article lends a measure of credibility to it by recognizing important information, data, or research techniques. Articles may also be cited because later authors disagree with an article's findings or authors may be citing themselves. Citations can be a gross measure of impact on a field or specialty, but a very good research article in a highly defined subspecialty may not be cited often or at all and still be a very valuable publication. The use of citation analysis for determining a journal's impact is discussed in more detail in Chap. 3.

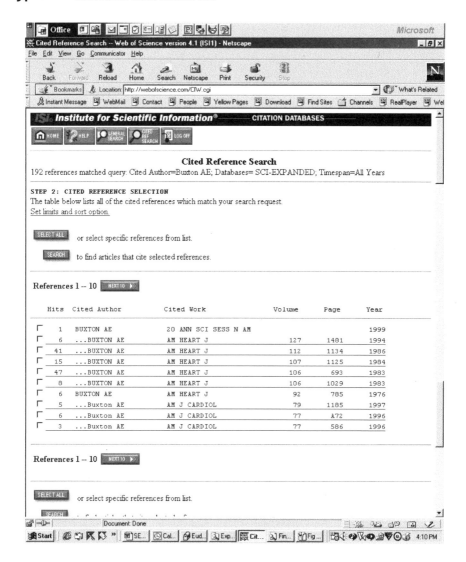

Figure 2-7 Example of a cited reference search by author name (appears as accessed on October 18, 2000).

The Web of Science record provides additional information. In recent years, the addresses of all authors of a particular article are provided in full. In the preceding example, all authors worked in 1998 at the National Institutes of Health (NIH) or the Food and Drug Administration, lending further credibility to the article. Web of Science, like PubMed, has new features added to it regularly including, increasingly, links to the full text of publications.

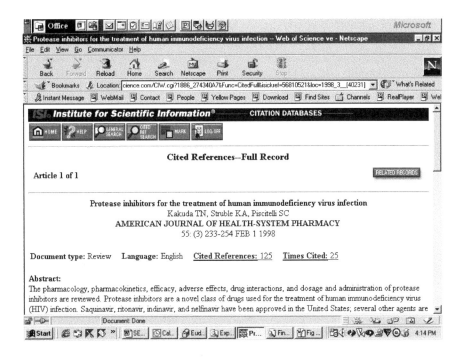

Figure 2-8 Example of a full record for a citation search (appears as accessed on October 18, 2000).

Search Strategies

To perform an efficient and effective search, knowledge of the basic principles of database searching needs to be combined with an understanding of the particular strengths of the major drug and medical databases. At times, a quick and precise search is required. Suppose a physician is interested in the use of fludrocortisone to treat subarachnoid hemorrhage. The component concepts are: fludrocortisone, subarachnoid hemorrhage, and treatment. Because Medline is the best database for finding references in support of clinical care, searching PubMed will be the best first step. The search can be entered into the PubMed query box as: *fludrocortisone AND subarachnoid hemorrhage AND treatment*. The results retrieved will consist of relevant articles. To achieve results that are even more precise, the words *fludrocortisone* and *subarachnoid hemorrhage* should first be entered into the MeSH browser. The subheading Therapeutic Use can be selected and automatically attached to *fludrocortisone* so that the resulting set is a highly precise seven articles.

Conversely, there are occasions when broader, more comprehensive searches are needed to ensure that all pertinent literature on a subject is retrieved. As highly indexed as Medline is, to be certain that all relevant records are retrieved, search statements should include synonyms and all possible text word variations. This is especially important for proprietary and generic drug names. For example, a search of the term *fluoxetine* produced 4496 results in Medline, whereas *Prozac* resulted in 3492 records. For comprehensiveness, it is also important to consider the review article, which summarizes a topic's literature. In Medline, a search can be limited to review articles only. A review article's references can be examined by finding the publication itself or its reference can be found in Web of Science. Once found, the Cited References link will lead to the review article's entire list of references. Clicking on Related Articles will introduce the searcher to additionally relevant articles. Taken together, the use of these strategies will assure that most publications on a topic will be found. For literature published prior to the mid-1960s (Medline) or mid-1970s (Web of Science), it is recommended that the pharmacist seek the assistance of a librarian.

Summary

This chapter has focused on the basic principles of reviewing and using Web-based drug and medical databases. Key points to remember include the following:

1. Web-based databases are searchable from any location with a computer, communications line, ISP, and a Web browser.

2. Major medical and drug databases such as Medline, Cancerlit, and Toxnet are available at no cost from U.S. government agencies.

3. Commercial database vendors offer access to the major databases as well as a number of more specialized databases.

4. Databases such as Toxnet are full-text databases and contain large amounts of data and publications. Bibliographic databases, such as Medline or Web of Science, contain mainly references but are increasingly supplying links to journal articles and other publications (when licenses or subscriptions are in place).

Advances in Web-based databases are rapidly being introduced to manage the monumental growth of drug, medical, and scientific publications. To assure that the student or pharmacist is comfortable using these databases in anticipation of future needs, it is important to explore the examples presented in this chapter and to regularly experiment with other topics of interest.

Study Questions

1. A patient has heard of a report concerning problems of taking St. John's wort with certain medications. What database can be used to help answer this question? What are two NLM services that can be used to search this database?

2. Access PubMed (www.nlm.nih.gov/pubmed) and use the Preview/Index function (see Fig. 2-9). How many articles are in Medline under the search terms *St.*

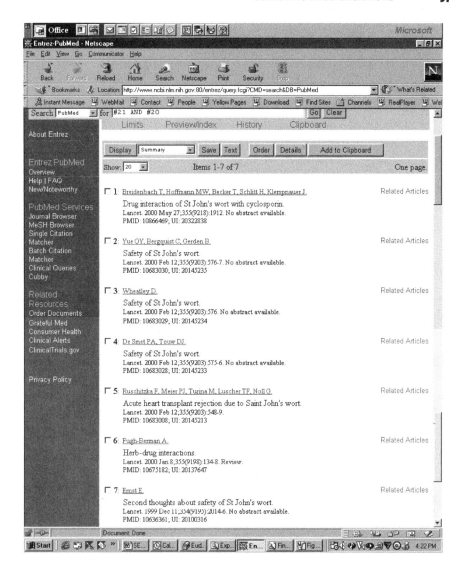

Figure 2-9 Results of search on drug interactions and St. John's wort.

John's wort and *hypericum?* Why is there a difference? Which is a free-text term and which is a MeSH term?

3. The patient shows you a *USA Today* article that refers to an article in the journal *Lancet.* Construct a search to identify the articles in *Lancet* that relate to drug interactions with St. John's wort. Provide a printout of the articles found.

4. In the preceding search, the article "Herb-drug interactions," by Fugh-Berman A, published in *Lancet* 355(9198):134–138, 2000, should be present. If possible,

access the Web of Science (http://webofscience.com) and perform a cited reference search for Fugh-Berman.

    a. How many citations for Fugh-Berman are listed?

    b. How many hits have occurred for this article?

    c. Provide the reference for one article that cites this article.

    d. Is this article suitable to answer this patient's question?

5. What limits could be provided to the aforementioned search such that primarily primary reference sources would be found?

References

1. *Physicians' Desk Reference.* Montvale, N.J., Medical Economics Co., 2001.

2. *Drug Facts & Comparisons 2000.* St. Louis, MO, Facts and Comparisons, 1999.

3. American Society of Health-System Pharmacists: *American Hospital Formulary
Service Drug Information 2000.* Bethesda, MD, ASHSP. (Also available in electronic formats as *Drug Information Fulltext.*)

4. Hardman JG et al: *Goodman & Gilman's Pharmacological Basis of Therapeutics.*
New York, McGraw-Hill, Health Professions Division, 1996.

5. Kakuda TN, Struble KA, Piscitelli SC: Protease inhibitors for the treatment of
human immunodeficiency virus infection. Am J Health-System Pharm 55:233–254,
1998.

Chapter 3

The Publication Process

David J. Edwards

OUTLINE

Goals and Objectives

Introduction

Why Are Papers Flawed?

The Review Process

Problems with Peer Review

Improvements to the Peer Review Process

Evaluation of Drug Literature: What to Look For

Selecting the Appropriate Journal

Authorship

Structure of Papers

Style Guidelines for Biomedical Writing

Study Questions

References

KEY WORDS

Peer review
Citation analysis
Impact factor
Lag time
Authorship

Goals and Objectives

The objective of this chapter is to familiarize readers with the evaluation process that manuscripts undergo prior to publication and to provide guidelines on journal selection, organization of papers, and writing style, which will help readers to evaluate drug literature. After reading this chapter, readers should:

1. Understand the process by which submitted manuscripts are examined and evaluated prior to acceptance for publication.

2. Understand the concept of peer review and recognize some of the common problems with this system.

3. Be familiar with the factors such as scope, citation analysis, impact factor, and lag time, which may influence the choice of journal to which a manuscript is submitted.

4. Be aware of the "Uniform Requirements for Manuscripts Submitted to Biomedical Journals" and the criteria for authorship suggested by these guidelines.

5. Be able to identify the individual parts (abstract, introduction, methods, results, conclusions) of a paper and know what information should be contained in each.

6. Understand the importance of accuracy, brevity, and clarity to the preparation of a quality paper.

Introduction

Most of the people who read the drug literature are practitioners who need to determine whether they should change the way in which they conduct their clinical practice on the basis of the results of a published study. The vast majority of readers have little experience themselves in the preparation and publication of manuscripts. This lack of understanding of the publication process may lead to a false sense of security on the part of the reader in terms of the quality of the research being reported. It is a relatively common misconception among students and practitioners in the health sciences that publication is in itself an assurance of quality and that there is little need for further critical analysis. If this were the case, books such as this, which provide guidance on how to evaluate biomedical literature, would be unnecessary.

Proof that not all published literature is of high quality comes from several sources. Many journals publish letters to the editor, which are often critical of recent papers. A quick glance at the letters section of a recent issue of a prominent journal, such as the *New England Journal of Medicine*, suggests that there may be considerable disagreement, often between highly trained experts in a field, over the appropriateness of the methods used or conclusions reached in published papers. Miller et al.[1] compared the effectiveness of chemotherapy either alone or in combination with radiotherapy for non-Hodgkin's lymphoma. The following excerpts are from letters published in response to this paper:

The median age of the patients was 59 years, which is old. Older patients tolerate intensive chemotherapy poorly, and it is difficult for them to complete the full course of treatment.[2]

The conclusions of Miller et al. that three cycles of CHOP followed by involved-field radiotherapy are superior to eight cycles of CHOP alone as treatment for localized stages of aggressive non-Hodgkin's lymphoma seem statistically misleading.[3]

Although the standard curative dose of radiotherapy for non-Hodgkin's lymphoma is approximately 4000 cGy, the majority of patients in the study received 4500 to 5000 cGy, which suggests that there was heterogeneity in the radiation doses.[4]

While the issues raised by letters such as these are not always valid and need to be examined carefully for bias on the part of the writer, they may identify flaws in study design or data analysis that were not detected prior to publication. This type of postpublication peer review can be very informative and a valuable source of information for anyone reviewing the literature on a particular topic.

Others have taken a more systematic approach to identifying problems with published literature. Papers from a particular journal or discipline are examined over a period of time in order to determine whether they meet appropriate standards with respect to adequacy of the study population, design of the study (e.g., controls, blinding, randomization, etc.), analytical methods, and appropriate use of statistical tests. For example, Welch and Gabbe reviewed the use of statistics in papers published in the *American Journal of Obstetrics and Gynecology* from January through June 1994.[5] They reported that only 30% of the articles could be classified as having appropriate usage of statistics with 27 of 46 articles having serious flaws.

Why Are Papers Flawed?

It is clear from the preceding discussion that not all published research is perfect and that the conclusions cannot always be accepted at face value. While it is unlikely that a researcher begins an investigation with anything other than the best of intent, the research may be compromised along the way for a number of reasons:

1. *Limited funding for research.* This forces investigators, particularly in the academic setting, to choose study designs that are less than ideal but that fit the investigator's budget. For example, the incidence of an adverse drug reaction may be best assessed through a study that includes a control group not receiving the drug in question and requires lab tests and other assessments specifically designed to detect the adverse reaction being studied. Much less expensive would be a review of the medical records of patients who have recently been treated with the drug. Although the information obtained from the latter design is less likely to yield valid, unbiased data, financial considerations may result in its use.

2. *Pressure to publish.* Researchers are often under significant pressure to get the results of their research published. Rewards such as promotion, tenure, and salary increases are frequently based on the publication record of scientists in universities. Unfortunately, it is easier to measure the quantity as opposed to the quality of publications. Researchers may have an incentive to publish two or three

mediocre papers rather than one excellent paper. Scientists working within the pharmaceutical industry may also be under pressure to publish. The successful marketing of a new drug may depend in part on the ability to refer health care professionals to papers published in well-known journals.

3. *Investigator or sponsor bias.* Researchers may be unwilling to admit or accept that a hypothesis that they may have spent years developing and studying is not supported by the results of their investigation. The conclusions of a study may tend to emphasize those aspects of the results that support the hypothesis while downplaying results that do not. Pharmaceutical manufacturers clearly have a vested interest in results that favor their product over those of a competitor. Although the vast majority of papers describing studies supported or conducted by drug companies accurately represent the results of the study, problems can result when a sponsor disagrees with the conclusions of the investigator. In a highly publicized case, the pharmaceutical company Boots forced the *Journal of the American Medical Association* (*JAMA*) to delay publication of a paper that was not favorable to the sale of the company's levothyroxine product.[6] Boots had sponsored the study but disagreed with the investigators over the interpretation of the results. The company threatened the University of California—San Francisco with a lawsuit based on a clause in the research contract stating that the results were not to be published without the consent of Boots. Although this was an isolated case and the results were eventually published in *JAMA*,[7] it illustrates the lengths to which a company may go to prevent the publication of findings that might jeopardize market share.

4. *Investigator incompetence.* Not everyone conducting research is necessarily qualified to do so. Health professionals are primarily trained as clinicians rather than scientists and may conduct research for the prestige of being published or because it is a requirement of their job. This may lead to poorly designed studies with too few subjects that cannot address the hypothesis being tested. Even scientists with extensive training in a particular technique or method may lack the statistical background to analyze their data appropriately. Issues related to study design and hypothesis testing are discussed in detail later in this book.

It is clear that published papers often contain minor flaws and occasionally have such significant problems that the paper is of little or no value. How is it that these papers escape detection prior to being published? A more detailed understanding of the specific process by which manuscripts submitted to journals undergo review may shed light on this issue.

The Review Process

Submitted manuscripts are initially examined by the editor to determine that the research fits within the scope of the journal and that the paper is of sufficient quality to warrant further review. The editor may also examine the paper to determine that it conforms to the style requirements of the journal. This information is published in the first issue of the year for most journals. In addition, it is increasingly available online (e.g., www.acponline.org/journals/resource/info4aut.html provides "Information for Authors" for *Annals of Internal Medicine*). In 1998, 21% of papers submitted to *Clinical Pharmacology and Therapeutics* were rejected by the editor without further review ("Annual Report 1998," Reidenberg MM, Reidenberg J).

In addition to providing an initial review, the editor has an important task in choosing appropriate peer reviewers for the manuscript. Most journals use two or three reviewers who are selected on the basis of their expertise in the area on which the research has been conducted. Some journals rely almost entirely on the members of the editorial board for reviews of submitted papers. The editorial board is composed of individuals who are well respected in the clinical or scientific field in which the journal publishes. The 1999 editorial board of the journal *Pharmacotherapy* lists 42 individuals with a mixture of Pharm.D., Ph.D., and M.D. training. Due to the large number of submitted manuscripts as well as the wide range of expertise required, most journals maintain a list of reviewers in addition to those on the editorial board who can be called upon for reviewing papers in their area of expertise. The contributions of these individuals are generally acknowledged in the last issue of the year. In the December 1999 issue, *Pharmacotherapy* lists 407 people who reviewed manuscripts in 1999 (Vol. 19).

KEY CONCEPT

Peer review is the process by which individuals with expertise in the problem under investigation evaluate submitted manuscripts to determine if they have sufficient validity and importance to warrant publication.

Problems with Peer Review

In principle, peer review should work. Experts decide on the merits of publication primarily based on the appropriateness of the methods, validity of the results, and the clinical or scientific significance of the conclusions. If the data is both valid and important, the paper is accepted. If appropriate standards are not met, the paper is rejected. However, in actual practice, peer review is less than a perfect system. Reviewers often have divergent views on the appropriateness of the methods used in addressing the hypothesis under study. In addition, what is important to one person may or may not be considered significant by another. Reviewers may have difficulty seeing the long-term significance of new ideas with the result that those rare papers that describe true breakthroughs in science often have more difficulty gaining acceptance than less important papers espousing more traditional theories.

A classic example of the vagaries of the system is provided in the autobiography of Kary Mullis, Nobel laureate and inventor of the polymerase chain reaction (PCR).[8] While a biochemistry student in 1968, Mullis submitted a paper to the prestigious journal *Nature,* entitled "The Cosmological Significance of Time Reversal." The paper was devoid of experimental results; indeed, the author had no experience or training in cosmology. It was based on Mullis's perception of the universe, a view highly influenced by his use of psychedelic drugs. Despite its shortcomings, the paper was accepted for publication. Fifteen years later, Mullis invented the PCR while working as a research scientist at Cetus Corporation. Again, a paper was submitted to *Nature,* but this time it was not accepted. Reviewers in this case failed to recognize the significance of an idea that led to a revolution in molecular biology and resulted in Mullis receiving the Nobel Prize for Chemistry in 1993.

Although examples such as this are hopefully rare, the peer review system is subject to a number of well-documented problems as described in the following:

1. *Reviewer bias or professional rivalry.* Peer reviewers are often selected because they are actively conducting research in the same area as the submitted paper. As a result, the reviewer may be a competitor of the author of the manuscript for the prestige and rewards associated with being the first person to publish a novel discovery. This results in a conflict of interest for the reviewer who may be motivated to reject the paper in order to enhance his or her own research reputation (see Chap. 14). Quality papers may be rejected or delayed in their publication. Even worse, ideas may actually be stolen during the review process. In a highly publicized case, a team of researchers funded by the biotechnology company Cistron submitted a paper to *Nature,* claiming to have isolated the human DNA coding for interleukin-1. The paper was reviewed and rejected by a scientist working for a rival company Immunex. In a lawsuit that eventually resulted in a $21 million out-of-court settlement, Cistron alleged that Immunex made improper use of the information obtained through the peer review process in its own attempts to sequence the DNA of interleukin-1.[9] A key piece of evidence in the case was that sequence errors in the original paper submitted by Cistron appeared in a patent application subsequently filed by Immunex.

2. *Lack of expertise by reviewers.* Journals make every effort to ensure that peer reviewers are experts in the subject that they are asked to review. However, in the increasingly specialized world of modern medical science, the review of submitted papers may require expertise in a very narrow area of subspecialization. For example, not every scientist with expertise in the general field of pharmacokinetics is qualified to review papers in specialized areas such as the molecular biology of drug metabolism or therapeutic drug monitoring. In addition, most reviewers have minimal training in statistics so that statistical errors frequently go undetected. Reviewers may be reluctant or unwilling to admit that they do not have the necessary expertise to provide a competent review of a particular paper. This results in situations where there is a significant difference of opinion between reviewers in their judgment concerning a paper and can lead to the acceptance of a paper with significant flaws. In an interesting examination of this problem, the editors of *Annals* *of Emergency Medicine* prepared a fictitious manuscript containing 10 major errors and 13 minor errors and sent it to all reviewers.[10] Many of the errors were obvious such as patients unaccounted for, missing figures, and duplicate data in tables. The test drug, propranolol, was even spelled incorrectly throughout the manuscript. Despite these rather obvious problems, two-thirds of the major errors were not identified, and over 40% of the reviewers recommended acceptance of the paper.

   3. *Bias against the null hypothesis.* Papers that conclude that the treatment under study has no effect on the outcome being measured are said to have "accepted the null hypothesis" (see Chap. 7 for a detailed discussion of hypothesis testing). Koren[11] has defined bias against the null hypothesis as the "systematic discrimination leading to decreased scientific presentation, peer-reviewed publication, and public dissemination of studies that show no or nonsignificant differences between or among the comparison groups." Stated more simply, papers that don't find a statistically significant difference in the outcome measure have a much harder time being published. Using the effect of maternal cocaine use on the neonate as an example, Koren found that abstracts submitted to the Society of Pediatric Research meeting that documented fetal or neonatal abnormalities were much likelier to be accepted than those that found no effect. Easterbrook et al.[12] reported that papers with negative findings were more than twice as likely not to be published.

   4. *Lack of time or motivation by reviewer.* Peer review is a voluntary system in which reviewers provide their services without pay or any other direct reward. While it may be gratifying to be recognized for one's expertise, well-known scientists or clinicians may find themselves receiving manuscripts on a regular basis from several different journals. A thorough review of a manuscript may take several hours and require a search of the literature and a trip to the medical library. Naturally, a reviewer who is busy managing patients in the clinic, conducting research, preparing a grant submission, teaching a course, grading papers, or all of the aforementioned may not be able to devote sufficient time to each submission to provide a quality review. Cursory review may result in the publication of papers whose merit is questionable. Reviewers may not even have the time or take the time to read instructions from the editor. As an experiment, the editors of *Obstetrics and Gynecology* included in their instructions to reviewers the following statement: "If you have read this and call or fax our office, we will send you a gift worth twenty dollars." These letters were sent to 122 reviewers over a 2-month period, and only 21 called to claim the gift, suggesting that less than a quarter of the reviewers read the instructions sent to them.[13]

Improvements to the Peer Review Process

There has been much discussion as to how the peer review process can be improved. In fact, this was a main focus of the International Congress on Biomedical Peer Review and Global Communications held in Prague, Czech Republic, in September 1997 (proceedings published in the July 15, 1998 issue of *JAMA*). Some problems appear to be easier to address than others.

Bias on the part of the reviewer could, in theory at least, be reduced by masking the author's identity from the reviewer. The current practice of most journals is to blind the authors of a submitted paper to the identity of the reviewers. Reviewers, however, are generally aware of the identity of the authors. Some editors have argued forcefully that it is inconsistent to contend that reviewers need anonymity in order to provide an "honest" review but that the same courtesy should not be extended to the authors of the paper. Journals such as the *American Journal of Health-System Pharmacy* require that submitted manuscripts have a title page that does not list any of the authors in an attempt to eliminate bias. Unfortunately, it is not always possible to maintain this masking since the institution at which the work was carried out is often identified in the "Methods" section of the paper. Consider the following statement from a paper by Lau et al.[14]:

> The study protocol was approved by the ethics committee of the faculty of medicine of the Chinese University of Hong Kong, and all patients or their next of kin provided written informed consent. From May 1998 to July 1999, all patients who were admitted to the Prince of Wales Hospital with upper gastrointestinal bleeding were treated jointly by a team of physicians and surgeons.

It is highly likely that anyone reviewing this paper would be able to identify the research group simply from this information in the "Methods" section of the paper. The author's identity may also be obvious from the type of research being conducted or the list of references, given the propensity of authors to cite their own work.

The editor of *JAMA,* Drummond Rennie, has argued for the opposite approach, that is, open peer review in which the identities of both authors and reviewers are known to each other.[15] Such a system would require reviewers to defend their decisions to accept or reject papers on the basis of objective criteria. It is hoped that it would also eliminate those occasional reviews that degrade into personal attacks on the authors, generally in situations where authors have challenged conclusions previously published by the reviewer. In an ideal world, open peer review would work fine. However, it is not a system favored by most reviewers who fear retribution should they be critical of a paper submitted by a prominent clinician or scientist in their field. In a study of this system, van Rooyen et al.[16] found that open peer review did not enhance quality of reviews or affect the probability of a paper being accepted or rejected, but it did result in significantly more reviewers declining to review papers.

Although the ethical issues associated with blinding and masking of the peer review process are complex, it is likely that the current system of blinding authors to the identity of the reviewers will remain in place for some time. The editor of the *Annals of Internal Medicine* has suggested that, by far, the biggest problem facing the peer review process is not bias but rather a lack of critical assessment skills on the part of reviewers.[17] It seems unlikely that this will improve dramatically given the limitations of the current system. However, technology may lead the way in developing new approaches to prepublication review of articles. The *Medical Journal of Australia* initiated a trial in which papers accepted for publication were published initially on the World Wide Web.[18] Readers were encouraged to submit comments, which the authors could then use to revise papers at their discretion. This opened up the peer review system to a wider audience and had the potential to improve the quality of papers eventually published in the journal itself. However, in practice, reader comments were few and brief. Only a small number of articles were actually changed as a result of the prepublication electronic review. The editors of the *Medical Journal of Australia* have subsequently initiated another Internet-based peer review experiment.[19] In this process, papers are posted on a closed Internet site and an online debate, moderated by the editor, is conducted between the authors, reviewers, and a consultant panel of six individuals with expertise in the field. Papers that are accepted for publication following this process are then posted on an open Internet site for review with the authors having the opportunity to revise the paper once more prior to final publication in the journal. This system has a number of advantages. Chiefly, the author gets a chance to interact directly with the reviewers and presumably clear up any misconceptions about the paper. One of the most common complaints of authors is that reviewers simply misunderstand the intent, methods, or conclusions of the study. Whether due to reviewer incompetence or a lack of clarity on the part of the author, these issues can be resolved through debate rather than the author simply receiving a rejection letter. In addition, one would hope that by expanding the process to involve a larger number of reviewers, the odds of a significant error in a paper escaping detection would be markedly reduced.

Evaluation of Drug Literature: What to Look For

So far in this chapter, it has been established that studies may contain flaws and that the peer review process does not always identify these problems or prevent the publication of substandard research. Even when a paper is rejected by one journal, another may still accept it. The fate of 350 manuscripts rejected by the *Annals of Internal Medicine* was examined by the editors who reported that 240 (69%) were eventually published elsewhere.[20] While one shouldn't infer that all of these papers were unworthy simply because they were rejected by one journal, it does point out the fact that a persistent author can usually find a journal somewhere that is willing to accept a paper that was deemed unacceptable by someone else.

The consequence of all of this is that the health professionals who make up the general readership of most biomedical journals must be capable of performing their own evaluations of published research. Although much of the rest of this textbook is concerned with fundamental issues such as study design and data analysis, this chapter will focus on basic questions such as:

• Has the proper journal for this research been selected?

• Who is deserving of authorship on a paper?

• What are the individual components of a research paper and what information should be contained in each section?

• Have the authors used a clear and concise writing style to accurately present their findings?

Selecting the Appropriate Journal

Authors should choose the journal to which a paper will be submitted before beginning to write the paper. Although most journals conform to the "Uniform Requirements for Manuscripts Submitted to Biomedical Journals,"[21] there are often requirements for preparation and submission that are unique to each journal. In addition, it is easier to write with a particular audience in mind. In some cases, the choice of journal may be relatively easy. There are only a small number of journals, for example, that publish research on the stability of intravenous drug admixtures (e.g., *American Journal of Health-System Pharmacy, Journal of Pharmaceutical Sciences, Annals of Pharmacotherapy*). However, in the case of a paper dealing with the clinical effects of a drug, the choice may be more difficult. The *1999 Science Citation Index* lists 175 journals in the category of Pharmacy and Pharmacology, 110 journals in General and Internal Medicine, and numerous others in medical sub-specialties.

The first step in selecting a journal is to determine whether the research fits the scope of the journal. The type of paper that the journal will publish can usually be found as part of the "Instructions to Authors." Some examples follow:

Pharmacotherapy. Devoted to publication of original research articles on all aspects of human pharmacology and review articles on drugs and drug therapy.

Clinical Pharmacology and Therapeutics. A monthly journal devoted to the publication of articles of high quality dealing with the effects of drugs in human beings.

A paper dealing strictly with drug effects in an animal model would likely be rejected by both of these journals. While both might be suitable for a paper describing the pharmacokinetics of a new antifungal drug, only *Pharmacotherapy* would be interested in a review article comparing the pharmacokinetics of currently available drugs of this class. In cases of doubt, a quick glance at the table of contents of recent issues will generally confirm whether the journal is likely to be suitable.

If there are several journals in a particular field to choose among, most authors would presumably like their paper to be published in the journal where it will receive the highest possible visibility. How can this be measured? One factor is the circulation of the journal. The circulation of several journals in medicine, science, pharmacy, and pharmacology is provided in Table 3-1.[22] The circulation of a jour-

TABLE 3-1. **Circulation and Impact Factor of Selected Journals in Medicine, Science, Pharmacy, and Pharmacology**

Subject	Journal Name	Circulation	Impact Factor
Medicine	New England Journal of Medicine	183,000	28.857
	JAMA (Journal of the American Medical Association)	3,705,000	11.435
	Lancet	45,000	10.197
	Annals of Internal Medicine	93,439	10.097
	British Medical Journal	115,000	5.143
Science	Nature	55,613	29.491
	Science	160,000	24.595
Pharmacy/	Clinical Pharmacokinetics	1,200	5.098
pharmacology	Clinical Pharmacology and Therapeutics	4,695	4.846
	Drugs	2,500	4.150
	Journal of Pharmacology and Experimental Therapeutics	2,074	3.300
	Drug Metabolism and Disposition	1,004	2.519
	British Journal of Clinical Pharmacology	1,570	2.545
	Journal of Pharmaceutical Sciences	5,400	2.270
	Journal of Clinical Pharmacology	1,925	1.827
	Annals of Pharmacotherapy	7,200	1.610
	Therapeutic Drug Monitoring	1,352	1.383
	Pharmacotherapy	4,717	1.376
	American Journal of Health-System Pharmacy	39,232	1.085

SOURCES: Circulation data from *Ulrich's International Periodicals Directory* (RR Bowker, New Providence, NJ). Impact factor data from the *Journal Citation Reports* (ISI, 1999).

nal is not always directly related to its popularity or importance. Many journals serve as the "official" journal of a clinical or scientific society. For example, *JAMA* is circulated to all members of the American Medical Association, *Science* to the American Association for the Advancement of Science, and *American Journal of Health-System Pharmacy* to everyone affiliated with the American Society of Health-System Pharmacists. Perhaps a more objective way of measuring the value of a journal is through citation analysis.

The *Science Citation Index* tracks the number of times a particular paper is cited in subsequent papers. From this information, the Institute for Scientific Information (ISI; www.isinet.com), the publishers of the *Science Citation Index,* produce *Journal Citation Reports.* This ranks journals on criteria such as impact factor [i.e., the average number of times that recent articles (in the previous 2 years) in a journal were cited in the year covered by the report]. If, for example, a journal published 100 articles in 1997 and 1998 and these papers were cited 400 times in total in 1999, the 1999 impact factor for that journal would be 4.0. Papers of little value are unlikely to be cited by other investigators while journals that publish a high proportion of important papers will have a higher impact factor than those that do not. Which journal has more impact, *New England Journal of Medicine* or *JAMA?* Although both rank highly, the 1999 *Journal Citation Report* lists an impact factor of 28.857 for the *New England Journal of Medicine,* first in the General and Internal Medicine category, while *JAMA* ranks second with an impact factor of 11.435.

KEY CONCEPT

Impact factor is a tool used for ranking the relative quality of journals and is based upon the number of times that published papers are cited in subsequent papers.

In comparing journals using citation analysis, it is essential to keep in mind that review articles or technical papers on methods (e.g., an assay or other technique) tend to be cited much more commonly than other types of research. Journals that publish these types of papers tend to have the higher impact factors. In 1999, the highest impact factor in the field of pharmacology and pharmacy was 21.175 for the journal *Annual Review of Pharmacology and Toxicology. Clinical Pharmacokinetics,* which publishes review articles on pharmacokinetics, has a higher impact factor than journals like *Clinical Pharmacology and Therapeutics* and *Journal of Pharmacology and Experimental Therapeutics,* which publish original pharmacokinetic research. In addition, the target audience for a journal plays a role in the impact factor. Journals that are aimed primarily at clinicians or other individuals who are not primarily engaged in research (e.g., *American Journal of Health-System Pharmacy*) will be at a disadvantage when rated by a parameter such as the impact factor. Authors must, of course, be realistic about which journal to prepare a paper for. While publishing a paper in the *New England Journal of Medicine* may be a worthwhile goal of many who are involved in clinical research, the odds of having a paper accepted in this journal are approximately 7%.

Another consideration in selecting a journal is the time delay between the submission of a manuscript to a journal and the publication of the accepted paper. There are two components to this delay. The first is the time required for the journal to arrive at a final decision regarding the acceptability of the paper for publication. This is typically from 2 to 6 months and is dependent on the efficiency of the editor, ability or willingness of reviewers to adhere to deadlines, as well as the speed with which authors respond to any concerns that arise as part of the initial review. The second component is the lag time between the time an article is accepted for publication and when it is actually published. Again, a delay of from 2 to 6 months is average. Prospective authors would be well advised to look at a recent issue of the journal in question to find out when they might expect to see their paper published. The dates of receipt and acceptance of papers are published on the title page in a number of journals. Perusal of the August 2000 issue of *Clinical Pharmacology and Therapeutics* indicates that the papers were received for publication between October 1999 and April 2000 and accepted for publication in May 2000. In cases where an investigator feels that it is important that a paper be published more quickly, some journals (e.g., *Drug Metabolism and Disposition*) offer an "Accelerated Communications" section in which papers of special significance may be published within 1 or 2 months of acceptance. In addition, journals such as *Life Sciences* and *Research Communications in Chemical Pathology and Pharmacology* specialize in the rapid dissemination of research results.

Readers should be aware of this time frame as they evaluate the literature. A review article on the treatment of congestive heart failure published today is unlikely to discuss or cite papers that have been published within the last several months. Lag times with textbooks tend to be significantly longer and often exceed 1 year. Authors may, in some cases, be given the opportunity to insert critical new information into a paper at the time that they receive galley proofs shortly before the manuscript goes to press. However, this practice adds to the cost of publication and is not always welcomed by publishers.

Authorship

A quick perusal of the table of contents of a recent issue of any medical or pharmaceutical journal will quickly reveal that most papers have multiple authors. In contrast, papers in the social sciences and humanities more commonly have only one or two authors. A sign of the trend toward increasing numbers of authors on scientific papers can be seen in the decision of the National Library of Medicine to list not just the first six authors in *Index Medicus,* but the first 24 plus the last author.

Who is deserving of authorship on a paper? The answer to this question differs depending on whether one is talking to a journal editor or a scientist. The International Committee of Medical Journal Editors has published guidelines for authorship. In the most recent edition of "Uniform Requirements for Manuscripts Submitted to Biomedical Journals,"[21] this group states:

> Authorship credit should be based only on substantial contributions to 1) conception and design, or analysis and interpretation of data; and to 2) drafting the article or revising it critically for important intellectual content; and on 3) final approval of the version to be published. Conditions 1, 2, and 3 must all be met.

However, most medical scientists are unaware of these guidelines and those that are aware do not necessarily agree with them. In one study, the staff at a university medical school was surveyed on criteria for authorship. Only 5 of 66 persons could name the criteria required by the International Committee of Medical Journal Editors and only one was aware that all three criteria had to be met.[23] When informed of this requirement, 62% disagreed with it.

It appears that scientists accept that authorship should involve a "significant" contribution to a paper, but the definition of *significant* differs widely. Most would agree that the concept of "gift" authorship, in which a department chair or other superior is listed as an author without having made any real contribution to the work, should be eliminated. Requiring authors to be actively involved with the entire research process would also help to eliminate some of the more blatant cases of scientific fraud. By specifying that authors must meet all three stated criteria, the guidelines are designed to ensure that each author can be held accountable for the entire content of the paper.

Unfortunately, the guidelines for authorship are at odds with the current methods by which medical science is conducted. Complex studies require multiple investigators, each responsible for a discrete portion of the overall study. A typical drug study may involve the following:

- *Statisticians.* Study design and data analysis
- *Physicians.* Patient recruitment, monitoring, and medical care
- *Nurses.* Medication administration, record keeping, and nursing care
- *Pharmacists.* Blinding, randomization of subjects, and formulation of test drugs
- *Analytical chemists.* Drug assays
- *Scientists and other trained personnel.* Laboratory testing and other assessments of drug effects

The study could not be completed without the contribution of each of these individuals, and yet there may be only one person overseeing all aspects of the study. If the guidelines of the International Committee of Medical Journal Editors were followed, few of these individuals would be deemed worthy of inclusion as an author. Statisticians would seldom be granted authorship despite the critical role of these individuals in ensuring the accuracy of the conclusions of many studies.

In view of these problems, Drummond Rennie has suggested that the current system of authorship be abandoned in favor of a system in which the contribution of each member of the research team is specifically identified.[24] In other words, this system would be similar to that used in the film industry, whereby each individual receives a credit for his or her role in the project. This system has been adopted in part by the medical journal *The Lancet,* where a section called "Contributors" has been added at the end of each paper outlining the contribution of each author. The paper by Tisdale et al.,[25] reporting on the use of high-dose cyclophosphamide in severe aplastic anemia, contains the following statements under "Contributors":

> John Tisdale was responsible for protocol design, writing, submission, screening of patients, follow-up, termination, and report preparation. Daniel Dunn contributed to protocol design and writing, early screening of patients, and consent. Nancy Geller designed the statistical section, shared in planning, endpoint definitions, and analysed the trial at termination. Michelle Plant arranged randomisation, etc. . . .

Structure of Papers

Papers reporting original research rarely deviate from a standard format that includes an abstract, introduction, methods, results, discussion, and references. These components are described in detail in the "Uniform Requirements for Manuscripts Submitted to Biomedical Journals."[21] This document was developed by the International Committee of Medical Journal Editors and provides instructions to authors on how to prepare manuscripts as well as information on acceptable criteria for authorship and appropriate methods for citing various types of information sources from traditional journal articles to textbooks to conference proceedings to newspaper articles.

The rigid structure of papers in the drug literature makes it easier for a reviewer to evaluate a paper since each section has a defined content and purpose that needs to be met if the paper is to be of value. The editors of the *Annals of Internal Medicine* reported that most of the problems with papers can be characterized as too much, too little, inaccurate, or misplaced information.[26]

KEY CONCEPT

A systematic evaluation of a paper requires that the reviewer examine each section in detail to ensure that the content is accurate and complete.

The following paragraphs provide a description of the purpose and content of each of the major sections of a typical research paper:

1. *Abstract.* The abstract provides a short (150- to 200-word) summary of the paper. The format is dictated by the journal and may be free-style or a structured miniversion of the paper itself with 1 or 2 sentences on background, methods, results, and conclusions (see Fig. 3-1).[27] The abstract is the most visible part of the paper, not only because it is the first thing that readers encounter but also because it is the only part of the paper available to those searching secondary literature sources such as Medline or *International Pharmaceutical Abstracts*. If the message is not clearly expressed here, there is little chance that most readers will take the time to obtain or read the rest of the paper. Reviewers also need to assess the abstract carefully to make sure that the results and conclusions are consistent with those in the body of the paper and not overstated by an overly enthusiastic writer.

2. *Introduction.* The introduction should provide the reader with enough background information to understand why the study was undertaken as well as

Abstract

Background. Opioid dependence is a chronic, relapsing disorder with important public health implications.

Methods. In a 17-week randomized study of 220 patients, we compared levomethadyl acetate (75 to 115 mg), buprenorphine (16 to 32 mg), and high-dose (60 to 100 mg) and low-dose (20 mg) methadone as treatments for opioid dependence. Levomethadyl acetate and buprenorphine were administered three times a week. Methadone was administered daily. Doses were individualized except in the group assigned to low-dose methadone. Patients with poor responses to treatment were switched to methadone.

Results. There were 55 patients in each group; 51 percent completed the trial. The mean ($\pm SE$) number of days that a patient remained in the study was significantly higher for those receiving levomethadyl acetate (89 ± 6), buprenorphine (96 ± 4), and high-dose methadone (105 ± 4) than for those receiving low-dose methadone (70 ± 4, $p < 0.001$). Continued participation in the study was also significantly more frequent among patients receiving high-dose methadone than among those receiving levomethadyl acetate ($p = 0.02$). The percentage of patients with 12 or more consecutive opioid-negative urine specimens was 36 percent in the levomethadyl acetate group, 26 percent in the buprenorphine group, 28 percent in the high-dose methadone group, and 8 percent in the low-dose methadone group ($p = 0.005$). At the time of their last report, patients reported on a scale of 0 to 100 that their drug problem had a mean severity of 35 with levomethadyl acetate, 34 with buprenorphine, 38 with high-dose methadone, and 53 with low-dose methadone ($p = 0.002$).

Conclusions. As compared with low-dose methadone, levomethadyl acetate, buprenorphine, and high-dose methadone substantially reduce the use of illicit opioids. (N Engl J Med 2000;343:1290–7.)

Figure 3-1 Example of a structured abstract. [*From Johnson et al. (27). Reproduced from N Eng J Med 343:1290–1297, 2000, with permission from the Massachusetts Medical Society.*]

what the study proposes to accomplish. In other words, what was the purpose of the research? A statement of purpose can generally be found in the final paragraph of the introduction. For example, in the paper by Molander et al.,[28] the introduction finishes with the following sentence: "The purpose of this study was to assess the pharmacokinetics of intravenously administered nicotine and its main plasma metabolite cotinine in healthy subjects and in patients with different degrees of chronic renal failure." Sometimes the purpose may be stated more in the form of a hypothesis (e.g., "We postulated that inhibition of P-glycoprotein with guinidine would increase entry of loperamide into the CNS with resultant respiratory depression.").[29] In either case, it is important that the reader have a clear idea as to the purpose and potential value of the information after having read the introduction.

3. *Methods.* The "Methods" section is critical to evaluating the validity of the results. Although the casual reader is likely to gloss over highly detailed procedures, a critical evaluation of a paper requires that close attention be paid to this section. The patient population must be described as well as the methods for recruiting patients. In clinical studies, it is particularly important that the criteria used for patient entry and exclusion be listed so that clinicians can determine whether the results and conclusions can be applied to their own patients. The study design must be apparent, including the primary and secondary outcome measures that were used to assess drug response. This section should also include a description of the statistical methods used to draw conclusions. This can be a difficult section to write as authors must balance the needs of reviewers and other investigators in the field for specific, often highly technical information with the wishes of publishers and many potential readers to keep it as brief as possible.

4. *Results.* The results of the experiments are described using a combination of text, tables, and figures. The "Results" section should be consistent with the "Methods" section; in other words, there should not be results for which no methods were described, and there should not be procedures mentioned under "Methods" for which there are no results. Patients should all be accounted for including those who failed to complete the study. This should be the most important part of the paper. Reviewers should be able to draw their own conclusions concerning the interpretation of the data free of any "slant" that the authors may try to put on the results in other parts of the manuscript. This is frequently the shortest section of many papers since it is devoted to simply reporting the facts, hopefully accurately and without embellishment.

5. *Discussion.* This section provides the investigators with an opportunity to comment on the results, relate the data to previously published work, discuss the limitations of the study, and make inferences as to value of the work. It is here that the reader must be aware of attempts on the part of the authors to minimize any flaws in the design of the study while exaggerating the significance of the results. It is critical that the conclusions stated in the discussion are supported by the data from the study. The discussion also may include ideas for future studies that have arisen from the findings of the current study.

6. *References.*   Although the references would seem to be a necessary but rather innocuous section of a paper, a careful reviewer will examine the citations in detail. Key is that the references are accurate, current, and complete. It is not an uncommon practice for authors to simply ignore papers that contradict or do not support the hypothesis being tested. In addition, a paper published in 1998 that has no citations more current than 1991, for example, should raise concerns about the completeness of the bibliography. Alternatively, if no one has published a paper on this subject in 7 years, is it really an important area for investigation?

Style Guidelines for Biomedical Writing

"It was a dark and stormy night. . . ." A nice start to a short story or novel but not to a scientific or medical paper. Medical writing, like other forms of technical writing, is a unique literary form. The main objective of the medical writer is not to entertain the readership but rather to inform. It is beyond the scope of this chapter to present a detailed style guide for biomedical writing. A number of excellent books exist on this subject, including the following:

Huth ER: *How to Write and Publish Papers in the Medical Sciences,* 2d ed. Williams and Wilkins, Baltimore, MD, 1990.

Byrne DW: *Publishing Your Medical Research Paper: What They Don't Teach You in Medical School.* Williams and Wilkins, Baltimore, MD, 1998.

Weiss-Lambrou R: *The Health Professional's Guide to Writing for Publication.* CC Thomas, Springfield, IL, 1989.

Iverson C (chair) et al: *American Medical Association Manual of Style: A Guide for Authors and Editors,* 9th ed. Williams and Wilkins, Baltimore, MD, 1998.

All of these texts stress several common principles that can be paraphrased as the "ABCs" (accuracy, brevity, and clarity) of effective writing:

1. *Accuracy.*   It is essential that all statements in a paper written for the pharmaceutical or medical literature be accurate. In the case of an original research report, care must be taken to ensure that calculations are made correctly and that the results are summarized accurately in tables and figures as well as in the text. It is all too common to find errors in published articles. In the paper entitled "Failure of Prophylactically Administered Phenytoin to Prevent Early Posttraumatic Seizures," published in the *Journal of Neurosurgery,*[30] 136 patients were randomized to receive phenytoin. However, in Table 1 of this paper in which the patient population is broken down by age, there are 6 patients listed as being between 0 and 4 years old, another 6 between 5 and 15 years, and 104 who are over age 15, for a total of only 116 patients. Since the table also states that 4.4% of the patients were between 0 and 4 years of age, while 19.1% were between 5 and 15 years, it appears that there were actually 26 patients aged between 5 and 15 years since this would be 19.1% of 136. Clearly 6 patients cannot represent both 4.4% and 19.1% of the total patient population. A similar mistake appears in the same table in listing the Glasgow Coma Scale scores for the patients. It is relatively easy to find the discrepancies in this table and, fortunately, they are not critical to the conclusions of this particular paper. However, this is not always the case. Errors such as these may be due to a mistake by the authors in preparing the paper or by the publishers in preparing the text for publication. In the latter case, the authors are still held responsible since they are given a proof copy of the paper prior to publication to review for errors.

Needless to say, careful preparation of a paper and attention to detail during the editing process will hopefully eliminate errors of accuracy. Some writers find that having written a paper and revised it several times, they have difficulty detecting errors that are obvious to the first-time reader. It may be helpful to have a colleague who is not involved with the paper review it for accuracy prior to submission.

2. *Brevity.*   Brevity and clarity go hand in hand. It is hard to have one without the other. Authors should try to avoid words, sentences, and paragraphs that are too long. The readership of pharmacy, pharmacology, and medical journals is certainly better educated than the average citizen. However, the writer should not assume that this is a license to show off by using every 12-syllable word in the dictionary. Similarly, sentences that are too long can lose focus and become difficult to understand at all. Paragraphs should also convey a distinct message and, typically, one train of thought from beginning to end. Subdividing a paper into appropriate paragraphs helps organize the paper for the reader. Unnecessary words should be eliminated and modifiers kept to a minimum. The reader doesn't need to know that a result is "highly" significant; the degree of significance should be clear from the data. Writers should also avoid redundancy. A common problem is the repetition of statements in the "Introduction" and "Discussion" sections. Brevity is not just a guideline for good medical writing; it is often a requirement. Many journals specify that manuscripts not exceed a specific word count (e.g., 2000 or 3000 words).

3. *Clarity.*   A common complaint of authors is that the reviewer misunderstood the objective, study design, or some other aspect of their paper. Given the previously outlined problems with the peer review process, this may indeed be true. However, it may also be the author who is at fault for not writing in a clear manner. There are a number of stylistic and grammatical guidelines that can enhance clarity and are covered in detail in the texts referred to at the beginning of this section. Some general principles for clear writing include the following:

a. *Organization.*   Writing can be technically accurate, but without organization, it may be impossible to glean the primary message. Writers need to ensure that material is placed into the appropriate section. It is not uncommon to find results in the "Methods" section or results for which the methods for data collection are not described in the paper. In addition, a poorly organized discussion can leave the reader wondering exactly what point the writer was trying to make.

b. *Appropriate use of abbreviations.* Abbreviations and acronyms are abundant in medical science but are frequently unique to a specific discipline. It can be very frustrating to read a paper filled with abbreviations that requires the reader to constantly refer to other parts of the paper for explanation.

c. *Effective use of tables and figures.* A table is often a much more effective and efficient way to present raw or summarized data than simply stating the results using prose. Given the adage "A picture is worth a thousand words," it makes sense that a figure in a paper can provide a dramatic visual representation of the result of an experiment. A figure or table can also be a useful way to provide a summary of the disposition of patients entered into the study or to describe a complex study design involving multiple interventions and test groups. Figure 3-2 illustrates the design of a study in which the pharmacokinetics of three different statins (cerivastatin, atorvastatin, and pravastatin) were studied in the same subjects before and after treatment with itraconazole.[31] After an initial screening period, subjects received the first statin followed by blood sampling over the next 3 days. On days 6 through 10, itraconazole was administered. A second dose of the same statin was given on day 10 with further blood sampling. After completing a 14- to 17-day washout period, subjects repeated the drug administration and blood sampling cycle with the second and third statin.

Care must be taken with tables and figures to ensure that units are consistent and make sense. Although tables and figures, if used effectively, can improve the clarity of a paper, it is not uncommon to see the same data presented in a table and a figure, in two different figures, or in both the text and a table. Excessive use of tables and figures is discouraged since they can be time-consuming to lay out and add to the cost of publication.

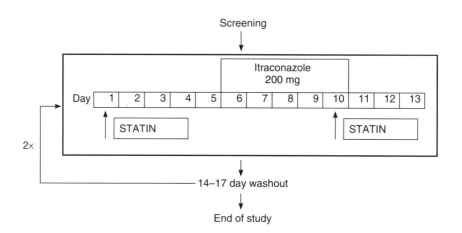

Figure 3-2. Use of a figure to illustrate a complex study design. [*From Mazzu et al. (31).*]

Study Questions

1. What is meant by the term *bias against the null hypothesis*? Why is this a problem?

2. Why is the *impact factor* a more objective measure of the quality of a journal than the circulation?

3. What information is contained in the document "Uniform Requirements for Manuscripts Submitted to Biomedical Journals"?

4. In which section of a manuscript should the reader find a summary of the demographic characteristics of the patients studied?

References

1. Miller TP, Dahlberg S, Cassady JR, et al: Chemotherapy alone compared with chemotherapy plus radiotherapy for localized intermediate- and high-grade Non-Hodgkin's lymphoma. N Engl J Med 339:21–26, 1998.

2. Machida U, Kami M, Hirai H: Treatment of intermediate-grade and high-grade Non-Hodgkin's Lymphoma. N Engl J Med 339:1475, 1998.

3. Mounier N, Gisselbrecht C, Lepage E: Treatment of intermediate-grade and high-grade Non-Hodgkin's Lymphoma. New Engl J Med 339:1476, 1998.

4. Decaudin D: Treatment of intermediate-grade and high-grade Non-Hodgkin's Lymphoma. N Engl J Med 339:1477, 1998.

5. Welch GE, Gabbe SG. Review of statistics usage in the *American Journal of Obstetrics and Gynecology*. Am J Obstet Gynecol 175:1138–1141, 1996.

6. Zinberg DS: A cautionary tale (editorial). Science 273:411, 1996.

7. Dong BJ, Hauck WL, Gambertoglio JG, Gee L, White JR, Bubp JL, Greenspan FS: Bioequivalence of generic and brand-name levothyroxine products in the treatment of hypothyroidism. JAMA 277:1205–1213, 1997.

8. Marshall E: Trial set to focus on peer review. Science 273:1162–1163, 1996.

9. Mullis K: *Dancing in the Mind Field*. New York, Vintage Books, 1998.

10. Baxt WG, Waeckerle JF, Berlin JA, Callaham ML: Who reviews the reviewers? Feasibility of using a fictitious manuscript to evaluate peer reviewer performance. Ann Emerg Med 32:310–317, 1998.

11. Koren G: Bias against the null hypothesis in maternal-fetal pharmacology and toxicology. Clin Pharmacol Ther 62:1–5, 1997.

12. Easterbrook PJ, Berlin JA, Gopalan R, Mathews DR: Publication bias in clinical research. Lancet 337:867–872, 1991.

13. Pitkin RM: The rewards of reading instructions from journal editors. N Engl J Med 339:1006, 1998.

14. Lau JYW, Sung JJY, Lee KKC, Yung M-Y, Wong SKJ, Wu JCY, et al: Effect of intravenous omeprazole on recurrent bleeding after endoscopic treatment of bleeding peptic ulcers. N Engl J Med 343:310, 2000.

15. Rennie D: Freedom and responsibility in medical publication: Setting the balance right. JAMA 280:300–302, 1998.

16. van Rooyen S, Godlee F, Evans S, Black N, Smith R: Effect of open peer review on quality of reviews and on reviewers' recommendations: a randomised trial. BMJ 318:23–27, 1999.

17. Davidoff F: Masking, blinding and peer review: The blind leading the blinded. Ann Intern Med 128:66–68, 1998.

18. Bingham CM, Higgins G, Coleman R, Van der Weyden MB: The *Medical Journal of Australia* Internet peer-review study. Lancet 352:441–445, 1998.

19. Bingham C, Van der Weyden MB. Peer review on the Internet: Launching eMJA peer review study 2. Med J Austr 169:240–241, 1998.

20. Ray J, Berkwits M, Davidoff F: The fate of manuscripts rejected by a general medical journal. Am J Med 109:131–135, 2000.

21. International Committee of Medical Journal Editors: Uniform requirements for manuscripts submitted to biomedical journals. Ann Intern Med 126:36–47, 1997.

22. *Ulrich's International Periodicals Directory*, 38th ed., New Providence, NJ, RR Bowker, 2000.

23. Bhopal R, Rankin J, McColl E, Thomas L, Kramer E, Stacy R, et al: The vexed question of authorship: Views of researchers in a British medical faculty. BMJ 314:1009–1012, 1997.

24. Rennie D, Emanuel L, Yank V. When authorship fails: A proposal to make contributors accountable. JAMA 278:579–585, 1997.

25. Tisdale JF, Dunn DE, Geller N, Plante M, Nunez O, Dunbar CE, et al: High-dose cyclophosphamide in severe aplastic anemia: A randomised trial. Lancet 356:1554–1559, 2000.

26. Purcell GP, Donovan SL, Davidoff F: Changes to manuscripts during the editorial process: Characterizing the evolution of a clinical paper. JAMA 280:227–228, 1998.

27. Johnson RE, Chutuape MA, Strain EC, Walsh SL, Stitzer ML, Bigelow GE: A comparison of levomethadyl acetate, buprenorphine, and methadone for opioid dependence. N Engl J Med 343:1290–1297, 2000.

28. Molander L, Hansson A, Lunell E, Alainentalo L, Hoffmann M, Larsson R: Pharmacokinetics of nicotine in kidney failure. Clin Pharmacol Ther 68:250–260, 2000.

29. Sadeque AJM, Wandel C, He H, Shah S, Wood AJJ: Increased drug delivery to the brain by P-glycoprotein inhibition. Clin Pharmacol Ther 68:231–237, 2000.

30. Young B, Rapp RP, Norton JA, Haack D, Tibbs PA, Bean JR: Failure of prophylactically administered phenytoin to prevent early posttraumatic seizures. J Neurosurg 58:231–235, 1983.

31. Mazzu AL, Lasseter KC, Shamblen C, Agarwal V, Lettieri J, Sundaresen P: Itraconazole alters the pharmacokinetics of atorvastatin to a greater extent than either cerivastatin or pravastatin. Clin Pharmacol Ther 68:391–400, 2000.

Chapter 4

Classification of Study Design— Observational Research

David J. Edwards

OUTLINE

Goals and Objectives

Introduction

Classification of Study Design

  Nature of Research

  Time Orientation of Research

  Investigator Action

Observational Research Designs in the Drug Literature

The Case Report

The Case-Control Study

The Cohort (Follow-Up) Study

Study Questions

References

KEY WORDS

Prospective	Experimental
Retrospective	Case-control
Cross-sectional	Cohort
Observational	Recall bias
Interventional	Attrition
Descriptive	

Goals and Objectives

The objective of this chapter is to introduce the reader to the terminology used to classify the design of a research study and to explore in detail observational research as represented by the case report, case-control study, and cohort study. After reading this chapter, readers should:

1. Understand the differences between descriptive and experimental research and the contribution of both to the drug literature.

2. Know the features that are required in order for a design to be considered experimental research.

3. Be able to identify a cross-sectional study and the differences between this design and others with respect to time orientation.

4. Understand the value of case reports as well as the disadvantages of this type of research compared with more rigorous study designs.

5. Be familiar with the features that distinguish case-control studies from cohort studies and be able to compare these designs with respect to their advantages and limitations.

Introduction

To students and clinicians who read and interpret the drug literature but are not actively involved in conducting research, the myriad of different study designs may appear bewildering. A large part of the problem is the jargon or terminology used to describe research designs and methods. Labels such as *crossover, parallel, cohort, case-control, retrospective versus prospective,* and *observation versus intervention* have little meaning to nonresearchers. While everyone is familiar with the traditional clinical trial, often considered to be the "gold standard" against which all other drug studies are compared, not all questions of interest can be addressed or are best examined with such a design.

In this chapter, the terminology used to describe and classify study designs will be defined. The role of observational studies in drug research will be discussed in detail with a focus on their relative advantages and disadvantages. Experimental research as exemplified by the clinical trial will be described in Chap. 5.

Classification of Study Design

The design of a study can be classified in a number of different ways. A useful model is that proposed by Burkett[1] in which the basic design of the study is assessed in three separate dimensions as illustrated in Fig. 4-1. This taxonomy suggests that the fundamental characteristics of any design can be described by a single term from each of the three categories. It should be noted that assignment of the study design in one dimension may or may not influence the categorization in another. For example, a study designated as *prospective* according to its time orientation can be either descriptive or experimental and may involve either observation of the patient or intervention in the patient's treatment. Retrospective studies, however, are always observational.

The choice of one design over another may be influenced by a variety of factors, including the availability of subjects, research funding, experience of the investigator, the nature of the problem to be studied, and ethical considerations.

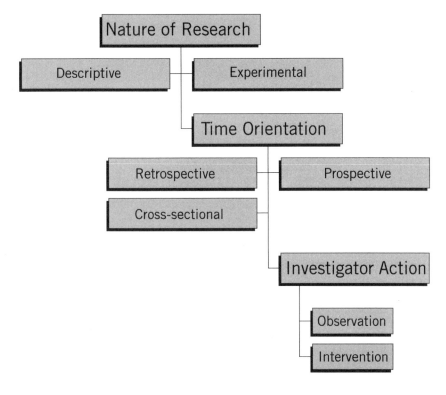

Figure 4-1. Classification of study designs in drug research.

Important information relevant to the use of a drug in a patient can be derived from any of the designs listed in Fig. 4-1. It should be recognized, however, that a hierarchy exists with respect to the level of confidence that is associated with the conclusions derived from particular designs. This hierarchy is illustrated in Fig. 4-2. According to this model, study designs at the bottom of the table merit the lowest level of confidence in the results while the highest level of confidence is reserved for the randomized, double-blind experimental study at the top of the table. While this may be a useful guide to the quality of research, readers should keep in mind that all designs are subject to bias and other confounding factors. A poorly designed and executed double-blind, randomized clinical trial will not necessarily yield more useful information than a well-done case-control study.

Nature of Research

Research can be classified according to the nature or objective of the study. Is the design sufficiently rigorous to allow for testing of a specific hypothesis? Studies in which causation or mechanism can be established represent the most rigorous designs and are variously referred to as *explanatory, analytical,* or *experimental* designs.

Level of Confidence in Conclusions	Control Group	Study Design	Blinding
↑	Randomized	Clinical Trial	Double-blind
	Nonrandomized	Cohort (Follow-up)	Single-blind
	None	Case-Control	None
		Case Report	

Figure 4-2. Hierarchy of research designs.

At the other end of the spectrum are studies designed to collect or gather information. These are classified as *descriptive, exploratory,* or *nonexperimental* designs.

Descriptive Studies. Descriptive studies are more commonly employed in the social sciences but, nonetheless, have a useful place in drug research. In contrast to experimental studies where hypotheses are tested, descriptive studies can be said to be "hypothesis-generating," in that the analysis of the collected data may suggest associations that lead to the formulation of a new hypothesis. For example, a survey was used to gather data concerning the usage of anticonvulsant medications in patients with preeclampsia and eclampsia.[2] The results suggested that the use of magnesium sulfate in eclampsia had increased from 2% in 1991 to 40% in 1996. Given the increasing and rather frequent use of magnesium sulfate in this condition, the investigators proposed that a clinical trial be conducted to test the hypothesis that magnesium sulfate is an effective anticonvulsant in these patients.

KEY CONCEPT

Descriptive research is necessary and valuable for a full understanding of the effects of drugs and may provide the background information for a hypothesis that can be tested by an experimental design.

While scientists sometimes consider descriptive studies to be second-rate, they provide valuable information to our understanding of human disease and its treatment. Investigators at the Centers for Disease Control in Atlanta reported on trends in the prevalence of drug-resistant tuberculosis in the United States.[3] This descriptive study provides clinicians in the field with data, which is directly useful in managing patients with this disease. Much of the research in the early phases of drug development can be classified as *descriptive* in nature. Pharmacokinetic studies measuring the clearance, volume of distribution, half-life, and routes of elimination of a drug are descriptive. These studies may involve small numbers of patients or may involve a large population; they examine the effect of disease states, body size, gender, and age on pharmacokinetic parameters. The descriptive nature of these investigations in no way detracts from their value in establishing rational dosing guidelines for patients.

Experimental Studies. In the laboratory, scientists are able to control a number of variables that could affect the validity of experimental results. This level of control is usually not possible in clinical research. Despite the limitations associated with studying patients, experimental drug research involves the formulation and testing of a hypothesis using a design that features the following elements:

1. *Manipulation of an independent variable (the drug treatment).* The effect of the treatment on one or more outcome measures (the dependent variable) is assessed. The dependent variable should ideally be a sensitive and specific indicator of the effect of the independent variable (see Chap. 6 for a discussion of measurement) whether it be a laboratory test (e.g., prothrombin time for assessing the efficacy of warfarin) or a more global measure of clinical outcome (e.g., 5-year survival of patients with breast cancer).

2. *Control of the experiment.* A variety of different methods for controlling an experiment are available and are discussed in more detail in Chap. 5. The goal is to ensure that a comparison can be made between two or more groups in which the only difference between the groups is the level of exposure to the drug treatment. For example, in a study examining the effectiveness of a new angiotensin II–converting enzyme inhibitor (ACE inhibitor) in treating hypertension, one group of subjects could receive the ACE inhibitor while another group receives a placebo.

3. *Randomization.* Randomization in an experimental study occurs at several levels. Individuals should be invited to participate in the study based on random selection from the patient population of interest. They should be randomly assigned to receive a particular treatment or, in designs where each subject receives multiple treatments, the order of treatment should be assigned at random.

True experiments are the only designs that can reliably answer questions as to mechanism or cause and effect (Does this drug cause the observed decrease in blood pressure?). Quasi-experimental designs are those that may contain some elements of a true experiment but at least one component (e.g., a control group) is missing.

Time Orientation of Research

Research designs can be classified according to the time when the data was generated relative to when the study was designed and initiated. Although all studies begin in the present, the answers to clinical questions may be found either by looking back at the work of others or by collecting new information.

Retrospective and Prospective Studies. The term *retrospective* can be defined as "directed to the past or contemplative of past events or experiences." In a retrospective study, the investigator examines past events and previously collected data (e.g., medical records, files in a database) to arrive at a conclusion regarding the problem under study. Drug usage patterns are commonly studied using a retrospective design. Bashford and coworkers[4] used a database with information on over 600,000 patients to examine prescribing patterns for proton pump inhibitors between 1991 and 1995. In a *prospective* study, the hypothesis is formulated a priori, that is, before setting out to collect data. In other words, the investigator has an idea for a study and subsequently generates the data to examine the problem.

Retrospective studies tend to be relatively inexpensive to perform because the data has already been generated. The investigator only needs to gather and analyze the information. Since new data does not have to be obtained, these studies can often be completed more quickly than prospective studies. However, because the events under study may have occurred several years previously, the investigator has no control over what data was collected, and information of interest may be missing (e.g., important laboratory tests, dietary habits of the subjects, socioeconomic status, or other important correlates). This should not be a problem in a properly designed prospective study where the investigator decides ahead of time what information to collect. In choosing a study design, a scientist must weigh the advantages of a retrospective study against the fact that the quality of data obtained prospectively will often be superior and allow for more confident conclusions regarding the study question. Case-control and cohort studies are designs frequently used to address the same types of research questions. They differ principally in that the former is a retrospective design, whereas the latter is usually prospective. The pros and cons of these designs are listed in Table 4-1 and are discussed in detail later in this chapter.

Cross-Sectional Studies. Whether a research design is retrospective or prospective, the data is typically generated over a period of time ranging from days to years.

TABLE 4-1. **Comparison of the Case-Control and Cohort Study Designs**

Parameter	Case Control	Cohort
Investigator action	Observational	Observational
Time orientation	Retrospective	Usually prospective
Outcome parameter	Odds ratio	Relative risk
Advantages	Less expensive, completed more quickly, fewer subjects required	Higher-quality data
Major limitation	Recall bias	Loss to follow-up

When research examines an issue at a specific point in time, the design is said to be *cross-sectional*. Patients may be surveyed regarding their medication use, compliance, or a myriad of other questions. Cross-sectional studies may use either previously collected or newly generated data, but in all cases, the data provides insight into the state of affairs at the time at which the data were collected. McAlister et al.[5] studied the use of digoxin in 2490 patients with atrial fibrillation. The data was obtained retrospectively from the medical records of 12 hospitals and six outpatient clinics in 1993 and 1994 and provides the reader with information concerning the prescribing patterns for digoxin at that specific time. Cross-sectional studies are widely used to establish the prevalence of diseases or drug usage. Schubiner and coworkers[6] used a cross-sectional design to assess the prevalence of attention-deficit/hyperactivity disorder (ADHD) in adults with chemical dependency. 28% of chemically dependent men were found to meet the diagnostic criteria for ADHD, a much higher percentage than that found in the general population.

KEY CONCEPT

Cross-sectional studies provide information concerning drug use at a specific point in time using data that has been generated either retrospectively or prospectively.

Trends can be examined by comparing cross-sectional studies conducted at different times. For example, teens are regularly surveyed regarding use of substances such as alcohol, tobacco, or illicit drugs. A comparison of data obtained in 2000 with similar data collected at various times over the previous 20 years can assist health care practitioners, social agencies, and legislators in addressing undesirable trends. Similar comparisons have been made in examining trends in the prevalence of HIV infection since the beginning of the AIDS outbreak approximately 20 years ago. Waldo et al.[7] studied a population of homosexual men in 1994 and 1995 and found that the seroprevalence for HIV was somewhat lower in the 15 to 17-year-olds compared with those aged between 18 and 22. However, the percentage of men engaging in unprotected sex (approximately 30%) was similar in both groups. The results can be compared with previous studies to determine whether infection rates are declining, as well as the effectiveness of education programs designed to promote AIDS awareness and prevention.

Cross-sectional studies are most useful if completed and published in a timely fashion. Although the study by McAlister et al.[5] provided accurate information on digoxin prescribing patterns in 1993 and 1994, the study was unfortunately not published until 1999 and may not be entirely relevant to current usage of the drug. Another potential problem with cross-sectional research can be confusion regarding cause-and-effect relationships. If subjects are observed to have impaired renal function and high drug levels in a cross-sectional study, which came first? Did high drug concentrations cause kidney damage or is reduced kidney function the cause of the high drug levels? Despite some limitations, cross-sectional designs are a valuable source of information (usually descriptive) and may lead to the development of new hypotheses that can be tested using prospective, experimental designs.

Investigator Action

The final criterion used to classify research design, according to Fig. 4-1, relates to the actions of the investigator.

Observational Studies. *Observational studies* are those in which the investigator is merely a passive observer and recorder of events and information. The investigator makes no attempt to intervene in the clinical course of the research subject. In retrospective studies, the events under study have already occurred prior to the formulation of the research hypothesis. Therefore, retrospective studies are always observational since there is no opportunity for intervention on the part of the researcher. The drug utilization review is an example of an observational, retrospective, descriptive study. This does not mean that all observational studies are retrospective, however. The cohort study discussed in detail later in this chapter is an example of an observational design in which patients are usually identified and followed prospectively.

Interventional Studies. In drug research, intervention is common. In *interventional studies,* patients receive a drug or perhaps laboratory or clinical testing that they would not otherwise receive if they were not participating in the research. These studies are, by definition, prospective. However, the nature of the research may be descriptive (patients required to take a new drug for the purpose of characterizing the pharmacokinetic properties) or experimental (patients required to take a new drug to test the hypothesis that it will lower blood pressure). This type of study design is represented by the clinical drug trial, discussed at length in Chap. 5.

Observational Research Designs in the Drug Literature

In reviewing the drug literature, the reader will come across a variety of different types of studies, some of which are unique to the use of drugs while others could be used to study other nondrug treatments (e.g., surgery, diet, lifestyle modification). Research designs specific to the use of drugs include the evaluation of drug stability and the pharmacoeconomic consequences of drug use. Studies examining the stability of drugs in various dosage forms are important to the practicing pharmacist. Physical and chemical stability must be ensured particularly when a product must be compounded or prepared by the pharmacist prior to administration, as is the case with many intravenously administered drugs.[8] In evaluating studies of this type, a key component is the use of a stability-indicating assay, that is, a method of analysis that will be sensitive enough to detect loss of drug as well as specific for the drug of interest and not subject to interference by the degradation products that may be formed. Pharmacoeconomic studies assess the economic impact of drug use and typically examine the balance between the costs of drug use (e.g., acquisition costs, compounding and dispensing costs, nursing costs, adverse events, etc.) and the benefits (e.g., reduced length of stay in the hospital, faster return to work, improved survival, etc.). As one would expect, assigning a monetary value to many of the benefits of successful drug therapy can be a difficult task.

Perusal of the major medical and pharmacy journals indicates that the majority of papers pertaining to the use of drugs can be classified as either *observational studies* or *experimental studies.* It has been suggested that the lack of randomization in observational research designs can lead to an overestimation of the treatment effect. However, two groups of investigators recently conducted a systematic review of studies published in the past 15 years looking at a variety of clinical treatments.[9,10] Both concluded that well-designed observational studies were not more likely to find a difference between groups than randomized clinical trials. For example, in comparing the mortality in patients treated with coronary artery bypass graft surgery versus medical treatment, observational studies and clinical trials were equally likely to conclude a benefit of similar magnitude for bypass surgery.[10] The remainder of this chapter focuses on the common types of observational research reported in the literature, and Chap. 5 is devoted to a discussion of experimental research.

The Case Report

Case reports are a primary and highly respected form of research in the social sciences. A cursory examination of the tables of contents of journals in the field of psychology or sociology, for example, will often reveal lengthy papers devoted to a discussion of a single patient. Neurologist and author Oliver Sacks has published a number of popular books describing the symptoms and behavior of individual patients with a variety of neurological disorders.[11] In-depth reports of the symptoms associated with rare but specific lesions of the central nervous system add much to our understanding of the function of the different regions of the brain.

In drug research, the case report does not enjoy the same status as more sophisticated research designs, such as the clinical trial, but it is nonetheless a potentially valuable source of information. In the hands of a skilled observer, the detailed description of the clinical course of a single patient or a collection of patients can be crucial to the identification of previously unreported side effects or interactions between drugs. An excellent example is the 1990 report by Monahan et al.[12] describing the occurrence of torsades de pointes in a patient taking the nonsedating antihistamine terfenadine. These investigators documented that repeated episodes of syncope and light-headedness in a patient were temporally associated with the use of ketoconazole for the treatment of vaginal candidiasis. Terfenadine had been previously found to produce cardiovascular toxicity only with an overdose. However, since ketoconazole was a known inhibitor of the cytochrome P450 enzyme responsible for terfenadine metabolism, the authors speculated that the drug combination could produce elevated plasma concentrations of terfenadine. This was confirmed by measured terfenadine concentrations that were much higher than expected. This report, along with several that followed shortly thereafter, led to the identification of torsades de pointes as a potentially fatal complication of terfenadine therapy and eventually resulted in the removal of this drug from the market.

Using the classification system previously described, the case report falls into the category of descriptive research. In addition, the vast majority can be said to be retrospective in that the subject or subjects of a case report are identified only after experiencing an unusual response to a drug. In some cases, the original observation may be followed up by a prospective study involving intervention. For example, patients may be rechallenged with a drug combination while being closely monitored in order to document that an effect is indeed due to a drug interaction. In the terfenadine case described previously, the investigators did not merely speculate as to the cause of the interaction but actually obtained a blood sample in order to confirm that terfenadine concentrations were abnormally high.

Although potentially valuable, readers should bear in mind a number of caveats in interpreting the findings in case reports:

1. Case reports often represent extreme rather than typical situations with respect to the effects of a drug. In 1987, Rybak et al.[13] described the case of an older male who experienced a threefold increase in theophylline concentration after beginning treatment with the fluoroquinolone antibiotic ciprofloxacin. The authors speculated that the patient's age may have played a role in the magnitude of the observed interaction. Subsequent controlled studies found that ciprofloxacin reduced theophylline clearance by an average of roughly 30% in both young and elderly subjects.[14] While it is important that clinicians be aware of the potential for large interactions such as the patient reported by Rybak et al.,[13] these are not typical and are not more likely in older individuals.

2. A report describing an adverse reaction to a particular drug may imply that the incidence of toxicity is much greater than it really is. The reader has no way of knowing, in most cases, the number of other patients receiving the same drug who showed no evidence of such toxicity.

3. Case reports are unable to establish a cause-and-effect relationship or mechanism for an observation due to the lack of a true experimental design. Investigators may have a plausible explanation for the observed patient symptoms, but proof is usually not forthcoming in a case report. Although the most unique feature of the patient whose theophylline concentrations were dramatically increased by ciprofloxacin appeared to be his age,[13] subsequent studies could not confirm that age was a factor in this interaction. On the other hand, given the strong evidence that torsades de pointes was caused by ketoconazole inhibiting terfenadine metabolism, a prospective study was conducted to test this hypothesis. Terfenadine was administered alone and in combination with ketoconazole to a group of healthy volunteer subjects and found to produce EKG changes that were consistent with the development of torsades de pointes.[15]

> **KEY CONCEPT**
>
> In evaluating a case report, readers should be aware that a more rigorous study design is usually required to accurately assess the incidence, significance, and mechanism of the observation.

The Case-Control Study

In drug research, epidemiological studies are designed to examine the relationship between the development of a particular disease state or adverse effect and the use of a drug or class of drugs. The two primary methods utilized in research of this type are the *case-control* and *cohort* designs. They are observational investigations in that the researcher observes or records information about the subjects without actively intervening in their drug therapy. In addition, they are classified as quasi-experimental designs because they are more rigidly structured than typical descriptive studies but lack at least one feature of a true experimental design, such as randomization of subjects. Although they cannot directly answer questions of cause and effect, the case-control or cohort designs are often the only feasible approach for investigating the link between drug use and adverse events that may be rare and take years or decades to develop. The similarities and differences between these designs are listed in Table 4-1.

Although the case-control study and the cohort study are both observational designs that may be used to answer the same question, they generally differ in the time orientation of the research. The case-control study is a retrospective design in which subjects are identified because they have already experienced the adverse effect or disease being studied (see Fig. 4-3). Czeizel, Toth, and Rockenbauer[16] examined the potential teratogenicity of clotrimazole, an antifungal compound applied topically for the treatment of vulvovaginal candidiasis. Like many drugs, the FDA rates clotrimazole as category C, meaning teratogenic risk cannot be ruled out. In this case-control study, 18,515 cases of pregnancies resulting in congenital abnormalities were compared with 32,804 control pregnancies in which no malformations at birth were observed. Mothers in each group were surveyed regarding use of drugs during pregnancy. To study this problem using a classic experimental design would be extremely difficult. The required administration of a suspected teratogen would be viewed as unethical by most observers, and recruitment of subjects for such a study would be next to impossible. In addition, the rigorous control and monitoring required in traditional clinical trials would be prohibitively expensive given the large number of subjects required to study a relatively rare event such as this. In this study, cases of mothers who had given birth to a baby with a congenital anomaly were already on record in the Hungarian Congenital Abnormality Registry.

In a case-control study, once the case and control groups have been selected, a retrospective review is conducted to determine whether differences exist between

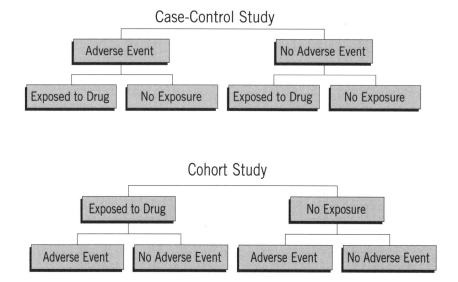

Figure 4-3. Case-control and cohort study designs.

the groups in the use of the drug in question. There are a number of drug surveillance programs in which large databases of patient information are used to conduct research of this type. The Boston Collaborative Drug Surveillance Program published numerous papers in the 1970s and early 1980s typically using a case-control design. A good example is the paper published in the journal, *Archives of Internal Medicine,* in which patients admitted to a hospital with serious gastrointestinal bleeding were found to be twice as likely to have a history of heavy, regular aspirin use compared with the control group of subjects admitted without gastrointestinal bleeding.[17] Note that the starting point for the investigation was the identification of patients who had already experienced the outcome (gastrointestinal bleeding) that was being investigated.

The conclusions of a case-control study are based on a parameter known as the *odds ratio.* This makes sense since the starting point for a case-control study is the occurrence of a particular adverse event or disease of interest. Therefore, the

KEY CONCEPT

The starting point for a case-control study is the identification of subjects who have experienced the effect of interest, whereas the starting point for a cohort study is the identification of subjects who are taking the drug of interest.

investigator is interested in knowing the odds of this event being associated with exposure to a drug as opposed to being a chance occurrence. The odds ratio is calculated by dividing the exposure rate to the drug under study in the subjects who have experienced the adverse event to the exposure rate in the control group:

$$\text{Odds ratio} = \frac{\text{drug exposure rate (cases)}}{\text{drug exposure rate (controls)}}$$

The odds ratio may be greater than, less than, or equal to 1. If the ratio is statistically greater than 1, then the odds of developing the effect under study are increased by exposure to the drug. Conversely, if the odds ratio is statistically less than 1, the drug reduces the probability. In the study examining the teratogenic potential of clotrimazole, the exposure rate was 7.1% in the mothers with malformed babies and 7.7% in the control group. The odds ratio was calculated by dividing 7.1 by 7.7 to give a value of 0.9. Since this was not statistically greater or less than 1, the odds of a congenital malformation occurring were not affected by exposure to clotrimazole. (The odds ratio is discussed in more detail in Chap. 9.)

The case-control study is a cost-effective method for obtaining timely information on drug effects, particularly those that occur rarely or after long-term exposure. This presumes, of course, that the data is available and accessible to investigators. Despite the advantages, case-control studies are subject to the same disadvantages as other retrospective designs. The validity of the conclusions depends on the answers to two primary questions:

1. Are differences in outcome caused by something other than differences in drug exposure?

2. Has the degree of drug exposure in the case and control groups been accurately determined?

It is critical that the criteria for inclusion in the case and control groups be carefully defined in order for the results of these studies to be of value. In the clotrimazole study described previously, the cases consisted of infants with malformations. However, it would not be appropriate to include infants with malformations clearly ascribed to some other cause (e.g., genetic disorder or documented exposure to another known teratogen) in the case group. This could lead to an underestimation of the potential problem since cases of malformations possibly due to clotrimazole become in essence diluted out by cases due to other causes. The control group must also be carefully selected. Key is that both cases and controls come from the same general population so that potential factors other than drug exposure are equally distributed. Because case-control studies sometimes examine rare or unusual events, the case group may be primarily patients who come to the attention of investigators at large urban teaching hospitals. In this situation, a control group selected from a more general population (e.g., patients admitted to community hospitals) may not be appropriate.

In assessing the incidence of exposure in the case and control groups, case-control studies often rely on the ability of the subjects to recollect past events. Recall bias occurs when there are differences between the case and control groups in their ability to determine whether they were exposed to the drug under investigation. Mothers with a malformed baby will undoubtedly be highly motivated to recall any event or exposure that could possibly have caused or contributed to their child's condition, whereas those in the control group with healthy babies are unlikely to be as diligent in examining past events. In this situation, the result could be an underestimation of drug exposure in the control group. A similar problem can occur if investigators are not equally diligent in searching medical records for evidence of drug exposure in both groups of subjects.

The Cohort (Follow-Up) Study

The fundamental difference between the cohort study and the case-control study is that the former begins by identifying potential subjects based on their use of the drug under investigation, not because they have already experienced an effect of the drug (Fig. 4-3). Because subjects are subsequently followed for weeks, months, or years to evaluate the development of specific adverse events or diseases, the term *follow-up study* is sometimes used to describe the cohort design. One of the most well-known examples of the cohort design is the Framingham Heart Study in which a cohort in Framingham, Massachusetts, has been followed for almost 50 years to examine the relationship between various risk factors and the development of cardiovascular disease.[18] Most cohort studies are prospective in nature since the study begins with the selection of the subjects and future events are recorded. However, it is possible to have a retrospective or historical cohort study. If accurate records are available, a cohort of subjects receiving a drug can be identified retrospectively and followed through their medical records, for example, to assess the development of the effects of interest. Sorensen et al.[19] used a retrospective cohort design in evaluating the risk of upper gastrointestinal bleeding due to the use of low-dose aspirin. The cohort was identified from a prescription database that was linked to a hospital discharge registry used to identify patients with gastrointestinal bleeding.

Cohort studies also differ from case-control studies in that the key measurement parameter is referred to as *relative risk:* the risk of development of a disease state or adverse event in those taking the drug under investigation compared with those not taking the drug as described by the following equation:

$$\text{Relative risk} = \frac{\text{adverse event rate (drug)}}{\text{adverse event rate (control)}}$$

As was the case with the odds ratio, the values for relative risk can be greater than, less than, or equal to 1. (The relative risk ratio is discussed in more detail in Chap. 9.) Beral et al.[20] used a cohort design to examine mortality associated with oral contraceptive use over a 25-year period. The cohort consisted of 46,000 women, half of which were using oral contraceptives at the time of entry into the study in 1968–1969. The results are summarized in Table 4-2. The risk of death

TABLE 4-2. **Relative Risk of Mortality from Various Causes Associated with Oral Contraceptive Use**

Cause of Death (ICD-8 code)	Standardized Mortality Ratio (No. of Deaths)		Relative Risk* (95% CI)
	Ever Users	Never Users	
All causes (000–999)	82 (945)	74 (654)	1.0 (0.9–1.1)
All cancers (140–209)	85 (474)	85 (355)	1.0 (0.8–1.1)
Colorectal (153–154)	62 (29)	108 (39)	0.6 (0.4–0.9)[†]
Liver (155)	126 (5)	34 (1)	5.0 (0.6–43.2)
Lung (162)	107 (75)	71 (40)	1.2 (0.8–1.8)
Breast (174)	87 (154)	81 (105)	1.1 (0.8–1.4)
Cervix (180)	115 (38)	57 (13)	1.7 (0.9–3.2)
Uterus (181–2)	22 (2)	83 (6)	0.3 (0.1–1.4)
Ovary (183)	49 (24)	83 (31)	0.6 (0.3–1.0)[†]
Other cancers	87 (147)	95 (120)	0.9 (0.7–1.1)
All circulatory diseases (390–458)	84 (237)	63 (143)	1.2 (1.0–1.5)
Ischaemic heart disease (410–414)	70 (98)	68 (79)	0.9 (0.7–1.3)
Other heart disease (420–429)	107 (19)	66 (9)	1.4 (0.6–3.1)
Cerebrovascular disease (430–438)	111 (87)	62 (38)	1.5 (1.0–2.3)[†]
Other circulatory	73 (33)	46 (17)	1.4 (0.8–2.5)
All digestive diseases (520–577)	85 (37)	74 (24)	1.1 (0.6–1.8)
Liver disease (570–573)	112 (23)	69 (10)	1.7 (0.8–3.6)
All other diseases (1–139, 210–389, 460–519, 578–799)	53 (95)	65 (89)	0.8 (0.6–1.0)
Violent or accidental causes (800–999)	111 (102)	68 (43)	1.6 (1.1–2.3)[†]
Suicide (950–959)	123 (39)	73 (16)	1.5 (0.8–2.7)

*Adjusted for age, social class, parity, and smoking.

[†]$p < 0.05$.

SOURCE: From Beral et al. (20). Reproduced from BMJ 318:96–100, 1999, with permission from the BMJ Publishing Group.

from all causes for subjects who had used oral contraceptives relative to those who had never used the product was found to be 1.0, suggesting that oral contraceptive use did not increase the risk of death. Analysis of specific causes of death indicated that the relative risk for development of ovarian cancer was reduced to 0.6 by oral contraceptive use (protective effect) while the risk of death from cerebrovascular disease was increased to 1.5.

The prospective nature of the cohort study makes it less susceptible to some of the problems typically associated with retrospective designs. Although there is no randomization of subjects, the control group can be carefully selected to ensure that it is well matched to the group exposed to the drug in terms of risk factors for the development of the adverse event or disease in question. This may not be possible in a case-control study where information on potentially important variables may be forgotten, not recorded, or unavailable. Cohort studies may still be susceptible to confounding factors, however. The oral contraceptive study reported that the risk of death from cervical cancer was higher in users of oral contraceptives.[20] However, users and nonusers were not matched with respect to other risk factors for cervical cancer. It is certainly possible that oral contraceptive users would be less likely to use condoms and likely to have more sexual partners than those who never used the birth control pill. This illustrates the need for careful selection of the control group in the cohort study to ensure that the use of the drug under study is the only significant difference between the patients under investigation.

Cohort studies have some other disadvantages compared with case-control studies. More subjects are generally required, particularly when studying drug effects that occur rarely. The risk of developing hereditary ovarian cancer with use of oral contraceptives was examined in a case-control study by Narod et al.[21] Although they reached the same conclusion as the cohort study conducted by Beral et al.,[20] namely that the use of oral contraceptives lowers the risk of developing ovarian cancer, the case-control study involved less than 400 women compared with 46,000 in the cohort study. Since the analysis of data from a cohort study is dependent on subjects developing a disease or adverse event (Fig. 4-3), uncommon drug effects will require the study of extremely large cohorts. Case-control studies can also be performed more quickly and at less expense since the data has already been collected and only has to be analyzed by the investigators. Contrast this with a cohort study that may be looking at adverse events that take years to develop.

The long-term follow-up required in many cohort studies can affect the relevance of the conclusions to current medical practice. The oral contraceptive cohort study[20] was initiated in 1968 and published in 1999, a delay of 31 years. Estrogen content and usage patterns have changed significantly during this period. While women are generally taking a lower-dose pill today, they also begin taking oral contraceptives at a much younger age compared with the 1960s. In addition, women are now much likelier to take the pill prior to having their first child, whereas 30 years ago, many women got married at an earlier age and only began using oral contraceptives after having one or more children. This could confound the conclusion that oral contraceptives do not increase the risk of death due to breast cancer.

Based on evidence that breast tissue may be more sensitive to carcinogens prior to giving birth, it is reasonable that the association between oral contraceptive use and the development of breast cancer can best be assessed by studying women who took the product before, not after, having children.

A final problem with the cohort design, and one of the most significant, is the attrition of subjects. Over the course of a study lasting many years, subjects may change physicians, move to another city or country, fail to respond to inquiries from investigators, or be lost to follow-up for any number of other reasons including death. In the oral contraceptive study, approximately 25% of the original cohort recruited in 1968 could not be located by 1976–1977.[20] These losses can bias the conclusions of a study, particularly if attrition occurs unequally in the groups. It is not hard to imagine the potential problem in a study in which subjects in the group exposed to the drug are more difficult to locate because they have died.

Despite these limitations, a well-designed cohort design can produce high-quality data and valid conclusions with respect to the effects of drugs. This design may be the best or, in some cases, the only option available to investigators who wish to study the risk of developing serious and relatively rare drug effects. Since most cohort studies are prospective, this design tends to have more in common with clinical trials than the case-control study. However, a key difference is that the clinical trial involves intervention rather than mere observation of events.

Study Questions

1. Why is a cohort study not considered to be a true experimental design?

2. What are the advantages and disadvantages of a retrospective study compared with a prospective study?

3. Leitzmann et al.[22] examined the link between drinking coffee and gallstone disease. Individuals who drank between 2 and 4 cups of coffee per day had a relative risk of developing symptomatic gallstones of 0.6. What type of study was this and how should the results be interpreted?

4. What is recall bias? What type of study design does it affect?

References

1. Burkett GL: Classifying basic research designs. Fam Med 22:143–148, 1990.

2. Gülmezoglu AM, Duley L: Use of anticonvulsants in eclampsia and pre-eclampsia: Survey of obstetricians in the United Kingdom and Republic of Ireland. BMJ 316:975–976, 1998.

3. Moore M, Onorato IM, McCray E, Castro KG: Trends in drug-resistant tuberculosis in the United States, 1993–1996. JAMA 278:833–837, 1997.

4. Bashford JNR, Norwood J, Chapman SR: Why are patients prescribed proton pump inhibitors? Retrospective analysis of link between morbidity and prescribing in the General Practice Research Database. BMJ 317:452–456, 1998.

5. McAlister FA, Ackman ML, Tsuyuki RT, Kimber S, Teo KK: Contemporary utilization of digoxin in patients with atrial fibrillation. Ann Pharmacother 33:289–293, 1999.

6. Schubiner H, Tzelepis A, Milberger S, Lockhart N, Kruger M, Kelley BJ, et al: Prevalence of attention-deficit/hyperactivity disorder and conduct disorder among substance abusers. J Clin Psychiatry 61:244–251, 2000.

7. Waldo CR, McFarland W, Katz MH, MacKellar D, Valleroy LA: Very young gay and bisexual men are at risk for HIV infection: the San Francisco Bay Area Young Men's Survey II. J Acquir Immune Defic Syndr 24:168–174, 2000.

8. Kowaluk EA, Roberts MS, Polack AE: Interactions between drugs and intravenous delivery systems. Am J Hosp Pharm 39:460–467, 1982.

9. Benson K, Hartz AJ: A comparison of observational studies and randomized, controlled trials. N Engl J Med 342:1878–1886, 2000.

10. Concato J, Shah N, Horwitz RI: Randomized, controlled trials, observational studies and the hierarchy of research designs. N Engl J Med 342:1887–1892, 2000.

11. Sacks O: *An Anthropologist on Mars.* New York, Alfred A. Knopf, 1995.

12. Monahan BP, Ferguson CL, Killeavy ES, Lloyd BK, Troy J, Cantilena LR: Torsades de pointes occurring in association with terfenadine use. JAMA 264:2788–2790, 1990.

13. Rybak MJ, Bowles SK, Chandrasekar PH, Edwards DJ: Increased theophylline concentrations secondary to ciprofloxacin. Drug Intell Clin Pharm 21:879–881, 1987.

14. Loi CM, Parker BM, Cusack BJ, Vestal RE: Aging and drug interactions. III. Individual and combined effects of cimetidine and cimetidine and ciprofloxacin on theophylline metabolism in healthy male and female nonsmokers. J Pharmacol Exp Ther 280:627–637, 1997.

15. Honig PK, Wortham DC, Zamani K, Conner DP, Mullin JC, Cantilena LR: Terfenadine-ketoconazole interaction. Pharmacokinetic and electrocardiographic consequences. JAMA 269:1513–1518, 1993.

16. Czeizel AE, Tóth M, Rockenbauer M: No teratogenic effect after clotrimazole therapy during pregnancy. Epidemiology 10:437–440, 1999.

17. Jick H: Effects of aspirin and acetaminophen in gastrointestinal hemorrhage. Results from the Boston Collaborative Drug Surveillance Program. Arch Int Med 141:316–321, 1981.

18. Culleton BF, Larson MG, Kannel WB, Levy D: Serum uric acid and risk for cardiovascular disease and death: The Framingham Heart Study. Ann Intern Med 131:7–13, 1999.

19. Sorensen HT, Mellemkjaer L, Blot WJ, Nielsen GL, Steffensen FH, McLaughlin JK, et al: Risk of upper gastrointestinal bleeding associated with use of low-dose aspirin. Am J Gastroenterol 95:2218–2224, 2000.

20. Beral V, Hermon C, Kay C, Hannaford P, Darby S, Reeves G: Mortality associated with oral contraceptive use: 25 year follow up of cohort of 46,000 women from Royal College of General Practitioners' oral contraception study. BMJ 318:96–100, 1999.

21. Narod SA, Risch H, Moslehi R, Dørum A, Neuhausen S, Olsson H, et al: Oral contraceptives and the risk of hereditary ovarian cancer. N Engl J Med 339:424–428, 1998.

22. Leitzmann MF, Willett WC, Rimm EB, Stampfer MJ, Spiegelman D, Colditz GA, et al: A prospective study of coffee consumption and the risk of symptomatic gallstone disease in men. JAMA 281:2106–2112, 1999.

Study Design— Experimental Research

David J. Edwards

OUTLINE

Goals and Objectives

Introduction

Validity of Clinical Trials: Internal Versus External Validity

Enhancing Validity

    Use of a Control Group

Blinding

Selecting an Appropriate Sample

Subject Attrition and Intention-to-Treat Analysis

Study Questions

References

KEY WORDS

Internal validity	Washout period
Confounding	Carryover effect
External validity	Period effect
Hypothesis	Blinding
Randomization	Sampling
Parallel	Attrition
Crossover	Intention-to-treat analysis

Goals and Objectives

The purpose of this chapter is to describe the study design characteristics that distinguish experimental research, as illustrated by the clinical trial, from other types of drug research. Methods for enhancing validity through the use of appropriate controls, randomization, blinding, and sampling will be discussed. After completing this chapter, readers should:

1. Understand the difference between internal and external validity and be able to identify factors that affect each.

2. Understand the importance of a control group and be able to distinguish between the different types of controls employed in clinical drug trials.

3. Be able to compare the advantages and disadvantages of parallel and crossover studies.

4. Understand the role of randomization in enhancing experimental validity.

5. Be aware of the potential influence of subject and investigator expectations on the outcome of clinical trials and the role of blinding in minimizing these effects.

6. Understand the effect of inappropriate sample selection on external validity.

7. Know how intention-to-treat analysis can be used to deal with the influence of subject attrition on the results of a clinical trial.

Introduction

The origin of the modern clinical trial can be traced to the use of streptomycin to treat tuberculosis in the 1940s,[1] and it has rapidly become the standard against which all other designs are compared. The clinical trial is a true experimental design in which a hypothesis can be tested and cause-and-effect relationships established. Using the taxonomy described in the previous chapter (Fig. 4-1), this design is classified as prospective and involves intervention on the part of the investigator. It exhibits all of the properties of an experiment—that is, manipulation of an independent variable (the drug treatment), control, and randomization. These characteristics are required so that the results of the study can be used to either accept or reject the hypothesis being tested.

Clinical trials begin with the formulation of a hypothesis. A *hypothesis* is a statement predicting the relationship between variables or a difference between treatments. The hypothesis must be clear and straightforward, not convoluted, and must be testable by the methods and techniques available to the investigator. In addition, a good hypothesis is based on prior scientific evidence. The results of the study should be of interest even if the data indicates that the hypothesis should be rejected. A hypothesis that a beta blocker such as propranolol is useful in the treatment of colon cancer would be a poor one if based purely on speculation and not on any scientific evidence to support such a hypothesis. If a study were to conclude that propranolol is not effective in treating colon cancer, the results would not be of much interest. Although there is clearly a bias in the literature against the publication of negative results (see Chap. 3), in some cases, these are studies for which there was little objective support for or interest in the hypothesis being tested.

An example of a well-conceived hypothesis can be found in the study by King et al. published in the *Journal of the American Medical Association*.[2] These investigators tested the hypothesis that the testosterone precursor androstenedione would

KEY CONCEPT

The results of a study based on a well-founded hypothesis will be of interest even if no significant differences are observed in any of the outcome measures (the null hypothesis is accepted).

affect serum testosterone concentrations and the response of skeletal muscle fibers to resistance training. The hypothesis was based on the widespread use and marketing of androstenedione as a "natural" anabolic steroid in the wake of the publicity associated with the use of the product by professional baseball player Mark McGwire as he chased the major league baseball home run record during the summer of 1998. The results of the study supported the null hypothesis; that is, androstenedione did not affect either free or total serum concentrations of testosterone and did not improve the response of subjects to training. The fact that there was no difference noted in these primary outcome measures in no way detracts from the value or level of interest in the results. A more detailed discussion of the concepts and limitations of hypothesis testing is presented in Chap. 7.

Validity of Clinical Trials: Internal Versus External Validity

The design of a clinical trial revolves around ensuring that the conclusions reached will be valid. Ideally, studies have both internal and external validity. *Internal validity* means that the changes in the dependent variable or outcome (e.g., blood pressure, plasma cholesterol concentration, healing of ulcers) can truly be attributed to the manipulation of the independent variable (the drug treatment). When the outcome is influenced by something other than the drug treatment, the effect is known as *confounding*. Suppose that newly diagnosed patients with non–insulin-dependent diabetes mellitus are entered into a study to test the effectiveness of a new oral hypoglycemic agent. However, at the same time, many of the patients alter their dietary habits, reducing their intake of carbohydrates and losing weight. In this situation, it would not be possible to attribute a decrease in blood glucose

KEY CONCEPT

A study has internal validity if the changes in the outcome under investigation are due to the study drug and not to confounding factors. A study has external validity if the results can be extrapolated from the subjects studied to the general patient population.

concentration to the drug treatment. The use of an appropriate control group is generally the most effective way of enhancing internal validity and reducing confounding in a clinical trial.

External validity refers to the ability to generalize the results from the subjects participating in the clinical trial to the patient population in general. If a drug lowers blood pressure in a study, will it have the same effect on other patients with high blood pressure? The participants in a clinical trial are invariably a small subset of the patient population for which the drug under study is intended. The results of a study will be of little use if they cannot be extrapolated beyond the study participants. In addition, the study conditions must be realistic. If a useful drug effect can be demonstrated only under such stringently controlled conditions that it cannot be duplicated when patients are treated in their usual environment, then the drug will be of little value. Liberal entry criteria with relatively few restrictions will allow a broad spectrum of a population to qualify for study and will improve the external validity of the results. However, if patients are allowed to participate who have numerous coexisting disease states and are being treated with several drugs, there is a greater chance that the outcome of interest could be affected by something other than the study medication.

A high degree of internal validity can, in some cases, be achieved only at the expense of external validity. In designing a study, investigators are often faced with a difficult task in attempting to achieve both. Studies that have tightly controlled criteria for entry combined with numerous exclusions with respect to disease states or medications other than the one being studied may provide the best opportunity to test the hypothesis under study. However, the resulting study population may be so unique that the results will not be of value to the average patient with the disease. Furthermore, it may be impractical to complete such a study. Recruitment of patients will be time-consuming since relatively few patients will qualify to participate. In addition, the restrictions placed on the subjects to improve the internal validity of the study may make it difficult or impossible to fully adhere to the protocol.

The study by Tilley et al.[3] examining the efficacy and safety of minocycline in treating rheumatoid arthritis offers a classic example of this problem. A valid assessment of the activity of minocycline could be made only if the placebo and minocycline groups were well matched with respect to the use of alternative antiarthritic medications. As a result, significant restrictions were placed on the patients and their attending physicians with respect to the use of disease-modifying drugs, steroids, and nonsteroidal anti-inflammatory drugs during the investigation. At the time of entry into the study, the placebo and treatment groups were well matched with respect to other medications. However, as the study progressed, more patients in the placebo group received an increase in dosage of concomitant oral corticosteroids and nonsteroidal anti-inflammatory drugs. In addition, 17% of these patients were given intra-articular corticosteroids during the study compared to only 6% in the minocycline group. The net effect of these protocol violations was that the response of the placebo group was significantly better than expected, and no significant difference could be discerned between minocycline and placebo with respect to disease activity as assessed by either patient or physician. It is difficult to fault either the investigators for attempting to restrict the use of concomitant medications or the patients' physicians for responding to their needs for symptomatic relief. However, the numerous protocol violations compromised the internal validity of the study and prevented a full assessment of the efficacy of minocycline.

Enhancing Validity

The specific methods used in drug research vary from study to study and from discipline to discipline. However, a number of standard techniques are employed in studies to ensure that the results will be valid. It should be noted that while these are desirable features, they are not always necessary. For example, drug interaction studies examining the effect of one drug on the clearance of another rarely blind the subjects to the treatment they are receiving. The assumption is that an objective parameter such as drug clearance is unlikely to be influenced by subject expectations. On the other hand, use of an appropriate control group is critical in such studies. When evaluating the drug literature, readers should always examine papers carefully to determine whether the following design features are present or necessary to ensure the validity of the conclusions.

Use of a Control Group

A control group is a group of subjects not exposed to the drug treatment being studied. Ideally, the control group is identical in every way to the treatment group with the exception that they do not receive the study drug. Whether due to the natural improvement of the disease without treatment or perhaps a temporary remission of symptoms, a review of published clinical trials suggests that it is not uncommon for 25 to 40% of patients who are not receiving any active treatment to show signs of improvement. A control group allows for a true comparison of the benefits of the test treatment. Jorenby et al.[4] examined the effectiveness of sustained-release bupropion, a nicotine patch, or both for smoking cessation. At 6 months, 21.3% of patients treated with the nicotine patch remained abstinent (see Table 5-1). While this result might suggest that the treatment was moderately effective, a comparison with subjects in the control group suggests a different conclusion. In patients given a placebo patch, 18.8% were also abstinent at the 6-month evaluation. Given the importance of patient motivation and other psychological factors in the ability of patients to quit smoking, it is easy to see how the frequent monitoring in a controlled trial might result in a significant rate of success even in patients receiving a placebo.

KEY CONCEPT

An appropriate control group is essential to ensuring the internal validity of a study.

TABLE 5-1. **Effectiveness of Sustained-Release Bupropion on Smoking Cessation**

Outcome	Placebo (N = 160)	Nicotine Patch (N = 244)	Bupropion (N = 244)	Bupropion and Nicotine Patch (N = 245)
No. evaluated at 6 months	86	159	178	195
Abstinence at 6 months—% (no.)	18.8 (30)	21.3 (52)	34.8 (85)	38.8 (95)
Odds ratio (95% CI)	—	1.2 (0.7–1.9)	2.3 (1.4–3.7)	2.7 (1.7–4.4)
P value				
For the comparison with placebo	—	0.53	<0.001	<0.001
For the comparison with patch	—	—	0.001	<0.001
For the comparison with bupropion alone	—	—	—	0.37

NOTE: Some of the patients in most studies will respond even when treated with a placebo. In this study, the number of subjects who were available for evaluation at 6 months was much lower with placebo compared to the other treatments.

SOURCE: From Jorenby et al. (4). Reproduced from N Engl J Med 340:685–691, 1999, with permission from the Massachusetts Medical Society.

Control groups are also critical to the assessment of adverse events, particularly when dealing with nonspecific symptoms such as nausea, diarrhea, headache, drowsiness, insomnia, or other effects that can be relatively common in the general population not taking any medication. An appropriate control was critical to the conclusions of a study examining gastrointestinal symptoms associated with ingesting snack foods containing Olestra, a nonabsorbable fat substitute. In their investigation, Sandler et al.[5] found that 38.2% of individuals reported at least one GI complaint while taking Olestra-containing products. This would appear to be a discouraging observation for the manufacturers of Olestra were it not for the fact that GI symptoms were reported by 36.9% of subjects in the control group.

Subjects in the control group of a clinical trial generally receive either an inactive treatment (a placebo) or treatment with alternative medication. Although a control group could receive no treatment, this would make it impossible to disguise the identity of the treatments. In other words, it would be obvious to everyone that certain subjects are controls. This type of design is appropriate only when there is no reason to expect that subject or investigator could influence the dependent variable (e.g., pharmacokinetic studies with objective measures such as drug clearance).

A placebo control is used in trials where there is no clearly established acceptable treatment or where the consequences of denying treatment to some of the participants in the trial are minimal (see Chap. 14 for a more detailed discussion of this issue). Niewoehner et al.[6] used a placebo control in assessing the usefulness of systemic glucocorticoids for treating exacerbations of chronic obstructive pulmonary disease. The rationale for the study was that glucocorticoids were being widely used for this indication despite the fact that there was little published data documenting that they were effective. Prasad et al.[7] used a placebo to evaluate the effectiveness of zinc acetate lozenges for alleviating symptoms associated with the common cold. The use of a placebo posed no ethical or therapeutic dilemma in this case since there is no established treatment for rhinovirus infection and numerous controlled trials examining the effectiveness of zinc for this indication had yielded conflicting results.

In other situations, it may be ethically and scientifically unacceptable to administer a placebo to patients who have an active disease. When an acceptable treatment for a disease exists, particularly a life-threatening disease such as cancer or AIDS, withholding such treatment merely to enhance the validity of a clinical trial is not reasonable. Furthermore, if the goal of the clinical trial is to improve the drug treatment of a disease, then the scientific question of interest is not "Does the study drug perform better than placebo?" but rather "Does the study drug perform better than currently available treatment?" Steiner et al.[8] conducted a clinical trial to examine the effectiveness of monotherapy with lamotrigine for the treatment of previously untreated epilepsy. Since effective treatments already exist for epilepsy, the use of a placebo control group would not have been reasonable. Control patients in this study received phenytoin, the standard treatment.

A number of different types of control groups are used in clinical trials as described next.

Randomly Assigned Control Group. The most common method of creating a control group is to randomly assign subjects participating in the study to independent groups. One group will not receive the active treatment and will serve as the control, and the other group or groups will receive the treatment under investigation. If the assignment to the groups is truly random and a reasonable number of subjects are enrolled, the groups should be similar with respect to important characteristics such as age, gender distribution, body size, duration of disease, and severity of symptoms. As a rule, the larger the number of subjects participating in a study, the more likely that the groups will be similar in important characteristics. In a randomized clinical trial involving two or more treatments, subjects should have an equal chance of being assigned to a particular treatment group.

Randomization is essential if bias is to be minimized or eliminated. As stated by Kunz and Oxman, randomization is "the only means of controlling for unknown and unmeasured differences between comparison groups as well as those that are known and measured."[9] These investigators identified 1211 clinical trials and found that nonrandomized studies were more likely to overestimate treatment effects, usually due to the assignment of sicker patients to the control group. Non-random methods of assigning subjects (e.g., by alternating or by time of admission to hospital) have the potential to produce unmatched groups for comparison.

KEY CONCEPT

Randomization is the only effective technique for ensuring that the treatment and control groups are similar with respect to both the known and unknown factors that may influence the outcome.

An example of this problem comes from a study investigating the relationship between the renal toxicity of aminoglycoside antibiotics and the time of drug administration.[10] The investigators concluded that patients who received the aminoglycoside from midnight to 7:30 A.M. were more likely to develop nephrotoxicity than patients who received the drug at other times of the day (see Table 5-2). These results would have been more convincing had the patients been randomly assigned to receive the drug at different times. However, the time of drug administration was based on time of admission to hospital. As one might expect, patients who were admitted in the middle of the night tended to be much sicker than patients who entered the hospital during the day. A significantly higher percentage of these patients were treated in the intensive care unit, and they were approximately four times as likely to receive high-dose furosemide. Differences between the groups in these important risk factors clearly confound the study and make it difficult to attribute increases in serum creatinine to the time of administration of the aminoglycoside.

Papers describing clinical trials generally provide a table or tables comparing the control and treatment groups. In the smoking cessation study discussed earlier, age, gender, level of education, number of cigarettes smoked, duration of smoking, and number of prior attempts to quit were examined for each of the groups (Table 5-3). In a quality study, there will be no statistically significant differences in any parameter that could potentially influence the outcome measure. It is rather obvious that it would be difficult to draw an accurate conclusion from the results if the subjects receiving placebo had a history of smoking twice as many cigarettes per day as those in the active treatment groups.

Several techniques are available for randomizing subjects to treatments. Subjects can be assigned on the basis of coin flips, although this is cumbersome when randomizing large numbers of subjects or when there are more than two treatment groups. More practical is the use of a random-number table, which can be found in many statistical texts or generated by a computer program. For example, subjects may be assigned to the control group if matched with an even number or to the active treatment if matched with an odd number. It should be noted that while it is preferable from a statistical viewpoint, it is not essential that the number of

TABLE 5-2. **Incidence of Nephrotoxicity and Distribution of Potential Risk Factors for Nephrotoxicity According to Time of Aminoglycoside Administration**

| | *Time of Administration* | | | |
	Midnight to 7:30 A.M.	*8 A.M. to 3:30 P.M.*	*4 to 11:30 P.M.*	*p Value*
No. of patients	26	56	97	
Nephrotoxicity	9 (34.6%)	7 (12.5%)	9 (9.3%)	0.004
Risk factors				
Age, years	60 (29–88)	61 (18–90)	60 (17–92)	0.73
Baseline CL_{CR}, ml/min	84 (15–209)	76 (20–234)	100 (20–318)	0.03
Trough, mg/L	0.5 (0–4.2)	0.4 (0–2.7)	0.5 (0–4)	0.46
Peak, mg/L	8.3 (5.6–14.0)	9.6 (3.7–19.1)	10.7 (3.6–26.8)	0.09
Duration of treatment, days	4 (1–11)	5 (1–23)	5 (1–20)	0.06
Gender (male)	20 (77%)	31 (55%)	65 (67%)	0.13
Admission to ICU	20 (77%)	11 (20%)	43 (44%)	<0.001
Hypotension	3 (12%)	3 (5%)	2 (2%)	0.11
Oliguria	2 (8%)	0 (0%)	1 (1%)	0.10
Liver dysfunction	14 (54%)	21 (38%)	55 (57%)	0.04
Toxic antibiotics	4 (15%)	3 (5%)	11 (11%)	0.31
High-dose furosemide	8 (31%)	5 (9%)	8 (8%)	0.005

SOURCE: From Prins et al. (10). Reproduced from Clin Pharmacol Ther 62:106–111, 1997, with permission from Mosby.

subjects randomized to each treatment be equal. In the smoking cessation study, 160 subjects were assigned to the placebo group, and approximately 250 subjects were assigned to each of the other three treatments. By randomizing a greater number of subjects to active treatment, more information can be obtained concerning the effects of the drug of interest, particularly when the total number of patients available for study is limited. The downside of the use of unequal groups is that the statistical power of a study is decreased. However, as long as the ratio of number of subjects in the treatment group to the number in the placebo group is less than 2:1, the loss of power is relatively small. For a detailed discussion of this issue, see Chap. 7.

TABLE 5-3. **Evaluating the Success of Randomization**

Characteristic	Baseline Characteristics of the Subjects			
	Placebo (N = 160)	Nicotine Patch (N = 244)	Bupropion (N = 244)	Nicotine Patch and Bupropion (N = 245)
Age, years	42.7 ± 10.2	44.0 ± 10.9	42.3 ± 10.2	43.9 ± 11.6
Female sex, %	58.8	51.6	51.6	49.4
White race, %	93.1	93.0	93.9	92.2
Weight, kg	74.2 ± 14.6	76.9 ± 17.4	76.5 ± 16.2	76.1 ± 16.1
Education, %				
High-school graduate or less	24.4	21.3	21.3	18.4
Some education after high school	48.1	51.2	46.3	48.6
College graduate or more	27.5	27.5	32.4	33.1
No. of cigarettes smoked daily	28.1 ± 10.6	26.5 ± 9.4	25.5 ± 8.8	26.8 ± 9.4
Years of smoking cigarettes	25.6 ± 9.9	26.8 ± 11.1	24.6 ± 10.5	26.7 ± 11.6
No. of previous attempts to quit	2.8 ± 3.0	2.7 ± 2.4	3.1 ± 4.7	2.5 ± 2.4
Expired carbon monoxide, ppm	30.2 ± 12.2	28.3 ± 9.9	28.4 ± 11.1	28.7 ± 11.1
Serum cotinine, ng/ml	358 ± 157	373 ± 204	357 ± 170	362 ± 165
Fagerström score	7.5 ± 1.8	7.4 ± 1.7	7.4 ± 1.6	7.3 ± 1.8
Other smokers in household, %	37.1	28.3	28.7	24.5
Previous use of nicotine patch, %	36.5	38.1	36.9	34.7
Previous use of nicotine gum, %	34.0	23.4	28.3	28.2
History of major depression, %	15.6	18.0	20.9	17.6
Beck Depression Inventory score	4.0 ± 4.4	3.9 ± 4.5	4.4 ± 5.1	3.5 ± 4.7

SOURCE: From Jorenby et al. (4). Reproduced from N Engl J Med 340:685–691, 1999, with permission from the Massachusetts Medical Society.

When the control and treatment groups are independent (separate groups of subjects), they can be studied concurrently. This is often referred to as a *parallel trial* and offers the advantage that the study can be completed in a reasonable period of time. In addition, any confounding factors related to timing of the study will be the same for all groups. For some diseases, symptoms, exacerbations, and remissions vary with season or time of year. If the groups are not studied concurrently, differences in response may be due more to the change in weather or season than to an effect of the drug being studied.

Matched Controls. An alternative approach to the random assignment of subjects to control and treatment groups is to create a group of matched controls. In such a design, investigators who have a patient in the active treatment group will attempt to include a patient who is similar in certain key respects (demographics, disease characteristics) in the control group. This type of design was used in a study evaluating the 5-year survival rate of patients with alcoholic cirrhosis following liver transplantation.[11] Because of the limited number of livers available for transplant, subjects cannot be randomly assigned to receive a transplant as opposed to more conservative treatment. Candidates for transplantation are typically selected on the basis of priority. Therefore, the investigators compared the survival of 169 men who received transplants with 169 controls who were matched with respect to age, severity of cirrhosis, and history of bleeding. While this approach was reasonable in this study and may be necessary in clinical trials in which the available number of subjects for study is small, it is generally difficult to match subjects on all of the important factors. In addition, the strength of randomization is that it can, if properly executed, control for both the known and the unknown variables that influence the effect of the drug.

Subjects Serving as Their Own Controls. Another approach to controlling a study is to have subjects serve as their own controls. Studies of this type are often referred to as *crossover studies* since the subjects cross over from one treatment to the next. In this design, each subject receives all of the treatments sequentially. The primary advantage of a crossover study is that variability is dramatically reduced. The control group truly is identical to the treatment group because both are composed of the same patients. The reduced variability associated with crossover studies increases the statistical power of the study, allowing investigators to detect smaller treatment effects. In addition, a smaller number of subjects can be studied, an important consideration in studying clinical issues where recruitment of subjects is difficult.

Crossover studies are widely used in pharmacokinetic research to evaluate bioequivalence or assess the degree of interaction between drugs. However, there are a number of potential problems that make this design impractical for many clinical trials. Clearly, a crossover design is not feasible if either the control or the treatment under study could cure the disease. For example, a comparison of the effects of two antibiotics on the treatment of pneumonia could not be made using a crossover design since the first treatment will likely result in successful resolution of the infection in many patients.

Another disadvantage is the length of time required to complete the study. Since subjects must complete each treatment sequentially, a crossover study involving two treatments (e.g., placebo, active drug) will take at least twice as long to complete as a parallel design. This can be a significant concern in studies involving several different treatments or where outcomes are measured months or even years after initiation of treatment. Morales et al.[12] studied the effect of 6 months of treatment with dehydroepiandrosterone (DHEA) on a variety of outcomes, including body composition, muscle mass, and circulating concentrations of sex hormones. The use of a crossover design in which subjects received 100 mg of DHEA for 6 months as well as 6 months of a placebo resulted in a study that took a full year to complete. Dropouts are also a serious concern in studies such as this. Subjects who do not complete all of the treatments cannot be included in the data analysis since the conclusions are based on the differences between treatments within each individual. Investigators may have invested several months in following a subject through the first treatment in the DHEA study only to have all of their work become fruitless when the subject withdraws from the study during the tenth month.

The time required to complete a crossover study is also increased by the need to incorporate a *washout period*. The washout period is a drug-free interval between treatments intended to eliminate carryover effects, a situation in which the outcome measure with one treatment is influenced by residual effects from the previous treatment. A washout is particularly important when studying drugs that have an extremely long half-life or long-lasting effects on the disease being treated. The antimalarial drug mefloquine, for example, has a half-life of approximately 15 days. In a crossover study in which the bioavailability of mefloquine was compared under fasting conditions and when administered with food, a washout period of 3 months between treatments was required.[13]

Another potential problem with the crossover design is the *period effect*. Since the treatments are not being studied at the same time (in parallel), seasonal fluctuation in the severity and symptomatology of some chronic diseases could be misinterpreted as an improved response to one treatment over another. Suppose, for example, that a crossover design is used to compare the effectiveness of ibuprofen to that of a new cyclooxygenase-2 (COX-2) inhibitor for the treatment of rheumatoid arthritis. If all patients receive ibuprofen first and the COX-2 inhibitor second, differences in response could be due to variation in the severity of the disease related to weather conditions or time of year rather than to differences between the drugs.

Period effects can be detected after a clinical trial has been completed by using statistical tests such as analysis of variance (see Chap. 8). However, the problem can be minimized by randomizing the order of treatments in a crossover study. In other words, in a study with two treatments, half of the subjects would receive Treatment A first and half would receive Treatment B first, as illustrated in Figure 5-1. Again, a random-number table can be used to assign the treatment sequence (e.g., odd numbers receive A first, then B; even numbers get B first, then A). Although generally preferred, the treatment order in crossover studies is not always randomized. Ducharme et al.[14] studied the effect of the anticonvulsant phenytoin on plasma concentrations of itraconazole. Subjects were given a single oral dose of itraconazole alone (control) and after 15 days of treatment with phenytoin (active treatment). In this case, randomizing the order of treatment would have substantially increased the time required to complete the study. Phenytoin is an inducer of cytochrome P450 enzymes, and the effect may take several weeks to wear off. If some subjects had received the phenytoin-itraconazole combination first, a prolonged washout period would have been required before administering itraconazole alone in order to obtain an accurate estimate of the baseline clearance of itraconazole.

Historical Controls. Although not commonly used, another type of control group is the historical control. In this design, a comparison is made between subjects currently receiving a treatment and a control group of individuals previously studied and available to the investigators either from the published literature or an accessible database. Horowitz et al.[15] used historical controls to compare tacrolimus to cyclosporine for immunosuppression in patients receiving bone marrow transplants. For the control group of patients treated only with cyclosporine, data was derived from the International Bone Marrow Transplant Registry (IBMTR) database.

The use of historical controls is justified when the availability of subjects for study is limited and the expected outcome of established treatment regimens is well known. This type of design is prevalent in the evaluation of new treatments for cancer where there is a substantial body of literature documenting outcomes (e.g., 5-year survival) with specific combinations of chemotherapeutic agents for

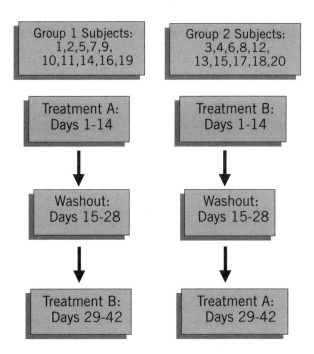

Figure 5-1 Crossover study design in which the order of treatment is randomized by assigning 20 subjects to two groups.

many types of cancer. In this situation, there is no need to subject patients in the control group to a regimen that may be known to be of limited efficacy.

In order for historical controls to be of value, the conditions under which the data was obtained must be similar for both the control and treatment group. Since the clinical treatment of most disease states is always evolving, there is often no assurance that the historical controls received similar treatment, monitoring, laboratory testing, or follow-up, and the medical records and databases from which this information is derived may not contain all of the relevant information. In addition, seemingly small differences in study populations or conditions can affect the outcome of treatment in a particular clinic, hospital, region, or country. Because of this problem, historical controls are of limited usefulness in testing many new drugs.

Blinding

It has been well established that the expectations of subjects and investigators can have a significant influence on the results of a clinical trial. The *Hawthorne effect* refers to the influence of subject expectations on outcome and derives its name from a study of worker productivity at the Western Electric Hawthorne Works in the 1920s. The investigators manipulated various factors such as heating and lighting and found that worker productivity was always improved over baseline. This was attributed to the fact that merely being under observation improves human performance. The analogous situation in drug research is that participating in a clinical trial may in itself lead to an improvement in patient symptoms. Clinical trials involve close monitoring and personal attention given to patients, along with a general atmosphere of excitement related to the possibility of a breakthrough in the treatment of a disease. Although the physiological reasons behind this remain unclear, it is evident that subjects in clinical trials frequently improve even when receiving no active treatment (a placebo). Subject expectations do not always produce a positive effect, however. The possibility that a subject may receive a placebo can reduce the overall response to the test drug. In two studies examining the efficacy of acetaminophen for the treatment of postpartum pain (Swartzman and Burkell), the analgesic effect of acetaminophen was less in the trial where the comparison was to placebo than when the control group received active drug (naproxen).[16] Since all other aspects of both studies were identical, the patients' expectation that they might receive a placebo presumably reduced the effect of the active drug.

The attitude of the investigator can also have an influence on the results of a study.[17] This phenomenon is referred to as the *Rosenthal effect*. It has been demonstrated that a positive study outcome is more likely when the investigator is an enthusiastic supporter of the treatment under study. Conversely, an investigator who is aware that the first several patients have failed with the active treatment may negatively affect the response of future patients. Although not due to overt bias, investigators may examine patients receiving the study drug more diligently for signs of a positive response or unconsciously rate the severity of symptoms differently. Both Rosenthal and Hawthorne effects tend to be more significant with subjective rather than objective outcome measures (see Chap. 6).

KEY CONCEPT

Blinding the identity of the treatments from subjects and investigators is an effective method for reducing the influence of expectations on the outcome of a clinical trial.

Blinding refers to the masking or disguising of the identity of treatments and is a potential solution to the problems posed by the Hawthorne and Rosenthal effects. If no one directly involved in the trial is aware of which drug is being administered, there should be no bias toward any particular treatment. Trials are said to be *single-blind* when either the subjects or investigators (usually the subjects) are unaware of which treatment they are receiving. In *double-blind* studies, both subjects and investigators are unaware of which treatment the subject is receiving. In this case, an independent third party with no direct interest in the results of the trial (often a pharmacist who must prepare the medication for administration) holds the key and is available to break the code should an emergency arise requiring that the patient's treatment be revealed. It is important that the key be held by someone not directly involved in the investigation. Otherwise, the unblinding of a single subject by the investigator will break the code for all subjects, effectively unblinding the entire study.

Blinding often requires that inert dosage forms be administered to the control group that are as identical as possible to the active formulation. With oral administration, products must be similar with respect to color, taste, and smell. This can be a challenge, particularly for compounds with distinctive characteristics such as a bitter taste. In some cases, multiple placebos are required in order to maintain blinding. Suppose the control group is receiving an active drug (e.g., the current drug of choice) and the treatment group is receiving a new drug. It is highly unlikely that these products will be visually or otherwise identical. In order to achieve blinding, subjects in the control group will have to take the standard therapy plus a placebo version of the new drug, while the treatment group will receive the new drug under study and a placebo copy of the standard treatment. In the smoking cessation study conducted by Jorenby et al., there were four groups of patients receiving two active treatments and two different placebos, as follows:

Group 1: Placebo patch, placebo tablet

Group 2: Nicotine patch, placebo tablet

Group 3: Placebo patch, bupropion tablet

Group 4: Nicotine patch, bupropion tablet

Blinding of both subjects and investigators may be difficult to achieve if the drug under investigation produces characteristic pharmacologic effects. For example, in a trial with a sedative-hypnotic drug, it may be impossible for subjects and investigators not to notice an effect such as drowsiness. An alternative approach in such a situation could be the use of an "active placebo," a placebo containing another drug, such as an antihistamine, that may partially mimic the effects of the drug without interfering with the pharmacologic effect being tested (Swartzman and Burkell). Despite the use of a placebo version of the nicotine patch in the smoking cessation study conducted by Jorenby et al., withdrawal symptoms were significantly greater in the patients who did not receive any active treatment. It is certainly possible that some of these individuals were able to recognize that they had been assigned to the placebo group, which may have affected their motivation to continue with the investigation. Indeed, the dropout rate in the placebo group was much higher than in the other groups—close to 50%.

The success of blinding is easy to assess. After the completion of the study, a survey can be administered to subjects and/or investigators in which individuals are invited to indicate which treatment they believe they were receiving. If a high proportion can accurately identify which treatment they were assigned, then the study was not successfully blinded. Bystritsky and Waikar[18] reported that 75% of patients enrolled in clinical trials with antidepressant medication were correctly able to identify whether they had taken placebo or active drug. In examining the usefulness of zinc acetate for the symptomatic relief of cold symptoms, Prasad et al. went to great lengths to ensure that patients were blinded. The subjective nature of the assessment of the severity of cold symptoms by the patients made it imperative that blinding be maintained to allow for a valid comparison between the treatment and control groups. Prior to the initiation of the actual study, a separate group of healthy volunteers were given both the zinc acetate and placebo lozenges for 1 week each using a crossover design. Only 5% of the subjects were able to accurately identify the lozenge containing zinc, and only 10% were correct in identifying the placebo lozenge. Participants in the clinical trial were asked to identify their treatment before and after the study. The ability of the subjects to correctly guess their treatment was not significantly better than expected by chance before or after treatment, suggesting that blinding was maintained throughout the study.

Unfortunately, while most published reports of clinical trials proudly proclaim in the methods that a double-blind study design was used, papers like the zinc acetate lozenge study that provide detailed descriptions verifying the success of blinding are the exception rather than the rule. One study examining this issue found that less than 5% of clinical trials published between 1973 and 1983 provided documentation regarding how well blinding was maintained.[19]

Selecting an Appropriate Sample

Sampling is the process of selecting a representative unit of a population for study. Since the subjects in a study represent a small fraction of the potential users of a drug, it is important for external validity that the sample be as typical as possible.

Sampling error is the difference between the sample mean and the true mean of the population (see Chap. 7) and is highly dependent on the number of subjects selected for study. A large sample is generally more representative of the population and can be more efficiently randomized into different treatment groups. However, investigators must weigh these benefits against the added costs of studying a larger number of subjects. While 100 patients with non-insulin-dependent diabetes are more likely to be representative of the population that could benefit from a new oral hypoglycemic agent, perhaps it would be sufficient to study 50 patients. Estimating the required sample size is one of the most important aspects of designing a study. The statistical power of a study to detect differences between treatment groups is highly dependent upon the number of subjects studied. The various factors that affect the calculation of power and sample size are discussed in Chap. 7.

Theoretically, every member of a particular population of patients should have an equal probability of being selected at random to participate in a clinical trial. Known as *probability sampling,* this offers the greatest likelihood of producing a truly representative sample. Unfortunately, investigators do not usually have access to the entire population, and convenience sampling is the norm. Subjects are asked to participate because they are known to the investigators or are geographically located near the site of the investigation. This may result in bias in some cases. The principal investigator in many clinical trials is typically affiliated with a large urban teaching hospital, which may receive a higher proportion of atypical or severely ill patients as a result of referrals from smaller centers. As a result, the patients available to the investigator may not be typical of the patients with a particular disease.

KEY CONCEPT

The external validity of a study is primarily dependent on the selection of a sample that is representative of the patient population with respect to key characteristics, including disease severity, age, gender, and race.

Convenience sampling may also result in samples that are unrepresentative with respect to factors such as age, gender, and ethnicity. Hypertension and cardiovascular disease, for example, are important therapeutic problems in African-American populations. There appear to be racial differences in both the etiology of the disease and response to treatment. Studies with antihypertensive drugs conducted primarily or exclusively in Caucasian patients are not necessarily relevant or of value to African-American patients. It has been well established that various racial groups show significant differences in the metabolic activity of several cytochrome P450 enzymes responsible for drug metabolism. The prevalence of the poor metabolizer phenotype for substrates of the CYP2C19 enzyme is approximately tenfold more common in Chinese subjects than in Caucasians, whereas in the latter population, deficient metabolism of CYP2D6 substrates is much more common.[20] Again, these differences in drug metabolism can affect the response of patients to drugs, making it imperative that the sample selected for study be representative of the population in which the drug will be used.

Females have historically been underrepresented in clinical trials due to concerns about the administration of drugs to women of childbearing potential and to a protective attitude of society in general toward female research subjects. It is clear, however, that gender-related physiologic differences mean that the results of studies performed in men cannot be assumed to be valid in women. Harris and Douglas[21] found that the enrollment of women in cardiovascular studies has increased significantly between 1965 and 1998 in studies funded by the National Heart, Lung, and Blood Institute. However, women continue to be underenrolled in studies of heart failure. It is incumbent upon the investigator designing a study to ensure that the sample includes males and females in proportions consistent with the prevalence of the disease.

Studies in which the subjects volunteer to participate also raise concerns about the appropriateness of the sample. Are subjects who volunteer to participate in a research study typical of the population as a whole? Perhaps differences in their attitude toward the likely success of treatment or the severity of their disease may make them more willing to participate. Regarding the smoking cessation study discussed previously (Jorenby et al.), it is tempting to speculate that the patients who volunteered to participate in the trial might be more highly motivated to quit smoking than the average smoker. This could result in an overestimation of the success of treatment compared to a more general population of smokers. A conscious decision must sometimes be made about whether the primary objective of the research is to address the study hypothesis (Does Drug A really cause Outcome B?) or to see the effects of a drug in the patients of interest. Drug interaction studies, for example, are often conducted in healthy volunteers who are free of disease and are not taking any other drugs. They are clearly not the population of interest since they don't require the drugs being tested. The fact that they have no potentially confounding diseases or alternative drug treatment may make them the best study subjects to determine whether or not one drug truly causes a change in the clearance of another. Interactions in patients may, however, be greater or lesser in magnitude than those in healthy subjects, and these studies must be conducted before a conclusion can be drawn that a particular drug combination is either safe or dangerous. The differences in drug response that can occur between healthy subjects and patients is illustrated by studies examining the development of "red man syndrome" with the intravenous administration of vancomycin.[22] More than 50% of healthy subjects experience this adverse reaction, suggesting that this would be an ideal population in which to study the mechanism. However, for reasons not yet clearly established, red man syndrome occurs in less than 10% of patients who receive the drug.

Subject Attrition and Intention-to-Treat Analysis

Another factor that can affect the validity of the results of a clinical trial is the attrition of subjects. Attrition refers to the failure of subjects to complete a study. In Chap. 4, the attrition of subjects was mentioned as being a significant problem for cohort studies, many of which take place over months or years. However, in clinical trials that involve seriously ill patients, that take a long time to complete, or that are very demanding (perhaps requiring numerous visits to the clinic and extensive laboratory testing), the attrition or dropout rate can also be significant. If fewer subjects than expected complete a clinical trial, this may result in inadequate statistical power for drawing conclusions. In addition, if the dropout rate in one group of subjects is higher than another, bias may be introduced. The treatment groups may no longer be well matched with respect to important confounding factors.

If subject attrition occurred randomly, it would tend to have little influence on the validity of the study results. However, attrition often occurs unequally due to either a lack of effectiveness or toxicity of a treatment. In the smoking cessation study referred to earlier in this chapter (Jorenby et al.), only 54% of the patients in the placebo group were available for evaluation at 6 months (see Table 5-1). This compares with 80% of those who were assigned to treatment with both bupropion and the nicotine patch.

> ### KEY CONCEPT
>
> Subject attrition can result in an overestimation of the benefits and an underestimation of the adverse effects of treatment. This can be minimized by an intention-to-treat analysis in which all subjects, even those who fail to complete the trial, are included in the final assessment.

One approach to dealing with this problem is to examine the data using a method known as intention-to-treat analysis. In this case, the data are analyzed based on the assumption that every subject who was assigned to a treatment completed the study. In the smoking cessation study, any subject who was not available for assessment at 6 months was assumed to be a treatment failure and included in the final analysis. As listed in Table 5-1, the abstinence rate using the intention-to-treat method was 30 out of 160 patients in the placebo group (18.8%) and 95 out of 245 (38.8%) in the subjects receiving both bupropion and the nicotine patch. If the dropouts are ignored and only those patients who remained in the study at the 6-month assessment are considered, the abstinence rate is substantially increased in the placebo group to 34.9% (30/86) but only marginally increased in the bupropion-nicotine patch group (95/195, or 48.7%). It is highly likely that the higher attrition rate in the placebo group was related to the lack of effectiveness, and failure to account for this in the data analysis would reduce the difference between placebo and active treatment.

A similar problem can occur with respect to assessment of adverse events. Subjects may drop out of a study if the study drug has a high incidence of significant side effects. If only subjects who complete the study are included in the final data analysis, differences between drug and placebo in adverse events may not be evident. By not ignoring those patients who fail to complete the study, biases related to lack of efficacy or drug toxicity can be minimized.

Study Questions

1. Can a study with poor internal validity have a high level of external validity?

2. How can the effectiveness of randomization be assessed?

3. In what type of study is blinding most useful?

4. The use of an intention-to-treat analysis in a clinical trial usually provides a more conservative estimate of the effectiveness of a treatment. Why?

References

1. Streptomycin treatment of pulmonary tuberculosis: a Medical Research Council investigation. BMJ 2:767–782, 1948.

2. King DS, Sharp RL, Vukovich MD, Brown GA, Reifenrath TA, Uhl NL, Parsons KA: Effect of oral androstenedione on serum testosterone and adaptations to resistance training in young men. JAMA 281:2020–2028, 1999.

3. Tilley BC, Alarcón GS, Heyse SP, Trentham DE, Neuner R, Kaplan DA, et al: Minocycline in rheumatoid arthritis: A 48-week, double-blind, placebo-controlled trial. Ann Intern Med 122:81–89, 1995.

4. Jorenby DE, Leischow SJ, Nides MA, Rennard SI, Johnston JA, Hughes AR, et al: A controlled trial of sustained-release bupropion, a nicotine patch or both for smoking cessation. N Engl J Med 340:685–691, 1999.

5. Sandler RS, Zorich NL, Filloon TG, Wiseman HB, Lietz DJ, Brock MH, et al: Gastrointestinal symptoms in 3181 volunteers ingesting snack foods containing Olestra or triglycerides. A 6-week randomized, placebo-controlled study. Ann Intern Med 130:253–261, 1999.

6. Niewoehner DE, Erbland ML, Deupree RH, Collins D, Gross NJ, Light RW, et al: Effect of systemic glucocorticoids on exacerbations of chronic obstructive pulmonary disease. Department of Veteran Affairs Cooperative Study Group. N Engl J Med 24:1941–1947, 1999.

7. Prasad AS, Fitzgerald JT, Bao B, Beck FWJ, Chandrasekar PH: Duration of symptoms and plasma cytokine levels in patients with the common cold treated with zinc acetate. Ann Intern Med 133:245–252, 2000.

8. Steiner TJ, Dellaportas CI, Findley LJ, Gross M, Gibberd FB, Perkin GD, et al: Lamotrigine monotherapy in newly diagnosed untreated epilepsy: a double-blind comparison with phenytoin. Epilepsia 40:601–607, 1999.

9. Kunz R, Oxman AD: The unpredicability paradox: review of empirical comparisons of randomised and non-randomised clinical trials. BMJ 317:1185–1190, 1998.

10. Prins JM, Weverling GJ, van Ketel RJ, Speelman P: Circadian variations in serum levels and the renal toxicity of aminoglycosides in patients. Clin Pharmacol Ther 62:106–111, 1997.

11. Poynard T, Naveau S, Doffoel M, Boudjema K, Vanlemmens C, Mantion G, et al: Evaluation of efficacy of liver transplantation in alcoholic cirrhosis using matched and simulated controls: 5-year survival. Multi-centre group. J Hepatol 30:1130–1137, 1999.

12. Morales AJ, Haubrich RH, Hwang JY, Asakura H, Yen SS: The effect of six months treatment with a 100 mg daily dose of dehydroepiandrosterone (DHEA) on circulating sex steroids, body composition and muscle strength in age-advanced men and women. Clin Endocrinol 49:421–432, 1998.

13. Crevoisier C, Handschin J, Barré J, Roumenov D, Kleinboesem: Food increases the bioavailability of mefloquine. Eur J Clin Pharmacol 53:135–139, 1997.

14. Ducharme MP, Slaughter RL, Warbasse LH, Chandrasekar PH, Vande Velde V, Mannens G, Edwards DJ: Itraconazole and hydroxy-itraconazole serum concentrations are reduced more than tenfold by phenytoin. Clin Pharmacol Ther 58:617–624, 1995.

15. Horowitz MM, Przepiorka D, Bartels P, Buell DN, Zhang MJ, Fitzsimmons WE, et al: Tacrolimus vs. cyclosporine immunosuppression: results in advanced-stage disease compared with historical controls treated exclusively with cyclosporine. Biol Blood Marrow Transplant 5:180–186, 1999.

16. Swartzman LC, Burkell J: Expectations and the placebo effect in clinical drug trials: Why we should not turn a blind eye to unblinding, and other cautionary notes. Clin Pharmacol Ther 64:1–7, 1998.

17. Rosenthal R: Interpersonal expectancy effects: a 30-year perspective. Curr Dir Psychol Sci 3:176–179, 1994.

18. Bystritsky A, Waikar SV: Inert placebo versus active medication. Patient blindability in clinical pharmacological trials. J Nerv Ment Dis 182:485–487, 1994.

19. Ney PG, Collins C, Spensor C: Double blind: double talk or are there better ways to do research. Med Hypothesis 21:119–126, 1986.

20. Bertilsson L, Lou Y-Q, Du Y-L, Liu Y, Kuang T-Y, Liao X-M, et al: Pronounced differences between native Chinese and Swedish populations in the polymorphic hydroxylations of debrisoquin and S-mephenytoin. Clin Pharmacol Ther 51:388–397, 1992.

21. Harris DJ, Douglas PS: Enrollment of women in cardiovascular clinical trials funded by the National Heart, Lung, and Blood Institute. N Engl J Med 343:475–480, 2000.

22. Rybak MJ, Bailey EM, Warbasse LH: Absence of "red man syndrome" in patients being treated with vancomycin or high-dose teicoplanin. Antimicrob Agents Chemother 36:1204–1207, 1992.

Data Measurement, Description, and Presentation

David J. Edwards

OUTLINE

Goals and Objectives

Introduction

Subjective Versus Objective Measures

Surrogate Measures

Validating the Measurement

    Accuracy

    Reproducibility (Precision)

    Sensitivity and Specificity

Types of Measurement Scales

    Nominal Measurement

    Ordinal Measurement

    Interval and Ratio Measurement

    Measurement Scales Used to Assess Outcome in Rheumatoid Arthritis

Discrete Versus Continuous Data

Description and Presentation of Data

    Nominal and Ordinal Data

    Interval and Ratio Data

    Measures to Describe Central Tendency: Mean, Median, and Mode

    Measures to Describe Variability: Range, Variance, Standard Deviation, and Coefficient of Variation

Degrees of Freedom

Study Questions

References

KEY WORDS

Subjective	Accuracy	Ordinal	Mode
Objective	Precision	Interval	Range
Surrogate	Sensitivity	Ratio	Variance
Discrete	Specificity	Mean	Standard deviation
Continuous	Nominal	Median	Coefficient of variation

Goals and Objectives

The objective of this chapter is to introduce the reader to the methods used to measure and describe the effects of drugs. The criteria used for validating measurements and tests are discussed and the different measurement scales used in drug research are presented. Finally, the descriptive statistics used to characterize the central tendency and variability in a sample are reviewed. At the completion of this chapter, the reader should:

1. Know the difference between a subjective and an objective measure and be aware of the value of each in assessing drug effects.

2. Understand the role of surrogate measures in drug research.

3. Understand how the accuracy, precision, sensitivity, and specificity of the measurement are used to assess the validity.

4. Be able to classify measurements as nominal, ordinal, interval, or ratio data.

5. Know the difference between incidence and prevalence.

6. Understand the advantages and disadvantages of mean, median, and mode as measures of central tendency.

7. Be able to assess the degree of variability in a sample by calculating and comparing the standard deviation and coefficient of variation.

Introduction

Measurement is the process of assigning numbers to the characteristics of living things, events, or objects. These characteristics are referred to as *variables* since they will typically assume at least two values. Whether it is gender, eye color, height, weight, blood pressure, or any number of other characteristics, there is at least some variation between living organisms. Variability in the development of disease and response to treatment may be due to a number of genetic or environmental factors. In order to quantitate the effects of a drug, scientists use a variety of outcomes that are based on several different measurement scales. Ultimately, investigators are always faced with the same question: What is the most appropriate variable to measure and how should it be measured?

Subjective Versus Objective Measures

The outcome of drug therapy can be assessed in a variety of ways. Some measures are termed *subjective* while others are classified as *objective*. The distinguishing characteristic is that instruments are used to quantify objective measures, whereas subjective measures are based on human ratings or evaluations. It is sometimes assumed that objective measures are best and that subjective measures are less reliable and to be avoided. This is certainly not always the case. Instruments may be improperly calibrated or simply inaccurate. Human error or negligence can play a role in poor instrument performance. In addition, an objective measure is of value only if it truly reflects the activity of the drug being evaluated. The white blood cell count is an objective measure, but by itself cannot be used to evaluate the effectiveness of antibiotic treatment since the white count can be influenced by many factors other than infection. Subjective measures are often the only way to evaluate the outcome of drug therapy, particularly in examining variables related to quality of life. Irrespective of the results of objective measurements, in many chronic diseases the question of most interest to both patient and health care provider is, "Does the patient feel better when taking this medication?" Because subjective measures require human ratings and evaluations, they are subject to bias from factors such as the Hawthorne and Rosenthal effects (discussed in Chap. 5). However, such problems can be minimized through appropriate study design and the use of techniques such as blinding.

> ### KEY CONCEPT
>
> While objective measures are less sensitive to bias than subjective measures, an objective measure of drug effect is not always available. Subjective measures can be valuable in assessing the effect of drugs on quality of life.

Surrogate Measures

It is not always possible or practical for researchers to measure the most interesting or clinically useful outcome. The goal of drug therapy is often to increase the survival rate or improve the quality of life of the patient. In the treatment of a life-threatening, acute illness such as a serious gram-negative infection, measurement of survival rate is an appropriate and practical endpoint. However, drugs are often used to treat chronic diseases where it may be years or decades before an improvement in survival is evident. In such cases, a surrogate measure may be used, one that reflects the activity of the drug being tested and is predictive of the clinical effect desired.

The presence of high concentrations of cholesterol in the blood is a risk factor for the development of cardiovascular disease. The goal of drug therapy with cholesterol-lowering drugs is to reduce the morbidity and mortality associated with cardiovascular disease. To actually test whether a new drug reduces the incidence of cardiovascular disease would take years, possibly decades. Therefore, cholesterol concentrations in the blood are measured instead. This is an inexpensive test that can be performed within weeks of initiating drug therapy and is assumed to be predictive of the development of heart disease.

A similar situation exists in the treatment of patients infected with HIV. Because the progression of the disease is slow, it may be years before the effectiveness of a new class of antiviral drugs is known. Lymphocyte counts, on the other hand, can be easily measured and provide an indication of the degree of immuno-deficiency that the patient is experiencing.

Bioequivalence testing is another example. In order to avoid duplicating the high costs of clinical trials, generic drugs are approved for use on the basis of measured concentrations of drug in the blood rather than on the clinical effects of the drug. Bioequivalence is a surrogate measure of therapeutic equivalence. Scientists are always looking for quality surrogate measures that are noninvasive, inexpensive, and can predict drug response rapidly. Clinicians must evaluate whether the conclusions reached using such a measure are valid.

Validating the Measurement

The quality of data depends on the reliability of the outcome measure. A good measurement must have all of the following properties.

Accuracy

It is easy to see that an inaccurate measurement would be of little value. Accuracy is related to the concept of measurement error, the difference between the true value and the measured value. Instruments that are outdated, poorly cared for, or improperly operated may yield results that are not accurate. The accuracy of objective measurements can be assessed through the use of calibrators or controls. For example, in drug analysis, the investigator may prepare or purchase samples containing known (true) quantities of the drug being assayed in order to evaluate the accuracy of the method being used for a particular study. Ideally, all samples in a particular study should be analyzed using the same instrument. This may be difficult in studies where samples are collected over a period of several years. In such studies, it is imperative that instrument performance be consistent throughout the study period. Again, control samples can be tested at regular intervals to ensure that no systematic changes (e.g., declining values) are occurring.

Reproducibility (Precision)

In order to be useful, a measurement must be not only accurate but also reproducible. The term *reproducibility* means that if the same measurement were performed multiple times on the same patient or sample, the result would be similar each time. With any instrument, there will be always be a certain degree of variability from measure to measure. For example, if a blood sample contains the antibiotic gentamicin at a concentration of 8.5 mg/L, it is highly unlikely that every measurement would yield a result of exactly 8.5 mg/L. The degree of variability will be dependent on the technology on which the measurement is based as well as on the expertise and experience of the laboratory personnel responsible for performing the measurement. Some laboratory measurements may be very reproducible with variability of less than 1%, whereas for others, variability of 10% or more may be the norm. The level of precision that is acceptable will differ depending on what is being measured. If a 10% change in a patient's potassium plasma concentration is clinically important, then an assay producing results that vary by as much as 20% will be of little value.

Reproducibility is just as important for subjective measures. Suppose pain is rated on a scale of 1 to 5. Does a patient with a constant level of pain rate that pain as a 2 on one occasion and a 3 at the next measurement time? This can be a difficult problem to detect since it is usually not possible for the investigator, or sometimes even the patient, to know whether pain has changed or not. Studies designed to assess central nervous system impairment often use the ability of patients to complete a task or test (a maze, puzzle, math problems, etc.) as the outcome measure. Even in the presence of a drug that should impair performance, some subjects may improve in their ability to complete the task as they become more familiar with it through repeated assessments. This is known as a *learning* or *practice effect* and can certainly compromise the usefulness of the outcome measure. A solution is to have subjects perform the test multiple times prior to the administration of the test drug. Only after any learning effects are maximized is the study drug given. Tests that are too long or tedious can have the opposite effect on the reproducibility of the outcome. Subject performance may decline over time due to boredom or lack of interest even if the drug being tested does not impair the subjects.

A related issue, particularly in multicenter studies, is interobserver reproducibility. Does the investigator at the site in Cleveland rate patient response the same as the investigator in Los Angeles? Buechler et al.[1] surveyed Level 1 trauma centers throughout the United States regarding usage of the Glasgow Coma Scale, a widely used predictor of patient prognosis and outcome following head trauma, and found that scoring varied widely from site to site. This would clearly be a problem in a multicenter study where all patients with the same score on the Glasgow Coma Scale are expected to have the same level of consciousness.

Sensitivity and Specificity

In instrumental analysis, *sensitivity* refers to the limit of detection, the lowest concentration of the compound of interest that can be reliably measured. It is often defined by the term *signal-to-noise ratio*. For example, the lowest concentration that can be measured may be the value that produces a signal that is twice the baseline noise of the instrument. *Specificity* refers to the ability of an assay to measure the compound of interest without interference from other components of the sample. Metabolites of a drug that are closely related to the parent in chemical structure, perhaps differing by only a methyl or hydroxyl group, may interfere with an immunoassay that employs an antibody that cross-reacts with both. Having a sensitive and specific analytical method for measuring drug concentration is critical in any pharmacokinetic study in order to allow for accurate calculation of parameters such as elimination half-life.

Sensitivity and specificity are also used to describe the usefulness of diagnostic tests. In this situation, sensitivity refers to the ability of the measurement to truly identify all of the subjects who have a particular condition. Suppose a pregnancy test is administered to 500 pregnant women. A positive result is obtained in 450 women. The sensitivity of the test can be calculated as 90% (450 out of 500).

The rate of false-negatives with such a test would be 10%. Specificity refers to the ability of the test to accurately identify those who do not have the condition. Using the pregnancy test example, if 500 nonpregnant subjects were tested and 25 tests were positive, then the specificity of the test would be 95% (475 out of 500 women correctly identified as not pregnant) and the false-positive rate would be 5%. This is illustrated in Fig. 6-1, with the rate of true-positives determining the sensitivity of the test and the rate of true-negatives the specificity.

KEY CONCEPT

A sensitive diagnostic test identifies those who have a disease or condition, whereas a specific test identifies those who do not have the condition. The sensitivity is determined by the rate of false-negative results, and the specificity depends on the rate of false-positives.

The acceptability of a particular test is dependent on the consequences of a false-positive or false-negative conclusion. Clearly, a pregnancy test that produced 10% false-negative results would not be of much clinical value. On the other hand, mammography is a widely used procedure that has relatively poor specificity. It has been reported that a 60-year-old woman who is screened annually for 10 years has a 50% chance of having at least one false-positive result.[2] Although the short-term stress associated with a false-positive test is not insignificant, women appear to be comfortable with a philosophy that it is better to be safe than sorry. According to one survey, a high percentage felt that as many as 10,000 false-positives was a reasonable price to pay if even a single life were saved.[3]

Whenever possible, researchers use measures or tests that have previously been validated by others and are widely accepted as an appropriate measure. Standard values are well established for many laboratory tests, and numerous rating

	Positive Tests	Negative Tests
Pregnant Subjects	450 (true-positives)	50 (false-negatives)
Nonpregnant Subjects	25 (false-positives)	475 (true-negatives)

Figure 6-1. Sensitivity and specificity of a diagnostic test.

scales have been developed and tested for assessing the severity of illness or reduction in organ function. The use of an outcome measure that has not been adequately validated or is not widely accepted by others will almost certainly lead to widespread skepticism or outright rejection of the conclusions of a study.

Types of Measurement Scales

Anyone reading the drug literature will quickly realize that a wide variety of measurements can be made in drug research. These may range from a global assessment (patient survives or does not survive) to a rating of the response (1 = excellent, 2 = good, 3 = fair, 4 = poor) to a quantitative measure (diastolic blood pressure = 94 mmHg in the control group versus 86 mmHg in the test group). These assessments involve different measurement scales. In evaluating the literature, a reviewer must be able to identify which type of measurement scale has been used, since this determines to a large extent which statistical test must be employed.

KEY CONCEPT

Different measurement scales are required to quantitate the effects of drugs. The choice of statistical test is dependent on whether the data to be analyzed is nominal, ordinal, or interval/ratio.

Nominal Measurement

This is the simplest form of measurement, in which numbers or labels are used to name or classify the values of a variable or outcome measure. Examples of nominal data include the classification of subjects by gender (male or female), response (yes, no), or disease state (pneumonia, sepsis, urinary tract infection). The outcome can be classified into any number of different categories. However, a key feature of nominal measurement is that no mathematical comparison can be made between the categories. All values within a particular category are assumed to be the same (e.g., all persons classified as responders to medication are assumed to be equal to each other, there are no gradations of response). Values in different classifications (e.g., male, female) are assumed to be unequal to each other. However, the level of inequality cannot be measured numerically. Even though numbers may be assigned to different categories (e.g., 1 = treatment failures, 2 = survivors), mathematical manipulations cannot be performed with the data. To be a survivor cannot be considered to have twice as much value as being a treatment failure because the assignment of numbers to the categories is completely arbitrary.

The analysis of nominal data typically involves counting the number of observations that fall into each category. For example, Sandler et al.[4] examined the frequency of gastrointestinal symptoms in volunteers ingesting snack products containing the fat substitute Olestra. Subjects were classified according to whether or not they had gastrointestinal symptoms. The number of subjects reporting symptoms in the Olestra group (619 out of 1620) was counted and compared to the number reporting symptoms in the placebo group (576 out of 1561). Once the number of observations in each classification has been counted, the data is commonly described using parameters such as rates, ratios, fractions, proportions, or frequencies. These are discussed in more detail later in this chapter.

Ordinal Measurement

Ordinal measurement uses a scale that permits the investigator to rank-order the values of the outcome measure. In other words, it can be stated that one value is better than or worse than another value. This contrasts with the nominal measurement scale, where the only statement that can be made is that the values are either equal or unequal to each other. Many ordinal measurement scales have been developed in order to rate the severity of a disease. For example, a patient with cancer may be assigned a number based on such attributes as the size of the tumor, histology of the tissue, presence or absence of involved lymph nodes, and the development of specific symptoms. A higher number may indicate a more serious form of the disease and a poorer prognosis. Some other common ordinal scales for rating severity of illness or impairment of function include the Acute Physiology and Chronic Health Evaluation (APACHE), Glasgow Coma Scale for head injury, Pugh Score for liver disease, New York Heart Association Classification for congestive heart failure, and Apgar scores for newborns. Drug response (e.g., pain relief) is often measured according to rating scales (e.g., 4 = excellent, 3 = good, 2 = fair, 1 = poor). In ordinal scales it can be stated that a response of 3 is better than a response of 2.

A key feature of an ordinal measurement scale is that the magnitude of the difference between units on the scale cannot be assumed to be equal, as represented schematically in Fig. 6-2. The difference between an excellent and a good response (4 versus 3), for example, is not necessarily the same as the difference between a good and a fair response (3 versus 2). This limits the calculations that can be made with ordinal scale data. Operations such as multiplication and division cannot be performed on the data since it cannot be stated that an excellent response has twice the value of a fair response even though they may be assigned values of 4 and 2.

Interval and Ratio Measurement

Interval and ratio scales represent a further advancement on the ordinal scale in that the data can not only be rank-ordered, but the distance between intervals on

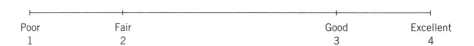

Poor	Fair	Good	Excellent
1	2	3	4

Figure 6-2. An ordinal rating scale illustrating that the magnitude of difference between values on the scale cannot be assumed to be equal.

the scale is equal. The distinction between interval and ratio measurement is that a ratio scale has a true zero point and an interval scale does not. The classic example of the interval scale is the thermometer. The distance from 10 to 20°C is the same as the distance between 30 and 40°C. However, a reading of zero on the Celsius scale does not indicate the total absence of heat (true zero) but is instead an arbitrary value equal to the freezing point of water. If a negative value can be obtained, the scale has an arbitrary zero point and the data will be interval rather than ratio. Many of the demographic parameters (height, weight, age) as well as outcome measures used in drug research (laboratory tests of biochemical parameters, drug concentrations, blood pressure, heart rate) are ratio measurements. Because ratio scales have a true zero point, all mathematical operations can be performed on the data. A drug concentration of 10 mg/L is truly twice as high as a concentration of 5 mg/L.

Measurement Scales Used to Assess Outcome in Rheumatoid Arthritis

Rheumatoid arthritis is a difficult disease in which to evaluate drug effectiveness. There is no single objective or subjective test or measurement that can be used to monitor relapses and remissions in the natural course of the disease or can tell investigators whether a drug is working. Tilley et al.[5] conducted a multicenter study to investigate the effectiveness of the antibiotic minocycline in the treatment of rheumatoid arthritis. A wide variety of measures with different scales were used to evaluate the outcome of treatment. Diarthrodial joints were examined for tenderness and swelling and labeled as present or absent. In addition, the presence of deformed joints and subcutaneous nodules was counted. These are examples of nominal measurement scales in that there is no rank ordering in these measures (e.g., subjects either have an affected joint or they do not). A number of different ordinal measures were used in this investigation. At each assessment point in the study, patients and examiners rated the activity of the disease according to the following scale: 1 = absent, 2 = mild, 3 = moderate, 4 = severe, 5 = very severe. In addition, patients completed the Modified Health Assessment Questionnaire in order to assess their ability to perform activities of daily living (0 = no difficulty, 1 = some difficulty, 2 = much difficulty, 3 = unable to perform). All of these scales permit rank ordering of the data. Certainly, a disease activity score of 4 is worse than a score of 2. However, a score of 4 does not indicate that the disease is twice as active. Measurements that could be classified as ratio included grip strength (assessed using a mercury strain sphygmomanometer) and laboratory tests such as erythrocyte sedimentation rate and IgM rheumatoid factor. A person with a hand-strength reading of 100 mmHg could be said to be twice as strong as a person with a reading of 50 mmHg.

This paper illustrates the difficulties that sometimes face investigators in evaluating drug response. Some of the outcome measures were clearly subjective (e.g., rating of disease activity), and others were objective (e.g., grip strength, erythrocyte sedimentation rate). The objective measures are not necessarily better than the subjective measures. Despite the fact that right-hand grip strength and erythrocyte sedimentation rate were statistically improved by minocycline treatment, there was no statistically significant difference between the placebo and minocycline groups in functional status or rating of disease activity by either the patient or physician. It would be difficult for a clinician to make a decision on whether to use minocycline for the treatment of rhematoid arthritis on the basis of this study since the various outcome measures do not all point to the same conclusion.

Discrete Versus Continuous Data

The data produced by the different measurement scales can also be classified as either discrete or continuous. Discrete measurements can assume only specific values, usually whole numbers, within a range and are typical of both nominal and ordinal data. The number of subjects responding to a drug treatment could be 3, 10, 20, or any other whole number, but 3.2 subjects could not respond. Similarly, most ordinal rating scales require the evaluator to limit responses to specific values. On the Apgar scale for evaluating newborn distress, heart rate must be classified as either 0 (absent), 1 (below 100), or 2 (over 100). No other choices are permitted. Patients may be asked to classify pain as 0 through 4 in order of increasing severity. The patient can choose 0, 1, 2, 3, or 4, but not 2.4. A continuous variable can assume any value within a range and is characteristic of interval and ratio measurement. The values that such data can assume are typically limited mainly by the analytical characteristics of the equipment employed for measurement.

Description and Presentation of Data

Rarely does the reader of a paper have the opportunity to view the raw data collected by the investigator. In most cases, the data has already been summarized and organized into tables or figures in order to make it more understandable. In a study investigating a drug interaction between a new antifungal drug and theophylline, the investigator may have measured theophylline concentrations 15 separate times in 20 subjects after administering theophylline alone and again in the presence of the interacting drug, generating approximately 600 data points. It would be prohibitively expensive for journals to publish all of this data—and of little interest to most readers, who wish to know only the effect of the interacting drug on the clearance and half-life of theophylline. In clinical trials involving hundreds or thousands of patients, the need to organize and summarize the data prior to publication is obvious. A variety of methods are available for describing and presenting data. The choice depends primarily on the measurement scale used to obtain the data. Nominal data does not have the same characteristics as ratio data and cannot be described using the same parameters.

Nominal and Ordinal Data

Little in the way of mathematical calculations can be performed on nominal and ordinal data. Generally, the investigator simply counts and tabulates the number of observations in each of the categories into which the data has been classified. The data can be summarized by calculating ratios, percentages, proportions, and rates.

Although related, there are differences between these calculations. Ratios are calculated by dividing the number of observations in one category by the number in a different category. For example, if a study involved 100 males and 50 females, the male:female ratio would be 2:1. Proportions and rates are calculated by dividing the number of observations in a category by the total number of observations. The proportion of males in the preceding study would be 2:3. Proportions are commonly expressed as the number of observations per 100—in other words, as a percentage. The percentage of males is 67% in the preceding example. Incidence and prevalence are rate calculations that are commonly used but not always clearly understood by readers. Incidence is used to describe the rate of occurrence of a disease or event over a specified period of time:

$$\text{Incidence} = \frac{\text{number of new patients with disease}}{\text{total population at risk}}$$

The incidence of an adverse drug reaction, for example, is a common calculation of this type. The term *prevalence* refers to the number of existing cases of a disease in a population:

$$\text{Prevalence} = \frac{\text{number of patients with disease}}{\text{total population at risk}}$$

In assessing trends in the development and treatment of disease, investigators may be interested in incidence, prevalence, or both. The incidence of AIDS, for example, declined dramatically in male homosexuals after 1984 due to efforts aimed at educating individuals about high-risk behavior (Fig. 6-3).[6] Prevalence, on the other hand, is affected by both the number of new cases and the length of time that patients with the disease survive. The prevalence of HIV remained relatively constant from 1984 through 1988 despite close to a tenfold decrease in incidence. Significant declines in the prevalence were not observed until several years after the drop in incidence.

Nominal and ordinal data may be presented in either tabular or graphic form. Pie charts are common since the number of observations in each classification can easily be presented as a fraction or percentage of the total (each percentage point represents 3.6° of angle). Bar graphs or histograms can be plotted with frequency or number of observations on the y axis and category label on the x axis. This type of plot is also known as a *frequency diagram*. The data reported in Table 3 of the paper by Sandler et al. in their investigation of the gastrointestinal side effects of Olestra can be presented in this manner (Fig. 6-4). Frequency diagrams such as this provide a convenient and effective method of presenting data. Hundreds of individual data points are summarized in this figure, and the reader can easily see how the treatment and control groups compare as well as which adverse events occur most commonly.

Interval and Ratio Data

The basic approach to summarizing nominal and ordinal data (i.e., counting the frequency or number of observations in each classification) is generally not useful

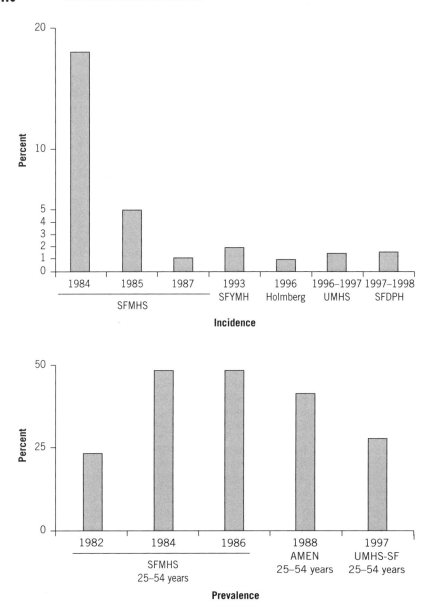

Figure 6-3. Incidence and prevalence of HIV from 1982 to the present as measured by a number of different studies. *[From Catania et al. (6). Reprinted with permission from Science 290:717, 2000. Copyright © 2000 by the American Association for the Advancement of Science.]*

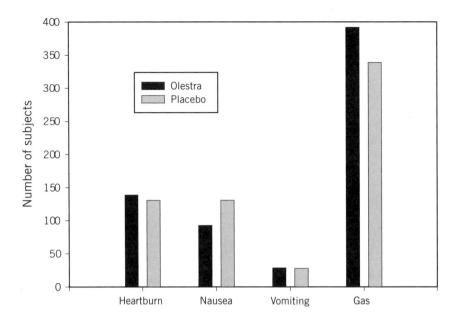

Figure 6-4. *Frequency diagram comparing gastrointestinal side effects of Olestra and placebo. [From Sandler et al. (4). Reproduced from Ann Intern Med 130:253–261, 1999, with permission from ACP-ASIM.]*

for interval and ratio data because the data is not discrete. Since interval and ratio measurement scales produce continuous data, the same value may not occur more than one time. Consider the values for plasma cholesterol concentration (mg/dL) in a randomly selected sample of 50 subjects (Table 6-1). The data has been organized by increasing value from left to right and top to bottom. The lowest observed value is 147 mg/dL and the highest 285 mg/dL. A quick perusal of the data indicates that, although several values occur twice, the most frequently occurring value is 193, which occurs only three times. Plotting the frequency of each observation would be of little value in summarizing this data since we have 39 different values among the 50 pieces of data, with the frequency of each value being either 1, 2, or 3.

With continuous data, a solution to this problem is to divide the data into class intervals, and 5 to 15 intervals are usually considered to be reasonable. The size or width of each interval is determined by the range of values to be summarized. In this example, the difference between the highest and lowest value is $285 - 147 = 138$. If we divide the data into 10 intervals, a convenient interval width to cover the entire range of data would be 15. Table 6-2 is a frequency table that has been created in this manner. By summarizing the data this way, several characteristics become evident. It is clear that most of the values (32 of 50) are in the range of 171 to 215 mg/dL, with values between 186 and 200 mg/dL being the most common.

TABLE 6-1. Cholesterol Concentrations in 50 Randomly Selected Subjects, mg/dL

147	150	154	156	165
165	169	173	174	177
178	178	182	182	183
183	186	186	187	188
192	192	193	193	193
195	195	195	196	196
202	203	205	206	208
211	214	215	215	223
224	225	241	243	252
264	273	275	284	285

There is, however, considerable variability in the data, particularly on the high end of the distribution. The properties of central tendency and variability are characteristic of most interval and ratio data. These characteristics can be visualized by inspection of Fig. 6-5, in which the data from Table 5-2 have been used to create a frequency diagram. Several descriptive statistics have been devised in order to quantify the central tendency and variability in the data and are discussed in detail in the following sections.

Measures to Describe Central Tendency: Mean, Median, and Mode

The three primary measures of central tendency are mean, median, and mode. The arithmetic *mean* is the most commonly used parameter and is the sum of the observed values divided by the number of observations. Mathematically,

$$\bar{x} = \frac{\Sigma X}{n}$$

where $\bar{x}$ is the mean and n is the number of observations. For the data in Table 6-1, the mean is 201 mg/dL. Although everyone is familiar with the calculation of mean, it is not always the best measure of central tendency. The primary disadvantage of this parameter is that it can be strongly influenced by extreme values, particularly when the number of observations is small. If the mean were calculated for the bottom row of numbers only (5 observations), the answer is 276 mg/dL. A change in the last value in the row from 285 to 385 mg/dL would increase the mean by 20 mg/dL, to 296 mg/dL.

TABLE 6-2. Frequency Table Illustrating the Relationship Between Plasma Cholesterol Concentration and Class Interval

Class Interval, mg/dL	Frequency
140–155	3
156–170	4
171–185	9
186–200	14
201–215	9
216–230	3
231–245	2
246–260	2
261–275	2
276–290	2

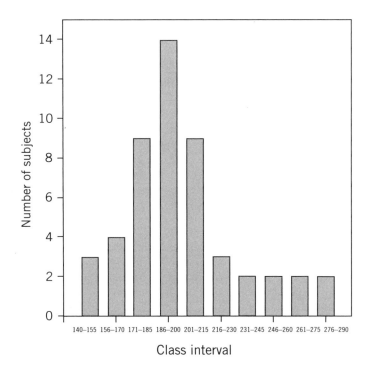

Figure 6-5. Frequency distribution of cholesterol data in Tables 6-1 and 6-2.

A measure of central tendency that is not influenced by extreme values is the median. The *median* is the value that half of the observations fall below and half lie above. In other words, the median value divides the distribution in half. It is also equal to the 50th percentile. In a set of data with an odd number of values, the median is the ranked value given by the following equation:

$$\text{Median} = \frac{n + 1}{2}$$

where n is the number of observations. For example, if the final value in Table 6-1 (285) is omitted, there are 49 remaining observations. The median is the 25th ranked value (193 mg/dL). When the number of data points is an even number, the median is the average of the two observations at the midpoint of the distribution. Using Table 6-1 with 50 observations, the median is the average of the 25th and the 26th observations. In this particular example, the 25th and 26th ranked values are 193 and 195 mg/dL, resulting in a median of 194 mg/dL. Since the median is dependent only on the relative ranking of the data points, extreme values have no influence on the calculation of this parameter. If the last value in the data set were increased from 285 to 385, the median would still be the average of the 25th and 26th ranked observations (194 mg/dL).

The final measure of central tendency is the mode. The *mode* is the most frequently occurring value or class interval, depending on whether the measurement is discrete or continuous. For the data in Table 6-1, the mode is the interval from 186 to 200 mg/dL (Table 6-2). The mode has several limitations as a measure of central tendency. It is dependent on the number of class intervals into which the data is divided, a process for which there are few hard-and-fast rules. The cholesterol data could have been broken down into 15 intervals of 10 mg/dL in width, creating a somewhat different mode. The frequency diagram for the cholesterol example clearly has a single mode (unimodal), as do many of the variables measured in drug research. However, other data sets may have two or more peaks in the distribution and are said to be *bimodal* or *multimodal.* Bimodal distributions often occur when the variability in the data is due to a single genetic or environmental factor.

An excellent example is the rate of metabolism of drugs that are substrates for the cytochrome P450 enzyme CYP2D6. In Caucasian subjects, approximately 90% have a fully functional form of this enzyme, and 5 to 10% of subjects have a mutated form with little activity. Debrisoquin is metabolized to 4-hydroxydebrisoquin by this enzyme, with the ratio of parent/metabolite concentration being much higher in subjects who lack the functional form of CYP2D. As illustrated in Fig. 6-6,[7] Swedish subjects exhibit a bimodal distribution for the metabolic ratio of debrisoquin/4-hydroxydesbrisoquin: a small peak representing the 5 to 10% of individuals with the mutated enzyme and a larger peak for those with the active enzyme. A bimodal distribution is not as evident for Chinese subjects because the mutated enzyme is much less common in this population.

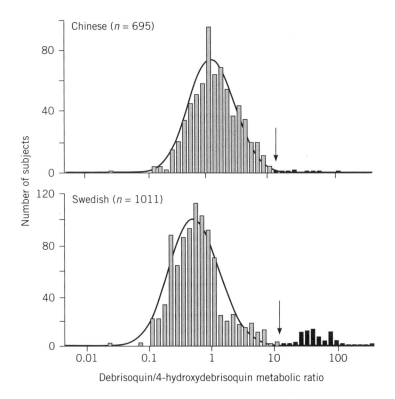

Figure 6-6. Frequency distribution for activity of the cytochrome P450 enzyme CYP2D6 in Chinese and Swedish populations. *[From Bertilsson et al. (7). Reproduced from Clin Phamacol Ther 51:388–397, 1992, with permission from Mosby.]*

In evaluating which measure of central tendency is most appropriate to use, an important factor is the symmetry of the frequency distribution. In unimodal distributions that are symmetrical, the mean and the median have the same value. Many data sets are not symmetrical, however, but are skewed toward either the high or low end of the distribution. Skewed data can be recognized by the presence of a tail in the frequency diagram. When the distribution tails to the right side of the diagram, it is referred to as *positively skewed,* and the mean will have a larger value than the median. *Negatively skewed* data tails to the left and has a mean that is smaller than the

KEY CONCEPT

When data are skewed or contain extreme values, the median is a better measure of central tendency than the mean.

median. The data in Table 6-1 has a slight tail to the right side (Fig. 6-5) It is positively skewed, as evidenced by a mean (201) that is larger than the median (194).

It is not uncommon for variables measured in drug research to be inherently skewed. Cholesterol concentration in plasma is one example. It is more common to see patients with high cholesterol concentrations than with low values. Renal function is an example of a negatively skewed variable. The majority of individuals have normal renal function, but glomerular filtration is reduced in a number of disease states as well as through the normal aging process. There are relatively few physiological or pathological conditions that increase the glomerular filtration rate. Since the number of patients with poor renal function far exceeds the number with increased renal function, the distribution is negatively skewed. The degree of skewedness can be measured by the magnitude of the difference between the median and the mean. Larger differences indicate that the data is more highly skewed, with extreme values at one end of the distribution or the other. With skewed data, the median is almost always a better measure of central tendency than the mean.

Measures to Describe Variability: Range, Variance, Standard Deviation, and Coefficient of Variation

All outcomes measured in drug research will exhibit some variability. Variability is an inherent feature of nature (biological variability) and is to be expected. Readers will commonly find references in the literature to intersubject and intrasubject variability. *Intersubject variability* refers to the variability that occurs from one patient to another and is also known as *between-subject variability*. If multiple measurements are made sequentially in the same subject, *intrasubject,* or *within-subject, variability* can be assessed. The variability between subjects tends to be greater than the variability within subjects for most measurements. Differences from one subject to another may be due to a host of genetic or environmental factors, whereas differences in the same subject over time may be related to physiologic or pathologic changes (e.g., diurnal variation in hormone concentrations). The procedures and instrumentation used for measurement add to the inherent variability in the data, but are likely to make up a larger fraction of the within-subject variability.

The simplest measure of variability is the range. *Range* is the difference between the highest value in the data set and the lowest value. More variable data will have a larger range. However, range is a poor parameter since it may be highly influenced by a single extreme value and tends to be dependent on the number of data points collected. As more data is added to the analysis, there is an increasing likelihood that an extreme value will occur and the range will increase. The range in the cholesterol distribution in Fig. 6-1 is 138 mg/dL (285 − 147). However, an increase in the largest value from 285 to 385 would almost double the range to 238 mg/dL. Despite the simplicity of calculation, the range is seldom used to assess variability because of the preceding disadvantages.

A more common and useful measure of variability is the *variance,* which refers to the difference between the individual values in a set of data and the mean. Variability is greater when the observations lie further from the mean. Differences between data points x and the mean $\bar{x}$ will be both positive and negative, and the sum of these differences will be equal to zero. Therefore, variance is calculated by first squaring the differences and then dividing the sum by the number of observations minus one:

$$\text{Variance} = \frac{\Sigma(x - \bar{x})^2}{n - 1}$$

The *standard deviation* is a parameter that is closely related to variance. It approximates the average amount of variation between individual data points and the mean. A simple average cannot be computed since, as previously stated, the sum of the individual deviations is zero. Since the deviations are squared to calculate variance, the standard deviation is calculated as the square root of the variance:

$$s = \sqrt{\frac{\Sigma(x - \bar{x})^2}{n - 1}}$$

The variance for the values in Table 6-1 is 1148, and the standard deviation is 34. The absolute value of the variance tends to have little meaning because each of the differences is squared. However, since standard deviation is calculated by first squaring the differences and then taking the square root, the units of standard deviation are the same as for the observations themselves.

The magnitude of the standard deviation is often compared to the mean of the observations through the calculation of the *coefficient of variation* (CV), also known as the *relative standard deviation*:

$$CV = \frac{s}{\bar{x}} \times 100$$

The result is usually expressed as a percentage (e.g., CV% for the cholesterol observations is 16.9%). The coefficient of variation allows the investigator and the reader to gain an appreciation of the degree of variability in the data and can be used to compare variability between studies or between different drugs or different measurements. For example, Adedoyin et al.[8] measured the plasma clearance of the S and R isomers of mephenytoin. S-mephenytoin had a clearance of 1986.9 ± 1878.4 mL/min (mean $\pm$ standard deviation) compared with 24.0 ± 10.6 mL/min for R-mephenytoin. The absolute values for the standard deviation are difficult to compare because that clearance is roughly 40-fold higher for S-mephenytoin. However, the coefficient of variation is 94.5% for S-mephenytoin clearance versus 44.2% for R-mephenytoin, suggesting that the clearance of the latter is less variable. Unusually high values for the coefficient of variation, particularly when compared with previously published values, may suggest problems with data collection and analysis. In addition, all other factors being equal, investigators would generally prefer to work with a less variable outcome measure since this will improve the power of the study (see Chap. 7).

> ## KEY CONCEPT
>
> Standard deviation has the same units as the measure itself and can be divided by the mean to obtain the coefficient of variation. This parameter can be used to compare the variability of measures where the magnitude of values is different or different units of measurement are used.

Degrees of Freedom

The use of $n - 1$ in the denominator of the equations for variance and standard deviation deserves mention. Since we are attempting to estimate the average degree of deviation of data points from the mean, why not divide by n rather than $n - 1$? The answer to this question relates to the fact that the standard deviation of a sample is meant to be an estimate of the standard deviation for the entire population. In order to account for the fact that the standard deviation from small samples (less than 30 observations) will generally underestimate the true standard deviation for the population, the denominator is reduced by 1, resulting in a larger and more realistic value for the standard deviation. From a practical standpoint, the use of n versus $n - 1$ makes little difference when the number of data points is greater than 30. The expression $n - 1$ is referred to as the *number of degrees of freedom* ν.

Statistics such as mean and standard deviation discussed in this chapter are used to describe the central tendency and variability of a sample. These values are estimates of the true mean and standard deviation of the entire population. The relationship between the sample and the population is explored in more detail in Chap. 7.

Study Questions

1. A new diagnostic test for screening blood for the presence of HIV has been developed. The test is administered to 985 individuals who have previously been diagnosed as HIV-positive and to 746 persons who are known to be HIV-negative. The following results are obtained:

	Positive Test	*Negative Test*
HIV-positive subjects	958	27
HIV-negative subjects	8	738

Calculate the sensitivity and specificity of this test.

2. It has been estimated that approximately 182,000 new cases of breast cancer will be diagnosed in the United States in 2000. Estimate the incidence of the disease expressed as number of new cases per million citizens.

3. McCune et al.[9] examined the effect of dexamethasone on the activity of the CYP3A4 enzyme as measured by two parameters: the erythromycin breath test (EBT) and the ratio of dextromethorphan (DM) to 3-methoxymorphinan (3MM). Using the baseline data in the following table, calculate the mean, median, standard deviation, and coefficient of variation for both parameters. Which of the two is the most variable parameter? Does the mean provide a reasonable estimate of the central tendency for the ratio of DM/3MM?

Subject	EBT	Ratio of DM/3MM
1	2.28	7
2	1.43	17
3	2.18	—
4	2.46	13
5	2.12	32
6	2.03	38
7	2.89	65
8	1.06	6
9	2.19	7.8
10	2.70	4.8
11	1.77	9.2
12	3.40	109

References

1. Buechler CM, Blostein PA, Koestner A, Hurt K, Schaars M, McKernan J: Variation among trauma centers' calculation of Glasgow Coma Scale score: Results of a national survey. J Trauma 45:429–431, 1998.

2. Elmore J, Barton M, Moceri V, Polk S, Arena P, Fletcher S: Ten-year risk of false positive screening mammograms and clinical breast examinations. N Engl J Med 338:1089–1096, 1998.

3. Schwartz LM, Woloshin S, Sox HC, Fischhoff B, Welch HG: US women's attitudes to false positive mammography results and detection of ductal carcinoma in situ: cross-sectional survey. Western J Med 173:307–312, 2000.

4. Sandler RS, Zorich NL, Filloon TG, Wiseman HB, Lietz DJ, Brock MH, et al: Gastrointestinal symptoms in 3181 volunteers ingesting snack foods containing Olestra or triglycerides. A 6-week randomized, placebo-controlled trial. Ann Intern Med 130:253–261, 1999.

5. Tilley BC, Alarcón GS, Heyse SP, Trentham DE, Neuner R, Kaplan DA, et al: Minocycline in rheumatoid arthritis: A 48-week, double-blind, placebo-controlled trial. Ann Intern Med 122:81–89, 1995.

6. Catania JA, Morin SF, Canchola J, Pollack L, Chang J, Coates TJ: US priorities—HIV prevention. Science 290:717, 2000.

7. Bertilsson L, Lou Y-Q, Du Y-L, Liu Y, Kuang T-Y, Liao X-M, et al: Pronounced differences between native Chinese and Swedish populations in the polymorphic hydroxylations of debrisoquin and S-mephenytoin. Clin Pharmacol Ther 51:388–397, 1992.

8. Adedoyin A, Arns PA, Richards WO, Wilkinson GR, Branch RA: Selective effect of liver disease on the activities of specific metabolizing enzymes: Investigation of cytochromes P450 2C19 and 2D6. Clin Pharmacol Ther 64:8–17, 1998.

9. McCune JS, Hawke RL, LeCluyse EL, Gillenwater HH, Hamilton G, Ritchie J, Lindley C: In vivo and in vitro induction of human cytochrome P4503A4 by dexamethasone. Clin Pharmacol Ther 68:356–366, 2000.

Concepts in Inferential Statistics: Distributions, Confidence Intervals, and Hypothesis Testing

David J. Edwards

OUTLINE

Goals and Objectives

Introduction

The Normal Distribution

   The z-Distribution

The Distribution of Sample Means and the Central Limit Theorem

   Standard Error of the Mean

   The t-Distribution

Confidence Intervals

   Confidence Interval of a Mean: Evaluating Bioequivalence

   Confidence Interval for a Difference Between Means

   Confidence Interval of a Proportion

Hypothesis Testing

   The Meaning of p-Values

   Statistical Versus Clinical Significance

   One-Tailed Versus Two-Tailed Testing

   Errors in Hypothesis Testing

   Factors Affecting Power

   Estimating Sample Size

Study Questions

References

KEY WORDS

Normal distribution	Confidence interval	Type II error
Sample	p-value	Power
Population	Statistical significance	Sample size
z-score	Clinical significance	
t-score	Type I error	

Goals and Objectives

This chapter explores the properties of the normal distribution and the use of the central limit theorem to assess the relationship between samples and populations. The calculation of the confidence interval is introduced as a method by which data from a sample can be used to draw inferences with respect to treatment effects in a population of patients. Hypothesis testing and errors associated with hypothesis testing are described. Finally, the factors affecting the power of a study to detect differences between treatments is discussed and the relationship between power and sample size examined. After completing this chapter, readers should be able to:

1. Calculate a z-score given an individual value from the population and use the z-score to determine how typical or atypical the value is.

2. Understand the difference between the standard deviation and the standard error of the mean.

3. Calculate and interpret the confidence interval for a mean.

4. Draw conclusions based on the calculated 95% confidence interval for differences between means and proportions as well as odds ratio and relative risk.

5. Understand the meaning of a calculated p-value and how the p-value is used to accept or reject the null hypothesis.

6. Understand the difference between statistical significance and clinical significance.

7. Distinguish between a Type I and a Type II error.

8. Identify the factors that affect the power of a study and understand the importance of selecting an appropriate sample size in designing a study with appropriate power.

Introduction

Chapter 6 discussed measures for describing the central tendency and variability in data. Parameters such as mean and standard deviation allow the reader to quickly gain an appreciation for the important characteristics of a sample without having to examine the raw data. It should be remembered, however, that the data obtained from a sample of patients participating in a study is of interest only if the results can be applied to the entire population who could benefit from the same treatment. It is not practical to include the whole population in a study since the population of potential users of a particular drug, for example, may be extremely large and mostly inaccessible to the principal investigator. Sample statistics such as mean $\bar{x}$ and standard deviation s are estimates of the true population mean and standard deviation represented by the Greek symbols μ and σ, respectively. Assuming that the sample is selected properly (see Chap. 6)—that is, sampling is random, unbiased, and includes a sufficient number of subjects—the sample statistics should provide a reasonable estimate of the population values most of the time.

The Normal Distribution

The distribution of data obtained from a sample is referred to as an *empirical distribution* and provides information about the underlying population. In Chap. 6, continuous data was presented in the form of a frequency distribution where the data range was divided into intervals and the number of data points within each interval counted and plotted on the y axis. The theoretical distribution depicts the distribution of data for the entire population. Since the number of data points is infinitely large, the data does not have to be divided into intervals, and a smooth curve is presented (see Fig. 7-1). A theoretical distribution may take any shape. However, experience has shown that when the variability in the data is a result of many independent factors, a unimodal distribution often results that is symmetrical about the population mean value of μ. This type of distribution is variously referred to as the *bell, gaussian,* or *normal curve.* The bell curve obviously derives its name from the shape of the distribution; the term *gaussian* refers to the German mathematician Carl Friedrich Gauss, whose work led to the discovery of the nature

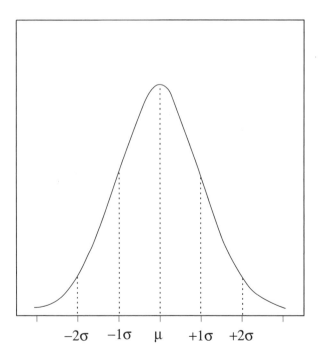

Figure 7-1. The normal distribution.

and significance of the bell-shaped curve. Because many variables in nature (e.g., height, blood pressure) follow a gaussian or bell-shaped distribution, this is also referred to as the *normal* distribution.

The precise shape of the normal distribution is determined by the population mean and standard deviation and differs from variable to variable. However, it is always true that approximately two-thirds (68%) of the area under a normal curve will lie within 1 standard deviation above or below the mean (Fig. 7-1). Similarly, 95% of the area under the curve lies within approximately 2 (actually 1.96) standard deviations of the mean, and 99% of the area is within 2.58 standard deviations. Another way of expressing this is to state that 95% of the observations in a normally distributed population will be within ± 2 standard deviations of the population mean. This also implies that 2.5% of observations will be more than 2 standard deviations below the mean and another 2.5% will be more than 2 standard deviations higher than the mean. This concept is sometimes used to define the so-called normal range for physical characteristics and common laboratory values. For example, if the average systolic blood pressure in the population is 120 mmHg and the standard deviation is 15 mmHg, then a normal range for systolic blood pressure can be calculated as $\mu \pm 1.96 \, (\sigma)$. In this case, normal values range from approximately 90 to 150 mmHg.

The term *normal* must be interpreted with caution. Generally, it is the range in which one would expect 95 out of 100 measurements to lie. Values outside the normal range are uncommon. They may or may not be associated with a specific disease state or clinical consequence. The definition of normal must also take into account factors such as the age, gender, and genetic background of the patient. A hemoglobin concentration of 13 g/dL in a 25-year-old male would be considered below normal, but a similar value in a 40-year-old female would not.

KEY CONCEPT

If data is normally distributed, approximately 95% of the observations can be found within 2 standard deviations of the mean. Values ranging from 2 standard deviations below the mean to 2 standard deviations above the mean are sometimes used to define the "normal" range for laboratory tests.

The *z*-Distribution

The shape of the normal distribution as defined by the mean and standard deviation will be different for every variable. However, all normally distributed variables can be standardized and compared by calculating standard values known as *z*-scores. The *z*-score is calculated for each individual measurement *x* using the following equation:

$$z = \frac{x - \mu}{\sigma} \tag{7-1}$$

The z-score, also referred to as the *standard normal deviate,* is equal to the number of standard deviations that a measurement lies from the population mean. The distribution of z-scores (z-distribution), the standard normal distribution, will have a mean of 0 (since the average difference between the individual measures and the population mean is 0) and a standard deviation of 1. z-Scores can be useful in drawing inferences about a specific measurement obtained in a patient. Using the example of systolic blood pressure again, suppose that the systolic blood pressure in a patient is measured and found to be 160 mmHg. Clearly, this is much higher than the mean population value of 120 mmHg, but how unusual is such a value? The z-score for the value of 160 mmHg can be calculated and is equal to +2.7. This indicates that a systolic blood pressure of 160 mmHg is 2.7 standard deviations above the mean. One can immediately assume that this occurs uncommonly, since 95% of values will be within 1.96 standard deviations of the mean. To find out the exact answer, a table of z-scores (see App. A) must be consulted. In this case, 99.3% of observations in a normally distributed population can be expected to be within 2.7 standard deviations of the mean, with 0.35% being more than 2.7 standard deviations above the mean. One would expect to encounter a systolic blood pressure of 160 mmHg or above between 3 and 4 times out of every 1000 observations.

The Distribution of Sample Means and the Central Limit Theorem

The calculation of z-scores allows us to draw conclusions about individual data points, but the mean and standard deviation of the population must be known in order to complete the calculation. This information is often not available and may differ substantially from the sample mean and standard deviation, particularly when the number of data points in the sample is small. Although the entire population cannot be sampled, information about the population mean and standard deviation can be inferred by collecting a number of samples and examining the distribution of the sample means.

The *central limit theorem* states that the distribution of the means of samples drawn from the same population will be normal, with a mean equal to the population value μ. The standard deviation of the distribution of sample means is referred to as the *standard error of the mean* (SEM) and can be expressed mathematically as follows:

$$SEM = \frac{s}{\sqrt{n}} \tag{7-2}$$

It should be noted that the population itself need not have a normal distribution in order for the distribution of sample means from the population to be normally distributed. However, the distribution of sample means will be normally distributed only if the size of each sample is reasonably large.

Standard Error of the Mean

The standard error of the mean is always smaller than the standard deviation of the sample. This is to be expected since the variability between the means of samples drawn from the same population should be smaller than the variability between individual observations within a sample. If systolic blood pressure were measured in 100 subjects, for example, it would not be unusual for individual values to range from 100 to 140 mmHg. However, if blood pressure were measured in several groups, each consisting of 100 patients, it is highly unlikely that any of the sample means would be as low as 100 mmHg or as high as 140 mmHg. The sample means would most likely not fall outside the range of 115 to 125 mmHg.

KEY CONCEPT

The appropriate statistic for describing the variability in a sample is the standard deviation. Use of the standard error of the mean for this purpose may provide a misleading underestimate of the degree of variability in a sample.

Everyone reading the medical literature should be aware of the difference between the standard deviation and the standard error of the mean, as both are sometimes reported in published papers. Authors may be tempted to use standard error in tables or figures since the standard error is always smaller and gives the appearance that the data are less variable than they really are. However, the standard deviation is the appropriate statistic for describing the variability in a sample. Standard error, on the other hand, is useful in measuring the relationship between the sample mean and the population value. The smaller the standard error, the more likely it is that the sample statistics are representative of the population. Looking at the equation for calculating standard error, it is clear that the value will be smaller if either the standard deviation of the sample is small or the number of observations in the sample is large. Both factors, little variability in the data and a large sample size, increase our confidence that the sample is an accurate reflection of the population.

The *t*-Distribution

The distribution of sample means referred to by the central limit theorem is known as the *t-distribution*. With individual sample means from a population, the *t*-score can be calculated according to the following equation:

$$t = \frac{\bar{x} - \mu}{\text{SEM}} \qquad (7\text{-}3)$$

Inspection of this equation indicates that it is identical to the calculation of the
z-score, with the exception that the denominator contains the standard error of
the mean. This is appropriate, of course, since the standard error of the mean is
equal to the standard deviation of the distribution of sample means. The characteristics of the distribution of sample means (t-distribution) are similar to the
distribution of z-scores (z-distribution). Since the differences between sample
means and the population mean will be both positive and negative, the distribution has a mean value of 0 and a standard deviation equal to 1. Irrespective of the
raw values or units for the sample mean and the population mean, the calculated
value of t will measure the deviation between the two in units of standard errors.
Since the distribution is normal, it can be predicted that 95% of sample means
obtained from the same population will lie between -1.96 and $+1.96$ standard errors of the population mean.

Up to this point, the calculation and interpretation of t-scores and z-scores
have been similar. However, there is an important distinction between the two.
Because the z-score measures the deviation between individual measures and the
population mean, there is only a single z-distribution. However, the deviation
between a sample mean and the population mean, as measured by the t-score, is
dependent on the number of observations (n) in the sample. The means obtained
from samples with a large number of measures will cluster more tightly around the
population mean and have a smaller standard error than means derived from samples containing only a few observations. Therefore, the distribution of t is different for each value of n. When the sample size—more correctly, the number of
degrees of freedom ($n-1$), see Chap. 6—is small, the t-distribution is more widely
spread. Consulting a table of t-scores (see App. B), it can be seen that with six subjects ($v = 5$), 95% of the differences between sample means and the population
mean will lie between -2.57 and $+2.57$ (Fig. 7-2). When the number of subjects
(observations) is increased to 16 ($v = 15$), the corresponding range is -2.13 to
$+2.13$. As the number of observations in the sample increases, the t-distribution
approaches a true normal distribution, and 95% of the calculated t-values will lie
within the range of ± 1.96.

Confidence Intervals

When observations are obtained from a population, it is not immediately obvious
to the investigator whether the sample mean is near the population mean. An important application of the t-score is in determining a range of values in which it is
highly likely that the true population mean lies. This range is known as the *confidence interval* of the mean. Different intervals can be calculated expressing differing levels of confidence. For example, we may be 90% confident that the mean

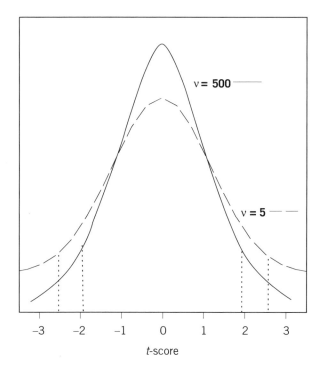

Figure 7-2. The t-distribution.

systolic blood pressure in the population is between 117.5 and 122.5 mmHg, 95% confident that it lies between 115 and 125 mmHg, and 99% confident that it is be- tween 110 and 130 mmHg. Notice that as the interval becomes wider, the level of confidence increases. Although varying levels of confidence can be calculated, it is the 95% confidence interval that is most widely accepted by the scientific commu- nity as providing a reasonable level of certainty. The general formula for calculat- ing the confidence interval (CI) of a mean is given by the following equation:

$$CI = \bar{x} \pm \left(t \times \frac{s}{\sqrt{n}} \right) \qquad (7\text{-}4)$$

It is clear from this equation that the confidence interval will be symmetrical about the sample mean $\bar{x}$, with the width dependent on the standard error of the mean $s/\sqrt{n}$. When the standard error of the mean is small, due to either a small value for s or a large n, the confidence interval will be narrow.

The value of t to be used in the equation depends on two factors. The first is the size of the sample and the second is the level of confidence that is being calcu- lated. If a sample consists of six observations ($v = 5$), it was previously mentioned that 95% of sample means will lie within ± 2.57 standard errors of the mean. Therefore, to calculate the 95% confidence interval for $v = 5$, the value of 2.57 is used for t in the equation. Similarly, if there are 16 subjects in the sample ($v = 15$), $t = 2.13$. The value of t always decreases as the number of observations increases, with a minimum value of 1.96 for an infinitely large sample. As the number of subjects in the sample increases, all else being equal, the range of values in which one is highly confident that the population mean lies will be smaller because the value of t and the standard error of the mean will both be lower. A t-table (App. B) must be consulted in order to obtain the correct value for t to be used in calculating the confidence interval for differing sample sizes and levels of confidence.

KEY CONCEPT

Both the standard error of the mean and the value of t decrease as the number of subjects studied increases. If the standard deviation remains constant, increasing the sample size will reduce the width of the confidence interval.

Confidence Interval of a Mean: Evaluating Bioequivalence

The calculation and analysis of confidence intervals is used by regulatory agencies around the world in determining whether generic drugs should be considered to be bioequivalent to brand-name products. In a bioequivalence study, the plasma concentrations are measured for both the generic drug and the innovator product in each subject participating in the study (crossover study design). Concentrations (peak as well as area under the concentration-time curve) obtained with the generic product are divided by those observed with the innovator product in the same subject to obtain a ratio. The mean ratio and standard error of the mean are then calculated for the entire sample. In a hypothetical study involving 20 subjects, suppose the mean concentration ratio was 0.95 with a standard deviation of 0.15. The 90% confidence interval can be calculated from this data. Standard error of the mean is $0.15/\sqrt{20}$, which is equal to 0.03354. The appropriate value for t (obtained from a t-table) is 1.729 for $v = 19$ and a level of confidence of 90%. Substituting these values into the equation $0.95 \pm (1.729 \times 0.03354)$ results in a 90% confidence interval ranging from 0.89 to 1.01. How should this be interpreted? The correct interpretation is that although the true ratio of concentrations for these products is unknown, one could predict with 90% confidence that it lies between 0.89 and 1.01. The U.S. Food and Drug Administration requires that in order for a product to be judged bioequivalent, the 90% confidence interval for the ratio must lie between 0.8 and 1.25. Given this data, the generic product would meet the bioequivalence standard set by the FDA.

Confidence Interval for a Difference Between Means

Other types of confidence intervals can be calculated to allow the investigator to draw inferences about the data. For example, Gorski et al.[1] studied the disposition of midazolam in men and women. After oral administration of midazolam to eight women, half-life averaged 2.6 h with a standard deviation of 1.3 h. In eight men, the average was 4.2 h with a standard deviation of 1.6 h. The calculation of the confidence interval for the difference between means is similar to calculating the confidence interval of a mean:

$$CI = \Delta \pm (t \times SE_{diff}) \tag{7-5}$$

In this case, the difference between the means Δ is equal to 1.6. The standard error of the difference between means SE_{diff} is a more complicated calculation than standard error of the mean since the variability in the two groups must be combined. A detailed description is beyond the scope of this chapter, but the value can be derived from the mean, standard deviation, and size of each of the samples. The result is equal to 0.73. The appropriate value for t from a t-table for 95% confidence and eight subjects per group is 2.145. Substituting these values into the preceding equation results in a 95% confidence interval of 0.04 to 3.16 h. In other words, it can be stated with 95% confidence that the true difference in half-life between men and women is somewhere between 0.04 and 3.16 h. Since this range does not include zero, a value that would indicate no difference, the conclusion can be made (with 95% certainty) that there is a difference in midazolam half-life related to gender. In this same study, the sleep time with midazolam was 48 min in women (SD = 18) compared to 43 min in men (SD = 28). Using the same approach, the 95% confidence interval for the difference in sleep time between men and women ranges from −20 to +30 min. Because the confidence interval includes zero, it cannot be concluded that there is any difference in sleep time related to gender.

Confidence Interval of a Proportion

The confidence interval approach to drawing conclusions is not limited to interval or ratio data that follow a normal distribution. In fact, the same principles can be applied to nominal data such as percentages, proportions, or frequencies. Perhaps the most common examples of this with which most people are familiar are the surveys that frequently appear in newspapers or magazines. A typical poll may indicate that 65% of voters favor a particular political candidate. Inspection of the

KEY CONCEPT

When the 95% confidence interval for the difference between two means or between two proportions includes the value of zero, the appropriate conclusion is that there is no difference.

fine print reveals that the poll is accurate within plus or minus 4%, 19 times out of 20. This is simply another way of saying that the 95% confidence interval for the percentage of voters favoring this candidate ranges from 61 to 69%. There are many examples of this type of data in drug research. In the report by Sandler et al.[2] (discussed in Chap. 6), 619 out of 1620 patients (38.2%) ingesting snack products containing olestra experienced gastrointestinal symptoms. Since this represents the frequency of side effects in this particular sample, it is of interest to know the range of values that contains the true rate of side effects with olestra. The confidence interval for a proportion can be calculated using the following equation:

$$CI = p \pm \left(z \times \sqrt{\frac{p(1-p)}{n}} \right) \tag{7-6}$$

where p is the sample proportion (0.382) and z is the z-score for the appropriate level of confidence. For a 95% confidence interval, a value of 1.96 should be used for z. With the olestra data, the 95% confidence interval ranges from 35.6 to 40.4%. This is a relatively narrow interval compared to previous examples primarily because of the large sample size in the study. With a large number of subjects, there is a high level of confidence that the true frequency of side effects with olestra in the population will be quite close to the mean in the sample studied.

Just as a confidence interval can be calculated for a mean as well as a difference between means, one can calculate a confidence interval for a difference between proportions. Without going through the rather complicated math, inspection of the paper by Sandler et al. reveals that the investigators have calculated the 95% confidence interval for the difference between the proportion of subjects with side effects in the olestra group (38.2%) versus the placebo group (36.9%). The difference in the proportion is 1.3%, with a 95% confidence interval of −3.6 to +6.2%. The appropriate conclusion is that there is no difference in the frequency of gastrointestinal symptoms between olestra and placebo since the 95% confidence interval for the difference includes the value of zero.

Finally, it is possible to calculate the confidence interval for a ratio of two proportions. Examples include the calculation of odds ratio and relative risk for case-control and cohort studies, respectively (discussed in Chap. 4). Relative risk is obtained by dividing the rate of adverse events in the group receiving the drug under study by the rate of adverse events in the control group. A value of 1 suggests that the risks are unchanged with the treatment under study. In the study by Beral et al.,[3] the relative risk of death in current users of oral contraceptives was compared to that of nonusers. Risk of death from any cause was 1.0, with a 95% confidence interval ranging from 0.9 to 1.2. Since the value of 1.0 was included in the confidence interval, it was concluded that oral contraceptive use did not increase the overall mortality risk. In the same study, the relative risk of ovarian cancer was 0.2 in current or recent users of oral contraceptives, with a 95% confidence interval of 0.1 to 0.7. Notice that the confidence interval does not contain the value of 1.0. Based on this, it can be stated with 95% certainty that there is a decreased risk of ovarian cancer in patients who are taking or have recently stopped taking oral contraceptives. Finally, the relative risk of dying from cerebrovascular disease was 1.9, with a 95% confidence interval of 1.2 to 3.1. For this adverse event, the confidence interval is entirely above 1, leading to the conclusion that oral contraceptive use increases the risk of dying from a stroke.

Hypothesis Testing

The use of confidence intervals to draw inferences or conclusions about data is one approach. The other is to use a specific statistical test to accept or reject a hypothesis at a predetermined level of probability. Although the hypothesis states the predicted relationship between variables or a predicted difference between treatments, it is the hypothesis of no difference, the null hypothesis, that is tested statistically. The null hypothesis H_0 states that the treatment under study has no effect on the outcome measure of interest. The alternative, or research, hypothesis H_1 states that the treatment has an effect. Generally, the alternative hypothesis is nondirectional, that is, it does not say that the treatment will have a positive effect or a negative effect. The decision to accept or reject the null hypothesis is dependent on a statistical analysis of the differences between the groups being studied.

The Meaning of p-Values

In any study in which the data from two or more groups is being compared, there will almost always be differences between the groups, even if they are merely due to random or biological variability in the parameter being measured. In other words, even if we measure blood pressure in two groups of subjects who are not receiving any active treatment, it is highly unlikely that the mean blood pressure will be exactly the same in both groups. This would be true even if we were to measure blood pressure in the same subjects on two different occasions. Intuitively, if the differences between groups, say a treatment group and a placebo group, are small, we conclude that the treatment has no effect and accept the null hypothesis. A large difference suggests that the treatment has an effect and that the alternative hypothesis should be accepted. Statistics allow us to quantify the magnitude of the difference and assess the probability that a difference is likely to be an effect of the treatment and not merely a chance occurrence.

Although a variety of statistical tests can be used depending on the study design and the type of data generated from the research, all statistical tests ultimately generate a p-value. The p-value gives the probability of the observed difference occurring if the null hypothesis is true. Values for p range from 0 to 1, with low values indicating that there is a small probability of finding the observed difference if the treatment has no effect. For example, a statistical result of $p = 0.03$ would indicate that there would be only a 3% chance of finding a difference of this size if the treatment had no effect. Stated another way, if the null hypothesis were true, 97 experiments out of 100 would find a smaller difference.

Investigators could simply state the calculated p-values and allow readers to draw their own conclusions about the meaning of the results. However, it is standard practice for the investigator to use the p-value to make a judgment about whether the null hypothesis should be accepted or rejected. If a low p-value means that there is a low probability that the observed difference could occur if the null hypothesis were true, then the logical conclusion is that the null hypothesis is not true and should be rejected. How low should the probability or p-value be before we reject the null hypothesis? A threshold value for p is set before beginning the experiment and, by convention, is generally 0.05. In other words, the investigator indicates prior to initiating the study that if the calculated p-value is less than 0.05, the null hypothesis will be rejected and the difference between treatments will be considered statistically significant. This is similar to the 95% confidence interval that is commonly calculated to provide a range that is highly likely to contain the "true" value. It is of historical interest that modern scientists are comfortable with the probability of being correct as seldom as 19 times out of 20. In his work on probability theory developed over 300 years ago, Jacob Bernoulli considered that in order to be "morally certain" of making the correct decision, an appropriate level of certainty would be 1000/1001, comparable to setting a threshold value of p less than 0.001. For an excellent review of the development of modern concepts of odds and probability, the reader is referred to the book *Against the Gods: The Remarkable Story of Risk* by Peter Bernstein.[4]

KEY CONCEPT

The p-value gives the probability of the observed difference between treatments occurring if the null hypothesis is true. If the probability is low ($p < 0.05$), then the null hypothesis is rejected.

The concept of hypothesis testing and the use of p-values to accept or reject the null hypothesis can be applied to the example of midazolam disposition discussed earlier in this chapter. The half-life of midazolam averaged 2.6 h (SD = 1.3) in eight women compared with 4.2 h (SD = 1.6) in eight men. In this case, the null hypothesis is that there is no difference in half-life between men and women. The specific statistical test used to test the null hypothesis depends on the nature of the data, but in this case, the appropriate test is the unpaired Student's t-test, discussed in detail in Chap. 8. Using this test, a calculated p-value of 0.046 is obtained. If there were no difference in midazolam half-life between men and women, a difference as large as that observed in this study would be expected only 4.6% of the time. Since there is a low probability (less than 5%) that the observed difference would occur if the null hypothesis were true, the null is rejected, and the alternative hypothesis—that there is a difference in midazolam half-life related to gender—is accepted.

Statistical Versus Clinical Significance

A statistically significant difference is one that would be unlikely to occur if the treatment had in fact no effect ($p < 0.05$). Statistically significant differences may or may not have any clinical significance or meaning to a patient. Consider the following statements from a paper studying the interaction between calcium channel blockers and theophylline.[5]

> Mean theophylline oral clearance decreased 18% and 12% after verapamil and diltiazem, respectively ($p < 0.05$). . . . The modest reduction in theophylline clearance observed after verapamil and diltiazem is unlikely to produce clinically significant increases in theophylline concentrations in most patients.

The investigators have concluded that verapamil and diltiazem have a statistically significant influence on theophylline clearance but that the effect is not clinically meaningful. Readers may or may not agree with the investigators' opinion regarding the clinical value of a statistically significant effect. It should be noted, however, that differences that are not statistically significant cannot be evaluated for clinical meaning since, by definition, there is a more-than-acceptable probability that there is no treatment effect (i.e., that the null hypothesis is true). This is a point that those evaluating the drug literature should keep in mind. In studies where the results approach but do not reach statistical significance, it is not uncommon for the authors of a paper to gloss over this fact and proceed with a discussion of what the clinical consequences would be if the result had reached statistical significance.

KEY CONCEPT

Statistically significant differences may or may not be clinically significant; differences that are not statistically significant cannot be evaluated for clinical significance.

The word *significant* is sometimes used very loosely in the biomedical literature. Wagner et al.[6] examined the effect of intravenous famotidine on gastric acid secretion in patients undergoing cardiopulmonary bypass surgery. The discussion section of this paper states, "We observed a significantly increased amount of gastric acid volume following CPB in the patients receiving placebo." It is unclear whether the authors mean statistical significance, clinical significance, or both. Inspection of the results reveals that gastric volumes were on average 24% lower with famotidine but that the result was not statistically significant ($p > 0.05$). The lack of statistical significance suggests that any further discussion of the significance of this finding is meaningless.

One-Tailed Versus Two-Tailed Hypothesis Testing

Statistical tests are usually accompanied by a statement that either a two-tailed or one-tailed test was used. The explanation for this can be found by examining the t-distribution depicted in Figure 7-2. The right and left ends of the distribution, representing uncommon values, are referred to as the *tails*. With a two-tailed test and a cutoff value for statistical significance of $p < 0.05$, the null hypothesis will be rejected if the difference between the groups falls in either the upper or lower 2.5% of the distribution. The dependent variable can be either increased or decreased by the experimental treatment or independent variable under study. For example, midazolam half-life could be either faster or slower in men than in women. With a one-tailed test, it is assumed that the difference between groups can occur in one direction only. If the experimental intervention can only increase the variable under study, then the null hypothesis can be rejected at $p < 0.05$ if the difference between groups is so large that it lies in the upper 5% (rather than 2.5% for a two-tailed test) of the distribution. Smaller differences between groups will be statistically significant with a one-tailed as opposed to a two-tailed test. In theory, a one-tailed statistical test can be used whenever it is highly likely that a difference between groups will occur in one direction only. However, in practice, most statisticians believe that a one-tailed test should be used rarely, if ever, and two-tailed statistical testing is much more common.

Errors in Hypothesis Testing

Type I Errors. When a decision is made to accept or reject the null hypothesis, that decision is based on a probability, not a certainty, of being correct. In other words, there is also the possibility of making an error. There are two errors associated with hypothesis testing, conveniently designated as *Type I* and *Type II errors*. When the conclusion is drawn that the null hypothesis should be rejected, the possibilities are as follows (see Fig. 7-3):

1. The conclusion is correct, and the treatment has an effect.

2. The conclusion is wrong, and the treatment does not have an effect.

A Type I error occurs when the null hypothesis is rejected when it should be accepted. In other words, the conclusion is made that there is a difference between treatments when in fact there is none. The chances of making a Type I error are directly related to the threshold value for p on which decisions are based. If $p < 0.05$ means that there is less than a 5% probability that a difference of this magnitude could occur if the null hypothesis were true, then the chances of making an error by rejecting the null hypothesis are also less than 5%. The symbol α is used to designate the possibility of making a Type I error. Given the traditional threshold value for $p = 0.05$, one can assume that a Type I error will be committed as many as 1 out of every 20 times the null hypothesis is rejected.

It should be noted that a Type I error is not necessarily obvious to either the investigator or a clinician who may be reading a paper. Experts in a discipline may be doubtful that a treatment effect exists under certain conditions, but only repeti-

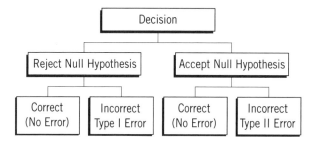

Figure 7-3. Errors in hypothesis testing.

tion of a study will verify whether the conclusions drawn are accurate or in error. For example, in the cohort study examining mortality associated with oral contraceptives discussed earlier (Beral et al.), one of the findings was that there was a statistically significant increase in the risk of violent or accidental death in women who had used oral contraceptives at some point. It seems likely that this was a Type I error since there does not appear to be a logical or rational explanation for such a finding and no other study has ever reported such an association. Readers (and investigators) should not, however, be too quick to categorize unexpected or unusual findings as Type I errors just because a logical explanation is not immediately forthcoming. Bailey et al.[7] reported in 1989 that an interaction between ethanol and the calcium antagonist felodipine occurred only in subjects who were given alcohol dissolved in grapefruit juice and not in individuals whose alcohol was mixed with orange juice. Although it may have been tempting to dismiss this as a Type I error, subsequent studies have confirmed that grapefruit juice is a potent inhibitor of the metabolism of these and other drugs metabolized by the cytochrome P450 enzyme CYP3A4.

KEY CONCEPT

A probability of making a Type I error exists whenever the null hypothesis is rejected. Type II errors are possible only when the null hypothesis has been accepted.

Type II Errors and Power. A Type I error can occur only if the decision is made to reject the null hypothesis. If the results of a study lead to the conclusion that the null hypothesis should be accepted, there are again two possibilities, as illustrated in Fig. 7-3. A Type II error occurs when the null hypothesis is accepted when it should be rejected. In other words, a treatment effect exists but the study concludes that there is none. The probability of making a Type II error is denoted by the symbol β and is associated with the concept of power. In reading the drug literature, clinicians will often come across references to the power of a study. *Power* is the ability of the study to detect a difference between treatments. Mathematically, power is inversely related to the probability of making a Type II error:

$$Power = 1 - \beta \qquad (7\text{-}7)$$

When designing a study, the investigator must make a decision regarding how much power is required. Stated another way, how much of a chance of making a Type II error is the investigator willing to accept? The minimal value for β in designing studies is generally considered to be 0.2; in other words, there should be at least an 80% probability of finding a treatment effect if one exists. In comparing the conventions for α (0.05) and β (0.2), it is clear that Type II errors will occur more frequently than Type I errors. Furthermore, scientists are more willing to accept the risk of making a Type II error. The implication of this statement is that the consequences of incorrectly concluding that there is a treatment effect when one doesn't exist (Type I error) are viewed as more serious than failing to find a treatment effect that does exist (Type II error). This may or may not be true, and individual studies may be designed to achieve a much higher level of power than 0.8 in order to reduce the odds of a Type II error occurring. In evaluating the treatment of a disease with a high mortality, failing to conclude, due to a lack of power, that a particular drug results in a small improvement in survival would have important clinical consequences.

The possibility that a Type II error has been made may be obvious to the reader. When an observed difference appears to be large enough to be of clinical significance but no statistically significant difference was observed, there is a possibility that a Type II error has been committed. Unfortunately, few studies actually report the power, even though it can be accurately calculated after the study has been completed. Type II errors occur for three main reasons:

1. More variability than expected in the outcome measure
2. Use of an inadequate number of subjects
3. Better-than-expected response in the comparison group

All of these factors reduce the power of a study and are discussed in further detail in the following sections.

Factors Affecting Power

The power of a study can be accurately calculated only after a study has been completed. However, an investigator has to make assumptions concerning the various factors that influence power prior to beginning in order to design the study appropriately. Power is a function of the following four factors:

1. *The size of the treatment effect.*   Since power is the ability of a study to detect differences between treatments, it stands to reason that it is easier to detect a large difference than a small one. If the difference between treatments is large, the likelihood of failing to find the difference will be small and power will be high. In designing a study, scientists must make a decision regarding the size of the difference between treatments that they would like their study to be able to detect. This is not an arbitrary decision. It is based on the investigator's opinion regarding the magnitude of treatment effect that would be clinically significant or meaningful. A new drug for the treatment of high cholesterol concentrations may be useful if it produces at least a 20% decrease in serum concentrations of cholesterol. There would be little point in designing a study so that reductions in cholesterol of only 5% could be detected, since such a small difference would have no clinical value. Everything else being equal, the chances of making a Type II error will be greater and the power lower when trying to detect a smaller difference between treatments.

A small difference between the active and control treatment is not always caused by the drug under investigation failing to produce the desired effect. It is also possible that the control group may exhibit a better-than-expected response. This may occur if the patient population does not turn out to be as sick or at as high a risk for the development of a disease as originally expected. For example, Lai et al.[8] studied the recurrence of duodenal ulcer in patients treated with antibiotics to eradicate *H. pylori* compared with treatment with a bismuth preparation. Prior to the study, they estimated that 30% of patients treated with bismuth would have a recurrence of bleeding ulcer and designed the study with the assumption that this would be reduced to 5% by antibiotic therapy. In fact, recurrence occurred in only 20% of the control group. This made it essentially impossible for the active treatment to achieve the 25% reduction in recurrence rate that was originally projected. In such cases, the power of the study is reduced, and the assumption that the drug under study has no effect may not be valid.

2. *The value of α.*   Although the threshold value for α is traditionally set at 0.05, a higher value could be used in theory. By setting a higher threshold value for α, differences between treatments would be more likely to be statistically significant. Power will be increased because it is unlikely that a difference between treatments will be missed. This is not a practical approach to improving power, however, since the investigator would be increasing power at the expense of increasing the probability of making a Type I error.

3. *Variability in the outcome measure.*   When the measure of a drug's effect is inherently highly variable, it will be more difficult to detect changes in the parameter. The chances of missing a treatment effect increase and the power of a study will be lower. Consider the data in Table 7-1 from a study by McCune et al.[9] in which the investigators examined the effect of dexamethasone on two different

TABLE 7.1. Influence of Variability in the Data on the Ability to Determine a Treatment Effect

Sub No.	Erythromycin Breath Test Result			Urinary Ratio of Dextromethorphan to 3-Methoxymorphinan		
	Baseline	Day 5	Percent Increase	Baseline	Day 5	Percent Decrease
1	2.28	2.56	12	7	12	71
2	1.43	2.13	49	17	10	41
3	2.18	2.22	2	ND	ND	ND
4	2.46	3.68	50	13	1	92
5	2.12	2.62	24	32	23	28
6	2.03	2.44	20	38	6.8	82
7	2.89	2.66	−8	65	1.97	97
8	1.06	1.8	.70	6.0	1.9	68
9	2.19	3.31	51	7.8	7.6	2
10	2.70	3.18	18	4.8	2.9	38
11	1.77	2.24	27	9.2	3.1	66
12	3.40	3.21	−6	109	7	93
Mean ± SD	2.20 ± 0.60	2.67 ± 0.55*	25.7 ± 24.6	28.11 ± 32.58	7.06 ± 6.40†	49 ± 50

Erythromycin breath test result and dextromethorphan to 3-methoxymorphinan ratio before and on day 5 of administration of 8 mg dexamethasone two times daily in 12 healthy volunteers.

Percent change = [Day 5 − baseline/baseline] × 100.

*p = .004.

†p = .06.

SOURCE: From McCune et al. (9). Reproduced from Clin Pharmacol Ther 68:356–366, 2000, with permission from Mosby.

measures of CYP3A4 activity: the erythromycin breath test and the ratio of dextromethorphan to 3-methoxymorphinan. Variability in the erythromycin breath test as assessed by the coefficient of variation was approximately 25%. With this degree of variability, the increase of approximately 21% with dexamethasone treatment was statistically significant ($p = 0.004$). In contrast, the urinary ratio of dextromethorphan to 3-methoxymorphinan was much more variable, with results varying from 4.8 to 109 before treatment and from 1 to 23 with dexamethasone. The standard deviation approaches or exceeds the mean in both cases. Despite the fact that the mean ratio was decreased roughly fourfold by dexamethasone, from 28.11 to 7.06, the difference was not statistically significant ($p = 0.06$).

4. *Sample size.* Power is directly related to the number of subjects studied; the larger the sample size, the higher the power. Of the four factors that influence the power of a study, sample size is the only one that can be controlled by the investigator in order to achieve a desirable level of power. The size of the treatment effect to be detected is dictated by the clinical characteristics of the drug under

KEY CONCEPT

The primary determinant of power that can be manipulated by the investigator is the sample size.

study. It is not reasonable to increase alpha in order to increase power, and the degree of variability in the outcome measure is typically dependent on physiologic and pathologic processes beyond the investigator's control.

Estimating Sample Size

The determination of an appropriate sample size is one of the most important decisions that investigators must make in designing a study. Tables and equations for calculating sample size can be found in the literature or in published textbooks (e.g., Bolton).[10] In addition, computer programs such as SamplePower 1.0 (SPSS Inc., Chicago) can be used to determine the required number of subjects for a variety of different study designs. In order to perform these calculations, the investigator must know the size of the treatment effect (Δ) to be detected and the expected degree of variability in the dependent variable (usually measured by the standard deviation). This information can be obtained either from the literature or from the results of preliminary studies that the investigator has conducted. In addition, a threshold value for alpha, a desired level of power ($1 - \beta$), and the study design must be specified since these influence the equations and algorithms used in the calculations.

Example 1: Sample Size for a Two-Sample Test of Means. Reducing plasma concentrations of cholesterol is presumed to lower the risk of developing coronary artery disease. How many subjects need to be included in a clinical trial comparing the effects of a new cholesterol-lowering drug to a placebo? An initial decision must be made with respect to the effect size to be detected. A search of the literature suggests that a reduction of less than 10% in total cholesterol would not have clinical value. Since most of the statin drugs currently on the market reduce cholesterol by at least 20%, it would be reasonable to design the study to detect a treatment effect of 20% or greater. Next, an estimate must be made of the variability in cholesterol concentrations in the population. This information is readily available from the many studies in the literature. The standard deviation for cholesterol concentrations is approximately 20%. Patients will be included in the study if they have cholesterol concentrations above 240 mg/dL. If the average cholesterol concentration is 280 mg/dL, a treatment effect of 20% would reduce the average concentration to approximately 224 mg/dL. Based on these assumptions, sample size can be calculated. Using a sample size table such as Table 7-2, the parameter s/Δ is equal to 1. For a power of 90% ($\beta = 0.1$) with alpha = 0.05, the table indicates that 23 subjects must be studied in each group. Inspection of

TABLE 7-2. **Number of Subjects Required per Group for $\alpha = 0.05$**

	Power			
s/Δ	*99%*	*95%*	*90%*	*80%*
4	588	417	337	252
2	148	106	86	64
1.5	84	60	49	37
1	38	27	23	17
0.8	25	18	15	12
0.67	18	13	11	9
0.5	11	8	7	6
0.4	8	6	5	4
0.33	6	5	4	4

SOURCE: Adapted from S Bolton: Sample size and power, Chap. 6 in Pharmaceutical Statistics: Practical and Clinical Applications, 2d ed. New York, Marcel Dekker, 1990, p. 196.

Table 7-2 suggests that more subjects are needed as the desired level of power increases (right to left) or the ratio of the variability to the size of the difference to be detected increases (bottom to top). A similar result is obtained using the computer program SamplePower 1.0 (Fig. 7-4).

Example 2: Sample Size for a Two-Sample Test of Proportions. There is considerable interest in new treatments for smoking cessation. While nicotine replacement therapy is of value in the short term, it has been demonstrated that most patients relapse without other forms of treatment. Antidepressant medication has been found to be of value in increasing the percentage of smokers who remain abstinent long term. How many subjects should be studied in assessing the effectiveness of a new antidepressant for smoking cessation? The study will be designed as a two-sample parallel study in which subjects receive either a placebo or the new antidepressant. The outcome measure will be the proportion of smokers who remain abstinent one year after treatment. In order to calculate sample size, estimations must be made regarding the proportion of smokers likely to be abstinent with a placebo as well as the size of the treatment effect that would be clinically meaningful. Jorenby et al.[11] examined the efficacy of bupropion in smoking cessation and found that approximately 15% of subjects receiving a placebo remained abstinent at the end of one year. In the bupropion group, 30.3% were abstinent. A reasonable assumption for the purpose of calculating sample size, therefore, is that 15% of the placebo group will respond and that doubling this proportion to 30% with treatment would be of clinical value. As illustrated in Fig. 7-5, the program SamplePower 1.0 estimates that 161 subjects would be required in each group to achieve a power of 90%.

t-Test for Two Independent Samples with Common Variance

	Population Mean	Standard Deviation	N per group	Standard Error	95% Lower	95% Upper
Placebo	280.0	56.0	23			
Treatment	224.0	56.0	23			
Mean difference	56.0	56.0	46	16.51	22.97	89.03

Alpha = 0.05, tails = 2, power = 0.91

Computational option: Variance is estimated (*t*-test)

Figure 7-4. Calculating sample size for a two-sample test of means.

Two-Sample Proportion

	Proportion Positive	N per Group	Standard Error	95% Lower	95% Upper
Population 1	0.15	161			
Population 2	0.30	161			
Rate difference	−0.15	322	0.05	−0.24	−0.06

Alpha = 0.05, tails = 2, power = 0.90

Power computation: Normal approximation (unweighted mean p)
Precision computation: Log method

Figure 7-5. Calculating sample size for a two-sample test of proportions.

It should be noted that in addition to estimating the required sample size, investigators must also estimate the dropout rate for a study. It is unlikely that all 161 patients treated with the new antidepressant will be available for assessment at 1 year. In the study by Jorenby et al. that was used to estimate the treatment effect, only 181 out of 245 subjects treated with bupropion and a nicotine patch were available for evaluation at the one-year assessment. Tilley et al.[12] examined the efficacy of minocycline in rheumatoid arthritis using a study design in which patients were required to undergo numerous assessments approximately every six weeks for 48 weeks. In calculating sample size for this lengthy and intensive study, the investigators predicted that the dropout rate would be 24%. This turned out to be an accurate estimate, since the actual dropout rate in the study was about 21%.

All of the calculations of sample size in this chapter have assumed that there will be an equal number of subjects in each group. As mentioned in Chap. 6, investigators may wish to randomize more subjects to the treatment groups and less to the placebo in order to gain more information about the treatment. Unequal numbers of subjects in the groups will decrease the power of a study. However, unless the groups are very unequal—for example, more than three times as many subjects in the treatment group as in the control group—the loss of power is relatively small. Consider the example presented in Fig. 7-6. For a study in which the baseline response in the control group is expected to be 40%, with the active treatment lowering the rate to 25%, 200 subjects are needed in each group for a power of 89.6%. If 150 subjects are randomized to the placebo and 250 to the active treatment, the power decreases to only 87.6%. With even more unequal groups (100 placebo, 300 treatment), power is decreased to 79.5%.

Two-Sample Proportion

Name	Prop(1)	Prop(2)	N_1	N_2	CI Level	Lower	Upper	Tails	Alpha	Power
Scenario 01	0.40	0.25	200	200	.950	0.06	0.24	2	.050	.896
Scenario 05	0.40	0.25	175	225	.950	0.06	0.24	2	.050	.891
Scenario 03	0.40	0.25	150	250	.950	0.05	0.25	2	.050	.876
Scenario 04	0.40	0.25	125	275	.950	0.05	0.25	2	.050	.847
Scenario 05	0.40	0.25	100	300	.950	0.04	0.26	2	.050	.795

Figure 7-6 Effect of unequal sample size on power.

Study Questions

1. The population mean for albumin concentration is 4.5 g/dL with a standard deviation of 0.5 g/dL.

   a. If an individual is randomly selected from the population, what is the probability that the albumin concentration will be less than 3.5 g/dL?

   b. The albumin concentration in 20 hospitalized patients is measured and found to average 3.5 g/dL. Is it likely that the hospitalized patients are typical of the general population?

2. Lilja et al.[13] reported that peak concentrations of simvastatin when given to 10 subjects 24 hours after treatment with grapefruit juice averaged 22.0 ng/mL with a standard deviation of 9.7 ng/mL.

   a. Calculate the 95% confidence interval for peak simvastatin concentrations with grapefruit juice.

   b. If the mean peak simvastatin concentration with water is 9.3 ng/mL, what conclusion can be drawn?

3. The following results were obtained in the smoking cessation study conducted by Jorenby et al.

Outcome	Placebo (N = 160)	Nicotine Patch (N = 244)	Bupropion (N = 244)	Bupropion and Nicotine Patch (N = 245)
No. evaluated at 6 months	86	159	178	195
Abstinence at 6 months—% (no.)	18.8 (30)	21.3 (52)	34.8 (85)	38.8 (95)
Odds ratio (95% CI)	—	1.2 (0.7–1.9)	2.3 (1.4–3.7)	2.7 (1.7–4.4)
P value				
For the comparison with placebo	—	0.53	<0.001	<0.001
For the comparison with patch	—	—	0.001	<0.001
For the comparison with bupropion alone	—	—	—	0.37

What conclusions can be drawn from the reported p-values? Which of the results could possibly represent a Type II error?

References

1. Gorski JC, Jones DR, Haehner-Daniels Bd, Hamman MA, O'Mara EM, Hall SD: The contribution of intestinal and hepatic CYP3A to the interaction between midazolam and clarithromycin. Clin Pharmacol Ther 64:133–143, 1998.

2. Sandler RS, Zorich NL, Filloon TG, Wiseman HB, Lietz DJ, Brock MH, et al: Gastrointestinal symptoms in 3181 volunteers ingesting snack foods containing olestra or triglycerides. A 6-week randomized, placebo-controlled trial. Ann Intern Med 130:253–261, 1999.

3. Beral V, Hermon C, Kay C, Hannaford P, Darby S, Reeves G: Mortality associated with oral contraceptive use: 25 year follow-up of cohort of 46,000 women from Royal College of General Practitioners' oral contraception study. BMJ 318: 96–100, 1999.

4. Bernstein PL: *Against the Gods: The Remarkable Story of Risk*. New York, John Wiley & Sons, 1996.

5. Sirmans SM, Pieper JA, Lalonde RL, Smith DG, Self TH: Effect of calcium channel blockers on theophylline disposition. Clin Pharmacol Ther 44:29–34, 1988.

6. Wagner BKJ, Amory DW, Majcher CM, DiFasio LT, Scott GE, Spotnitz AJ: Effects of intravenous famotidine on gastric acid secretion in patients undergoing cardiac surgery. Ann Pharmacother 29:349–352, 1995.

7. Bailey DG, Spence JD, Edgar B, Bayliff CD, Arnold JM: Ethanol enhances the hemodynamic effects of felodipine. Clin Invest Med 12:357–362, 1989.

8. Lai K-C, Hui W-M, Wong W-M, Wong BC-Y, Hu WH, Ching C-K, et al: Treatment of *Helicobacter pylori* in patients with duodenal ulcer hemorrhage—A long-term randomized, controlled study. Am J Gastroenterol 95:2225–2232, 2000.

9. McCune JS, Hawke RL, LeCluyse EL, Gillenwater HH, Hamilton G, Ritchie J, et al: In vivo and in vitro induction of human cytochrome P4503A4 by dexamethasone. Clin Pharmacol Ther 68:356–366, 2000.

10. Bolton S: *Pharmaceutical Statistics: Practical and Clinical Applications,* 2d ed. New York, Marcel Dekker, 1990.

11. Jorenby DE, Lieschow SJ, Nides MA, Rennard SI, Johnston JA, Hughes AR, et al: A controlled trial of sustained-release bupropion, a nicotine patch, or both for smoking cessation. New Engl J Med 340:685–691, 1999.

12. Tilley BC, Alarcón GS, Heyse SP, Trentham DE, Neuner R, Kaplan DA, et al: Minocycline in rheumatoid arthritis: A 48-week, double-blind, placebo-controlled trial. Ann Intern Med 122:81–89, 1995.

13. Lilja JJ, Kivisto KT, Neuvonen PJ: Duration of effect of grapefruit juice on the pharmacokinetics of the CYP3A4 substrate simvastatin. Clin Pharmacol Ther 68:384–390, 2000.

Chapter 8

Evaluating Statistical Results: Parametric Tests

Richard L. Slaughter

OUTLINE

Goals and Objectives

Introduction

Paired t-Test

   Summary

Unpaired t-Test

   Summary

Analysis of Variance (ANOVA)

   One-Way ANOVA

Repeated Measures ANOVA

Multiple Factorial ANOVA

Summary

Study Questions

References

KEY WORDS

ANOVA
Crossover design
Data
Parametric
Hypothesis testing
Multifactorial ANOVA

Null hypothesis
Paired *t*-test
Parallel design
Repeated measures ANOVA
Unpaired *t*-test

Goals and Objectives

The goal of this chapter is to discuss and demonstrate how common parametric statistical tests are used and evaluated when reading primary drug literature sources. The specific objectives are:

1. To be able to understand, based upon study design considerations, when it is most appropriate to use the following parametric tests:

 a. Paired t-test
 b. Unpaired t-test
 c. ANOVA
 d. Repeated measures ANOVA
 e. Multifactorial ANOVA

2. For each of the discussed parametric tests, to be able to understand the relationship between the factors that influences that test and the statistical result (t-statistic or F-statistic). These factors are:

 a. Difference in mean values
 b. Variance
 c. Subject number

3. To understand how a p-value is obtained from a statistical result (t-statistic or F-statistic) through the use of the appropriate statistical table.

4. To understand the relationship between the p-value obtained from a parametric test and the null hypothesis.

5. For an ANOVA procedure, to be able to identify when it is appropriate to use a post hoc test.

6. Be able to discuss the difference between a one-way ANOVA and a multifactorial ANOVA.

7. Given parametric results from the drug literature, to be able to make an assessment concerning whether the result will or will not be statistically significant and to be able to relate that to your clinical evaluation of that result.

Introduction

The previous chapters have discussed the types of data that are presented in drug studies, characteristics of that data, and distributional properties of data. The next several chapters will show the reader how to make comparisons of data using appropriate statistical tests. These chapters will build on concepts of hypothesis testing, errors associated with hypothesis testing, and power as discussed in Chap. 7. In general, there are two major categories of statistical tests: parametric (e.g., interval/ratio data) and nonparametric (nominal/ordinal data). The first two chapters dealing with evaluating statistical results (Chaps. 8 and 9) are organized along these divisions.

Parametric data may be of either the interval or ratio scale and is typically presented in the form of the mean and a variance measure such as standard deviation. Chapter 6 discusses concepts related to the characteristics of parametric data, including measures of central tendency (mean, median, and mode) and measures of variance (standard deviation, coefficient of variation). Concepts pertaining to confidence intervals are provided in Chap. 7. Finally, a basic assumption that is applied to all parametric tests is that the data analyzed will follow a normal distribution as described in Chap. 7.

This chapter reviews the common parametric statistical tests encountered in drug literature. The specific tests discussed are the t-tests (paired and unpaired) and analysis of variance (ANOVA). A t-test is used when two groups are being compared and the ANOVA when more than two groups are compared. When a crossover design is used, data obtained is analyzed using a paired t-test and repeated measures ANOVA. When a parallel design is used, an unpaired t-test and ANOVA is employed. In all situations, the goal of this statistical test will be to determine that data obtained from the groups being compared is from the same or different populations. A simple algorithm, shown in Fig. 8-1, can be used to decide which is the most appropriate test to use based on the study design employed. In making this assessment for parametric tests, three factors or questions require evaluation. No matter which statistical procedure is used, these factors will be the same:

1. How different are the mean values?
2. How variable is the data?
3. How many subjects were analyzed?

This chapter emphasizes how to apply these factors to the theory and equations used for these procedures.

Paired *t*-Test

A paired t-test compares data points that arises from the same subject and in this sense are considered to be paired. Most typically, the data will come from a

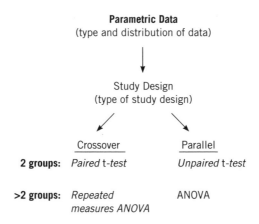

Figure 8-1. How to determine the most appropriate parametric test from study design.

KEY CONCEPT

Parametric tests determine the probability that data that follows a normal distribution is from the same or different populations.

crossover-designed study whereby each subject serves as its own control (see Chap. 5). Differences observed should therefore be a reflection of the conditions on the two study periods as opposed to differences inherent in the individual. In other words, the individual is constant (i.e., the study is performed on the same person), but the conditions under which the individual subject is tested are different. These are the study conditions in which a paired t-test is used. A paired t-test assesses the differences in observations within each subject and how similar these differences are. The paired t-test relates the mean value of differences between two observations D_m to the standard error of the mean of these differences SEM_d. The equation for the paired t-test is as follows:

$$t = \frac{D_m}{SEM_d} \qquad (8\text{-}1)$$

Evaluation of this equation indicates that the t statistic will get large when D_m is large in relation to SEM_d. This happens when each paired observation shows a difference and this difference is consistent within each data pair. The other factor involved is the number of paired observations. The value for SEM_d is inversely proportional to the number of observations, as would be the case for any standard error of the mean measurement (see Chap. 7). Therefore, as the number of paired observations increases, the value for SEM_d gets smaller and the t statistic gets larger. The following factors can influence the value of the t-statistic:

1. How observations change within the same subject as a function of the treatment

2. The consistency of this change between the subjects studied

3. The number of subjects studied

Once the t-statistic is obtained, the probability estimate is obtained from a t-table (see App. B). This provides the probability that the null hypothesis statement is true. For almost all clinical studies, when the p-value is less than 0.05, the null hypothesis statement is rejected and it is concluded that the two groups compared are from different populations. Note that this provides a statistical guess about the likelihood that data from the groups compared is from the same or different populations. As with all guesses, there is a chance you are right and a chance you are wrong. When a statistical conclusion is reached that the data from two groups are different based on a p value of <0.05, there is always a chance that the conclusion reached is wrong (i.e., a Type I error has occurred). When a p value is >0.05 and the null hypothesis is accepted, again this is based on a guess and there is always a chance the conclusion reached is wrong (i.e., a Type II error has occurred). See Chap. 5 for a discussion of statistical probability and Type I and II errors.

KEY CONCEPT

A paired t-test is used when a crossover study design is used that employs two study periods on the same group of subjects. It is influenced by the following:

1. How observations change within the same subject
2. Consistency of the change in observations
3. Number of subjects

CASE STUDY

The pharmacokinetics of cyclophosphamide and its metabolites were characterized in bone marrow transplant patients with the purpose of identifying the mechanism that causes the increase in the active metabolite 4-hydroxycyclophosphamide after two days of therapy with cyclophosphamide.[1] Eighteen patients who were scheduled to receive bone marrow transplants received a 1-hour intravenous infusion of 60 mg/kg cyclophosphamide for two days. Blood samples were obtained, and the pharmacokinetic profile of cyclophosphamide and its metabolites were characterized in each subject on days 1 and 2. The AUC values on days 1 and 2 of 4-hydroxycyclophosphamide and phosphoramide mustard are shown in Table 8-1. The null hypothesis statement H_0 to be answered is as follows:

There is no difference in the AUC of the metabolites 4-hydroxycyclophosphamide and phosphoramide mustard on day 1 and day 2 of cyclophosphamide therapy.

The research or alternative hypothesis is that the AUC values are different on day 1 and day 2.

A review of the data for both 4-hydroxycyclophosphamide and phosphoramide mustard indicates the AUC data for both metabolites is interval/ratio nature and is described by a mean and standard deviation, and the data appears to follow a normal distribution. Each subject was evaluated on two occasions (day 1 and day 2). It would be appropriate to use a paired t-test to determine the probability that the null hypothesis statement was true or the research hypothesis is false. Visual evaluation of the 4-hydroxycyclophosphamide data indicates that in

TABLE 8-1. **The AUC of Two Metabolites of Cyclophosphamide on Days 1 and 2 of Cyclophosphamide Infusion**

Patient No.	4-Hydroxycyclophosphamide, $\mu mol/(L \cdot h)$			Phosphoramide Mustard, $\mu mol/(L \cdot h)$		
	Day 1	Day 2	Difference	Day 1	Day 2	Difference
1	61.9	179	117.1	269	231	−38
2	74.3	79.9	5.6	231	192	−39
3	68.1	132	·63.9	329	308	−21
4	94.6	174	79.4	756	1010	254
5	ND*	ND		261	375	114
6	56.8	65.2	8.4	394	262	−132
7	83.4	134	50.6	ND	ND	
8	68.7	89.2	20.5	876	831	−45
9	61.7	86.5	24.8	353	431	78
10	88.8	93.1	4.3	419	468	49
11	117	134	17	314	335	21
12	81.4	99.5	18.1	479	485	6
13	ND	ND		ND	ND	
14	66.1	75.5	9.4	348	398	50
15	79.3	83.2	3.9	ND	ND	
16	61.5	66.7	5.2	489	476	−13
17	51.5	78.9	27.4	534	430	−104
18	29.2	97	67.8	230	399	169
Mean ± s	71.5 ± 19.9	104 ± 35.7	32.7 ± 33.4	419 ± 187	442 ± 216	21.8 ± 97.8

*ND = not detected.

each subject the AUC value is higher on day 2 than on day 1, indicating accumulation of the active metabolite of cyclophosphamide. The increase ranged from 4.3 to 117.1 $\mu mol/(L \cdot h)$. The mean of the difference D_m between day 2 and day 1 was 32.7 $\mu mol/(L \cdot h)$. The fact that the AUC value in each subject increased and that the increase was fairly large suggests that statistical difference might be achieved

and that the t-statistic would show a low probability of the null hypothesis statement being true. In this example, the t-statistic is calculated as follows:

$$t = \frac{D_m}{SEM_d} = \frac{D_m}{s/\sqrt{n}} = \frac{32.7}{33.4/\sqrt{16}} = \frac{32.7}{8.36} = 3.91 \qquad (8\text{-}2)$$

Once the t-statistic is calculated, the probability that the null hypothesis statement is true can be determined. This is determined using a t-table, which provides
probabilities for one- and two-tailed tests from the number of degrees of freedom
for the data set being analyzed. The degrees of freedom v are determined from the
number of observations analyzed, which in this case is the number of pairs evaluated. For a paired t-test:

$$v = \text{number of pairs of observations} - 1 \qquad (8\text{-}3)$$

In this case, the null hypothesis states no directional change; it states only that
there is no difference. Similarly, the research hypothesis states that there is no directional change when AUC values are compared on days 1 and 2. That is, the
AUC value could be either higher or lower on day 2 than on day 1. This is the case
with almost all research studies, so in most cases a two-tailed test is appropriate.
Once the t-statistic and number of degrees of freedom are known, the t-table can
be used. Look at the t-table in App. B. This table provides probability estimates for
a one-tailed (p) and two-tailed ($2p$) test (see the top horizontal headers) for the degrees of freedom v in the data set being tested (see far left vertical column). In this
example, v is 15 and the t-statistic is 3.91. In the t-table this value is greater than
2.95, the last t-value in the row for 15 degrees of freedom. Looking up the column
to the header for $2p$ shows that the probability is less than 0.01 (0.5%). This indicates that there is less than a 1% chance that the AUC values on days 1 and 2 are
the same and a greater than 99% chance that they are different. Since this is under
a p-value of 0.05, the null hypothesis statement is rejected and the alternative/re-
search hypothesis accepted—that the AUC values are in fact different. It is concluded that the active metabolite of cyclophosphamide does accumulate after two
days of administration.

   In contrast, look at the phosphoramide mustard AUC data in Table 8-1. There
is no consistent change from day 1 to day 2. Seven subjects showed a decrease in
AUC, and eight had an increase in AUC. The change ranged from −132 to 254
μmol/(L·h), the mean of the differences D_m was 21.8 μmol/(L·h), and the SEM_d was
24.5 μmol/(L·h), a value greater than D_m. In this situation, the AUC values for phosphoramide mustard are very similar between days 1 and 2, and we would expect that
the t-statistic would show that the null hypothesis statement is true. In this case,
there are 15 paired observations ($v = 14$), and the t-statistic of 0.89 falls between the
probability values of 0.3 and 0.4, so there is greater than 30% chance but less than
40% chance that the null hypothesis statement is true. Thus, the statistical conclusion that there is no difference in phosphoramide mustard AUC between days 1 and
2 matches the visual observation that there is no change in these values.

Summary

Note that for a paired t-test, a high t-value occurs when the average difference D_m is large and the variability in this difference SEM_d is small. If there is a large change and this change is consistent with each paired observation, a high t-statistic will occur. Also note the inverse relationship between the number of paired observations and SEM_d, which reveals a direct relationship with the t-statistic. As the number of paired observations increases, the t-statistic will increase, or will have a more likely chance to be significant. A low t-value will occur when either the change is small or the change is inconsistent between subjects. When evaluating the results of a paired t-test, look not only at the magnitude of the difference in the mean values being tested, but also at the individual data points to see if this change is consistent in each subject.

KEY CONCEPT

When a paired t-test is used, it's helpful to see how the data changes within each individual subject. Do not rely on only the mean and standard deviation, but also look at how each subject behaves.

Unpaired t-Test

The unpaired t-test is used when comparisons are made between two groups of subjects in a study employing a parallel design. This test will determine the probability that the mean values are the same between the two groups compared. The test will use the difference in the means, variance in each group, and number of observations analyzed. The equation to determine t-statistic is as follows:

$$t = \left(\frac{\bar{x}_i - \bar{x}_2}{\sqrt{s_1^2/n_1 + s_2^2/n_2}} \right) \qquad (8\text{-}4)$$

where $\bar{x}_i$ and $\bar{x}_2$ are mean values, s_1 and s_2 the standard deviations, and n_1 and n_2 the number of observations for the data from two respective samples. The number of degrees of freedom v is determined from:

$$v = n_1 + n_2 - 2 \qquad (8\text{-}5)$$

where n_1 and n_2 are the number of subjects in the two groups being compared. Evaluation of the preceding equation indicates the conditions that will result in a large or small t-value. A large t-value that may lead to a statistical difference occurs when the numerator is large relative to the denominator. Looking at those conditions that lead to a large numerator and a small denominator, you will readily understand the conditions that lead to a statistically significant result:

1. A large difference in mean values (results in a larger numerator)

2. Small s^2 values or a small variance (results in a small denominator)

3. Large n (results in a small denominator)

This provides the basis for evaluation of the t-statistic. The following specific criteria should be met to use the unpaired t-test:

1. The data should be parametric in nature.

2. The data should follow a normal distribution.

3. The variances of the groups being compared should be about equal.

Again, once the t-statistic is determined, the p value is obtained from the t-table in App. B.

KEY CONCEPT

An unpaired t-test is used when a parallel study design is used in two independent subject groups. It is influenced by the following:

1. Differences in mean values
2. Variance in the sample groups
3. Number of subjects

CASE STUDY

Consider the following study[2] that compared the oral bioavailability of odansetron administered as two extemporaneously prepared suppositories and the commercially available 8-mg tablet in men and women. Sixteen healthy subjects (eight men and eight women) received an 8-mg oral odansetron tablet and 16-mg suppository prepared using Fattibase and Polybase. The pharmacokinetic parameters obtained included AUC_{inf}, C_{max}, T_{max}, half-life, $C1/F$, and V_d. Data for AUC_{inf} in men and women is shown in Table 8-2. The null hypothesis is as follows:

> There is no difference in odansetron AUC_{inf} between men and women following the administration of odansetron as a tablet, Fattibase, or Polybase suppository.

The data shown in Table 8-2 is parametric in nature (i.e., described by a mean and SEM), and the AUC values in men and women are independent from one another, so it would be appropriate to consider using an unpaired t-test to determine the probability that the null hypothesis statement is true. Variance measurements be-

TABLE 8-2. Odansetron AUC$_{inf}$ [Mean (SEM)] following the Administration of Odansetron Tablets and Two Suppository Formulations

	Tablet, 8 mg	Fattibase Suppository, 16 mg	Polybase Suppository, 16 mg
Men ($n = 8$)	167.9 (25.7)	275.2 (82.3)	319.4 (138.1)
Women ($n = 8$)	393.3 (54.7)	589.5 (122.0)	811.4 (138.1)
t-statistic	3.72	2.13	2.52
p-value	<0.01	>0.05	<0.025

tween the two groups should be compared using the coefficient of variation (CV) that is determined from the following equation:

$$CV = \frac{s}{\bar{x}} \cdot 100 \qquad (8\text{-}6)$$

In this case, s needs to be calculated from the SEM as follows:

$$s = SEM \cdot \sqrt{n} \qquad (8\text{-}7)$$

Table 8-3 shows the CV values for the data presented in Table 8-2. Variance in AUC$_{inf}$ is similar in women between all groups studied. The variance in AUC$_{inf}$ is also similar between men and women following the administration of the tablet, with great variability seen in men following the administration of both suppositories. A possible conclusion could be reached that the variances are not equal and that a non-parametric test should be used. If a parametric test is used, the high variances, particularly in the Polybase group, will reduce the ability or power of the statistical procedure to detect a difference. This could result in a Type II error (see Chap. 7 for information on Type II errors). When using an unpaired t-test, the three factors to be considered are the difference in the mean values, variance, and number of subjects. In this example, the AUC$_{inf}$ values are more than twofold higher in women than in men, indicating that women will have more than twice the exposure to odansetron for a given formulation studied compared to men. Therefore, based on the difference in mean values, it would be expected that the unpaired t-test would indicate that there is a low chance that the null hypothesis statement is true. This is countered by the low number of subjects ($n = 8$ in each group) and the high variances observed in men who received the suppository formulations. The variances following the tablet formulation were similar in both genders. When these factors are accounted for, it would be expected that a difference would be detected following the tablet formulations, but possibly not after the suppositories (because of the high variance in men).

TABLE 8-3. **Comparison of CV Between Men and Women Following Administration of Odansetron**

	Tablet	*Fattibase Suppository*	*Polybase Suppository*
Men ($n = 8$)	43.3%	84.6%	122.3%
Women ($n = 8$)	39.3%	58.5%	48.1%

The t-values indicate that following the administration of the tablet and Polybase suppository, there is a low probability that the AUC_{inf} values are the same ($p < 0.01$ and $p < 0.025$, respectively), so the null hypothesis is rejected and it is concluded that they are different. However, the AUC_{inf} values following the Fattibase suppository show that there is a greater than 5% chance that the null hypothesis statement is true, so in this case it would be concluded that there is no statistical difference, despite the fact that the mean AUC_{inf} values were 214% higher in women. Since a difference was observed with the tablet and Polybase suppository, it is expected that a difference would be seen after the Fattibase suppository. A Type II error could be occurring. In fact, by reducing the variance in the men by only 10% (i.e., decreasing SEM from 82.3 to 75.0), the statistical conclusion will change. When small manipulations in the data can change a result from being statistically insignificant ($p > 0.05$) to being statistically significant ($p < 0.05$), the presence of a Type II error should be considered. This is particularly true if your clinical experience suggests that a difference should be present. As a general rule, statistical conclusions should be in agreement with clinical conclusions.

Manipulating statistics is easy to do; designing studies to make statistical conclusions is easy to do. There is no truer statement than that there are lies and then there are statistics. What is important is what you think about the result. Ask yourself, when no differences are reported, does the data look like a difference exists? Does my clinical judgment lead me to think a difference should exist? If the answers to these questions are yes, then a Type II error may exist. The other side of this issue arises when a statistical difference is reported. Always ask yourself, does the reported difference make sense? Is this a result that I would have expected based on my clinical judgment? If the answers to these questions are no, look for a possible Type I error. Remember, it is your judgment and interpretation that are important!

Summary

For an unpaired t-test, statistical significance is achieved when the difference in the values of the means from the two groups being compared is large and the variability in the two groups is small. The t-statistic is also directly related to the number of subjects studied in each group. When evaluating data compared using the t-test, look for the magnitude of the differences, the variability of the data, and the number of observations included in the results.

Analysis of Variance (ANOVA)

ANOVA procedures are used when a comparison of mean values from more than two groups is desired. A one-way ANOVA involves evaluating the effect of one independent variable, such as treatment group. A factorial ANOVA assesses more than one factor, such as treatment group and study design. ANOVA tests the likelihood that the mean values between three or more groups are similar or come from the same population. When a parallel study design and ANOVA procedure is used, this is analogous to the unpaired t-test. When a crossover design is used, a repeated measures ANOVA is used, which is analogous to the paired t-test. Conceptual understanding of how ANOVA functions is more complex than for a t-test; however, it is helpful to review the concept of how ANOVA procedures are performed to appreciate how the ANOVA procedures come to the conclusions they do.

Understanding ANOVA procedures requires analyzing the factors that influence the experimental variance of the dependent variable. This is depicted in Fig. 8-2. Variance is presented as the sum of square (SS) for the term discussed. Total variance SS_{tot} is the sum of within-subject variance SS_{wit} and between-subject variance SS_{bet}. That is to say, study variance comes from the variance seen within the study participants and the variance seen between the groups or subjects being compared. Between-subject variance can be further divided into variance caused by the treatment and variance that is not related to treatment effects. If a treatment causes an effect, then treatment variance will increase in proportion to the residual variance within subjects. In a parallel-designed study, the treatments are given to different subjects. If the treatments cause an effect, then the variance observed between the subjects will increase. Expressing total variance as a ratio of the variance observed between subjects and that observed within subjects serves as the basis of an ANOVA. A repeated measures ANOVA evaluates data obtained when different treatments are given to the same subject (as would occur with a crossover design). This procedure evaluates only within-subject variance. It expresses within-subject

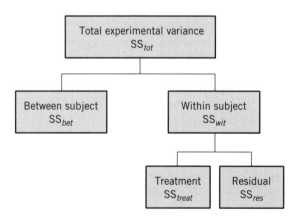

Figure 8-2. Partitioning of experimental variance.

variance as a ratio of the variance caused by the treatments used to the variance SS_{res} that is not related to the treatment. A multifactorial ANOVA assesses the influence of two or more factors on treatment variance. Understanding the relationships shown in Fig. 8-2 will assist in conceptually understanding the analysis of variance.

One-Way ANOVA

ANOVA procedures are used to determine the similarity of mean values from more than two groups using a ratio called the F-statistic:

$$F = \frac{SS_{bet}}{SS_{wit}} \qquad (8\text{-}8)$$

where SS_{bet} is the variance that is estimated from the sample means and parameter SS_{wit} estimates the variance within each sample group. Theoretically, both parameters are measures of the population variance such that if all samples came from the same population, the ratio of these two variance measures would be equal to 1. The

KEY CONCEPT

ANOVA procedures analyze experimental variance caused by the treatments compared to variance that is not related to treatment conditions.

ANOVA will test for a difference in the F-statistics from 1.0. If the mean values differ from one another, then SS_{bet} will get large; if the variances within each group are small, the SS_{wit} is small. If this is large in comparison to SS_{wit}, then it would be concluded that the mean values come from different populations and are in fact different from one another. The null hypothesis statement would be rejected. If the mean values are all similar to one another, then the F-statistic will be small, and the null hypothesis is accepted. This should sound similar to the unpaired t-test discussed earlier. The variance between means is calculated as follows:

$$SS_{bet} = \Sigma\,(\bar{x}_i - \bar{X})^2 \cdot n \qquad (8\text{-}9)$$

where $\bar{x}_i$ is the mean value from an individual group of observations, $\bar{X}$ is the grand mean of the mean values for each group of observations, and n is the number of groups compared. This term increases as $\bar{x}_i$ becomes more different from $\bar{X}$ or as the difference in mean values increases and as the number of groups that are being compared increases. The variance within each group SS_{wit} is determined as follows:

$$SS_{wit} = \Sigma\,(x_i - \bar{x})^2 \qquad (8\text{-}10)$$

where x_i is each individual value. Once the F-statistic is determined, the probability that the mean values are from the same population is determined from the F-table.

The procedure for using the F-table is very similar to that of the t-table. An F-table is given in App. D. The F-statistic is determined from the degrees of freedom v_n determined between the groups (numerator), defined as the number of groups compared m minus 1, $v_n = m - 1$, and the within-group comparison (denominator) $v_d = m \cdot (n - 1)$, where n is the number of observations in each group. Critical F-values required to achieve a p-value of <0.05 or <0.01 are given for a given set of v_n and v_d.

KEY CONCEPT

A one-way ANOVA determines the probability that the mean values from three or more groups come from the same population.

Post Hoc Tests. As stated, an ANOVA will determine whether multiple mean values are from the same or different populations. The procedure does not indicate where specific differences exist. This is accomplished using a post hoc test. A post hoc test is performed only if the ANOVA test shows statistical significance. When differences are being assessed between multiple mean values (e.g., >2), several post hoc tests can be used. Most post hoc tests are variations of the t-test. Examples include Tukey's HSD (honestly significant difference), Bonferroni's t-test, and the Student-Neuman-Keuls (SNK) test.

The procedure used when multiple mean values are being compared is to compare highest to lowest, highest to next lowest, second highest to lowest, and so on. For example, if four mean values (1, 2, 3, 4) are being compared, and 4 is the highest and 1 is the lowest, the comparison would be done as follows: 4 to 1, 4 to 2, 4 to 3, 3 to 1, and 3 to 2. If multiple mean values are compared to a single control value, as may occur when two or more drug treatments are compared to a single control, then Bonferroni's t-test and Dunnett's t-test can be used.

KEY CONCEPT

Post hoc tests are used when an ANOVA is statistically significant to determine which specific mean values differ from one another.

CASE STUDIES

Two examples will be shown: one that illustrates no difference between groups and another that shows a difference between the groups compared. Consider the following baseline cardiac index data from a study that compared the effects of quinapril in low, medium, and high doses to placebo.[3] Data from this study is shown in Table 8-4. The null hypothesis statement is as follows:

TABLE 8-4. **Cardiac Index in Patients with Congestive Heart Failure After Placebo and Low, Medium, and High Doses of Quinilaplat**

Group	N	Cardiac Index, $L/(min \cdot m^2)$	CV
Placebo	13	2.3 ± 0.3	13.0%
Low dose	12	2.6 ± 0.7	26.9%
Medium dose	13	2.2 ± 0.2	9.1%
High dose	12	2.1 ± 0.4	19.0%
Average of groups	4	2.3 ± 0.20	8.7%

There is no difference in the baseline cardiac index in patients who received placebo, low-dose, medium-dose, or high-dose quinapril.

Note that the null hypothesis statement addresses only whether a difference exists or does not exist. This is what the ANOVA procedure tests for. It does not determine which groups are different from one another. It assesses only whether a difference between groups exists. ANOVA tests the chance or probability that this statement is true—in other words, the chances that the data from these four groups comes from one population as opposed to coming from different populations. ANOVA compares the variance estimate for the average of the four mean values SS_{bet} to the average of the individual variance estimates for each group SS_{wit}.

The key to evaluating an ANOVA test is to compare how similar the mean values appear and how small or large the variance estimates are within each group. In the preceding example, the mean values are all similar to one another (i.e., 2.3, 2.6, 2.2, and 2.1), so the between-group variance estimate is small (i.e., $s = 0.20$, CV = 8.7%). In this example, the between-group variance is smaller than the variance estimates within each group (CVs are 13.0%, 26.9%, 9.1%, and 19.0%). Since the between-group variance is small relative to the within-group variance, it is expected that the ANOVA procedure will determine that there is no difference between cardiac indexes in these groups. This is what is reported, and the null hypothesis is accepted. A post hoc test is not performed because no differences were detected.

The following example illustrates a case in which an ANOVA procedure rejects the null hypothesis statement. The data comes from a study that compared the pharmacokinetics of prednisolone in the following categories of women.[4]

- Group A: 6 premenopausal women
- Group B: 6 postmenopausal women
- Group C: 6 postmenopausal women taking estrogen replacement therapy
- Group D: 6 postmenopausal women taking estrogen and progesterone therapy

The null hypothesis statement is as follows:

There is no difference in the pharmacokinetics of prednisolone when comparing premenopausal women to postmenopausal women who are not taking replacement therapy, to those who are taking estrogen only, and to those who are taking estrogen and progesterone therapy.

Prednisolone clearance values for each group are shown in Table 8-5. In this example, the means are somewhat different from one another. There is a 70% difference between the lowest and highest mean value (1.53 versus 2.59). The between-group variance (CV = 24.6%) is also higher than the variance estimates within each group (CVs in individual groups were 14.3%, 15.7%, 19.6%, and 18.0%). Thus, one would expect the F-statistic to possibly show a low probability that these groups are from the same population. In fact, the ANOVA shows a p-value of <0.01, so there is less than a 1% chance that prednisolone clearance is the same in these four groups of women, and the null hypothesis statement is rejected. Note that the ANOVA does not tell which groups are different from one another. This is done using a post hoc test. There are many different post hoc tests, but they all serve the same purpose, which is to identify exactly where differences exist. In this example, a Student-Newman-Keuls test is the post hoc test used to determine that the clearance value in the premenopausal women is differ-

TABLE 8-5. **Prednisolone Clearance in Pre- and Postmenopausal Women and Postmenopausal Women with Estrogen and Estrogen and Progestin Replacement Therapy**

Group	Clearance, ml/(min · kg)	CV
Premenopausal	2.59 ± 0.37	14.3%
Postmenopausal	1.84 ± 0.29	15.8%
Postmenopausal—estrogen	1.53 ± 0.30	19.6%
Postmenopausal—estrogen and progestin	1.66 ± 0.30	18.1%
Average of the mean of four groups	1.91 ± 0.47	24.6%

ent from that in those in the other three groups. This post hoc test can be used because the comparison is made between all four groups and not with a single control group.

Repeated Measures ANOVA

When a crossover design is used, with each subject receiving more than two treatments, it is a goal to identify the effect that the treatments have on each individual and then determine whether this effect is statistically significant. The procedure that allows this to be done is the repeated measures ANOVA. This test is analogous to the paired t-test. When each subject is given a different treatment, total variability in the study can be divided into three major components: variability between all subjects, variability within the subjects in each treatment group, and variability that is caused by the treatment. Recall from the preceding ANOVA discussion that total variation SS_{tot} within a study can be defined as the sum of the variation between subjects SS_{bet} and the variation that occurs within subjects SS_{wit}. Within-subject variance can further be broken down into the variation that is caused by the treatments SS_{treat} and the variation that is not related to the treatments, or residual variation SS_{res}. The F-statistic for a repeated measure ANOVA is determined as follows:

$$F = \frac{MS_{treat}}{MS_{res}} \tag{8-11}$$

where MS_{treat} is determined from the ratio of variance due to treatment effects SS_{treat} to the degrees of freedom associated with treatments $v_{treat} = m - 1$, where m is the number of treatments. MS_{res} is determined from the ratio of SS_{res} to v_{res}. Remember from the previous discussion that SS_{wit} is the sum of SS_{treat} and SS_{res}, so that

$$SS_{res} = SS_{wit} - SS_{treat} \tag{8-12}$$

and v_{res} is determined from

$$v_{res} = (n - 1)(m - 1) \tag{8-13}$$

The F-value obtained from a repeated measures ANOVA compares the factors that influence within-subject variance, which are the variance caused by the treatment and residual variance. When a treatment effect is seen, then values within a subject between the various treatments will differ. This means the variance caused by treatments will be large relative to the residual variance. If there is no effect, then the values for different treatments within a subject should be similar, resulting in a small variance caused by the treatment, meaning a smaller F-value. Finally, the equation for F can be rearranged as

$$F = \frac{SS_{treat}}{SS_{res}} \cdot (n - 1) \tag{8-14}$$

indicating the direct relationship between F and the number of subjects. Thus, a repeated measures ANOVA is influenced by the following:

1. The effect that a treatment would have within each subject tested
2. The variability of the data observed within the subjects studied
3. The number of subjects studied

KEY CONCEPT

A repeated measures ANOVA determines the effect that three or more treatments have in the same individual.

CASE STUDY

The cytochrome P450 enzymes are responsible for the metabolism of a large number of drugs. This family of enzymes is divided into specific isozymes that metabolize drugs that have affinity for that isozyme. Examples of isozymes include the CYP2D6, CYP3A4, and CYP1A2, which metabolize the majority of drugs eliminated by the cytochrome P450 system in humans. The CYP2E1 isozyme metabolizes alcohol, anesthetics, and analgesics including acetaminophen. Chlorzoxazone is a substrate that is used to determine the level of activity of the CYP2E1 isozyme. This isozyme is also inhibited by isoniazid. A study[5] titled "Inhibition of Chlorzoxazone Metabolism, a Clinical Probe for CYP2E1, by a Single Ingestion of Watercress" evaluated the effects of watercress ingestion compared to isoniazid on the pharmacokinetics of chlorzoxazone. Ten healthy volunteers (six men and four women between the ages of 26 and 55) received in sequential fashion chlorzoxazone alone (day 1), chlorzoxazone after watercress ingestion (day 7), and chlorzoxazone after isoniazid ingestion (day 14). The primary endpoint was the area under the curve (AUC) of serum concentration versus time of chlorzoxazone. The null hypothesis was as follows:

> There is no difference in the AUC of chlorzoxazone when administered alone or after watercress ingestion or after the administration of isoniazid.

In this study design, the pharmacokinetics of chlorzoxazone was evaluated in each subject after three treatment periods (alone, watercress, and isoniazid administration). The treatment effects (watercress and isoniazid) were compared within each subject to their own control values. In this study, the following conditions make it acceptable to use a repeated measures ANOVA:

1. Each subject serves as its own control to which the effects of watercress and isoniazid pharmacokinetics are compared.

2. More than two groups are being compared.

3. The data, AUC, is parametric in nature and is normally distributed.

Data for the AUC of chlorzoxazone is shown in Table 8-6. Evaluation of this data indicates that chlorzoxazone AUC increases in every subject after both watercress and isoniazid administration. The average increase after watercress is 53.8% and ranges from 18.4 to 83.2%. A greater change in AUC is seen after isoniazid, with chlorzoxazone AUC increasing on average by 131.3% (range, 81.4 to 234.9%). Recall that the repeated measures ANOVA analyzes the factors that influence within-subject variance SS_{wit}, or how much of the within-subject variability is influenced by the treatment conditions. Comparing the treatment variance SS_{treat} to the residual variance SS_{res} does this. Since the AUC values between the three treatment groups differ within each subject, it is expected that within-subject variance would be high and that variance caused by the treatments (watercress and isoniazid) would account for most of this within-subject variance. Such is the case with this

TABLE 8-6. AUC of Chlorzoxazone When Taken Alone (Day 1), After Watercress (Day 7), and After Isoniazid (Day 14)

Subject	Day 1	Day 7	Day 14	Subject Mean
1	40.22	61.7	76.5	59.5
2	50.6	92.7	113.1	85.5
3	38	62.5	77.3	59.3
4	34.6	56.9	115.9	69.1
5	34.5	61.3	87.8	61.2
6	36.5	43.2	103.1	60.9
7	54.6	68.6	103.5	75.6
8	65.7	87.3	119.2	90.7
9	76.2	113.2	167.0	118.8
10	36.6	61.9	85.4	61.3
Treatment mean	46.7	70.9	104.9	

SOURCE: Adapted from Table 1, "Effects of Watercress and Isoniazid on Chlorzoxazone AUC (0–∞) and Plasma Elimination $t_{\frac{1}{2}}$," in Leclercq et al. (5). Reproduced from *Clin Pharmacol Ther* 64:144–149, 1998, with permission from Mosby, Inc.

example. SS_{wit} is calculated to be 19,207.52 and SS_{treat} 17,059. Therefore, 88% [17,059/(19,207.52 · 100)] of within-subject variance of chlorzoxazone is accounted for by the effects of watercress and isoniazid. The calculated F-statistic is 71.48, which shows a p-value of 0.001, indicating that there is less than a 0.1% chance that the AUC values are similar across treatment groups. It is concluded that watercress and isoniazid increase chlorzoxazone AUC.

Multiple Factorial ANOVA

In the previous examples the analysis involves a one-way experimental design that categorizes all subjects in one way. There is no differentiation of subjects by factors such as gender, age, presence/absence of disease, and so on. Often a study is designed such that two or more factors are manipulated at the same time. A multifactorial ANOVA allows for the simultaneous analysis of several independent factors (e.g., age, gender) on a dependent variable (e.g., AUC, blood pressure response). The multifactorial ANOVA is quite complex since it involves evaluating the influence that several factors have on a single variable.

As an example, a drug interaction study is performed evaluating the effects of a low dose and a high dose of one drug (Drug A) on the pharmacokinetics of another (Drug B), with the primary endpoint being AUC. In a randomized crossover design, subjects receive Drug B alone, followed by a low dose of Drug A and a high dose of Drug A, after which the AUC of Drug B is determined. The null hypothesis is as follows:

> The AUC of Drug B is the same when administered alone or after a low or high dose of Drug A.

A one-way repeated measures ANOVA would be used to determine the probability that the null hypothesis statement is true. A one-way procedure is used because all of the subjects are treated alike. Suppose it is known that gender significantly influences the disposition of Drug B and that the effect of Drug A on Drug B may be influenced by gender. The null hypothesis would then be changed to the following:

> The AUC of Drug B is the same in men and women, and the AUC of Drug B is the same after low and high doses of Drug A in both men and women.

A two-way ANOVA could be used to answer this null hypothesis statement. It is called a two-way ANOVA because the effects of two independent factors (dose and gender) are being evaluated on the dependent variable (AUC of Drug B). The two-way ANOVA also evaluates the possible interaction between the two factors. This process can be broken down into three clearly separate components:

> **1.** *First factor:* Determining if the AUC of Drug B is the same in men and women.

2. *Second factor:* Determining if the AUC of Drug B is the same after low and high doses of Drug A.

3. *Interaction:* Determining if the response of men and women to the effects of Drug A (for both low and high doses) is the same.

A multifactorial (or in this example a two-way) ANOVA will provide a p-value for each of the preceding scenarios. The procedure used is similar to other ANOVAs in that total variance SS_{tot} is

$$SS_{tot} = SS_{treat} - SS_{res} \qquad (8\text{-}15)$$

Treatment variance SS_{treat} is the sum of the variances due to the factors evaluated and the interaction between these factors, as follows:

$$SS_{treat} = SS_{gender} + SS_{dose} + SS_{gender/dose} \qquad (8\text{-}16)$$

Once the variance terms are known, they are converted to mean square (MS) terms using the appropriate degrees of freedom for that factor. The mean square for residual variance MS_{res} is also calculated. The F-statistic is calculated from the appropriate treatment MS term to MS_{res}. As with other ANOVAs, if a treatment effect is observed, the variance term caused by the treatment will be high in relation to residual variance.

Summary

Analysis of variance procedures are used when determining if the mean values from more than two groups are from the same population. Conceptually, the procedures are more complex than the t-test and require a higher level of understanding factors that influence variance in an experimental study. These procedures are commonly used and can provide very useful information concerning the effects observed in studies that compare data from more than two groups. The procedures analyze variance parameters obtained and compare the variances that are caused by the study treatments to variances inherent in the individuals studied. A one-way ANOVA is used when a parallel study design is employed and is analogous to the unpaired t-test. When a treatment has a significant effect, the variance between subjects (an estimate of treatment variance) will be large relative to the variance within subjects (variance not influenced by treatment). When a crossover study is used, a repeated measures ANOVA is employed and is analogous to the paired t-test. The repeated measures ANOVA compares only within-subject variance and compares the variance caused by the treatments to the residual variance, which is not related to the treatment. A multifactorial ANOVA can be very useful in assessing the effects of multiple factors on a single variable. This procedure is also complex, but will allow a deeper understanding of factors than may influence how a given variable may respond to a given treatment. The key with ANOVA procedures is to understand how the variance terms are related to one another. Finally, no matter how complex a parametric procedure appears, remember that only three basic factors are involved in the evaluation of each procedure:

1. How similar or different are the mean values
2. How large or small are the variances
3. How large is the subject number

Bringing the evaluation of any parametric procedure back to these three points greatly simplifies each procedure and enhances the understanding of the concepts behind the procedure.

Study Questions

1. A study titled "St. John's Wort: Effect on CYP3A4 activity" published in *Clinical Phamacology and Therapeutics* (67:451–471, 2000) reported the results of a study that assessed urinary 6-β-hydroxycortisol/cortisol ratio in 13 subjects before and after 14 days of therapy with St. John's wort, 300-mg tablet, reagent grade, standardized to 0.3% hypericin. The following table shows the data for urinary 6-β-hydroxycortisol/cortisol ratio.

Subject Number	Baseline Urinary 6-β-Hydroxycortisol/Cortisol Ratio	Posttreatment Urinary 6-β-Hydroxycortisol/Cortisol Ratio
1	8.0	16.7
2	3.8	13.7
3	9.5	11.3
4	6.3	20.3
5	8.8	12.9
6	20.8	15.5
7	5.0	5.7
8	4.8	7.4
9	4.4	14.2
10	4.9	9.2
11	6.1	20.9
12	6.5	14.9
13	3.2	6.4
Mean ± s	7.1 ± 4.5	13.9 ± 4.9

Name the most appropriate statistical test to use to determine the probability that the following null hypothesis statement is true: "There is no difference in baseline and posttreatment with St. John's wort values of urinary 6-β-hydroxycortisol/cortisol ratio." Explain why the test you chose is the most appropriate test.

2. For the table in Question 1, determine the difference in urinary 6-β-hydroxycortisol/cortisol ratio between the baseline and posttreatment period for each subject. Does the urinary 6-β-hydroxycortisol/cortisol ratio change in a consistent manner in all subjects?

3. In the following table, indicate whether the associated factor (degree of change, consistency of change, and subject number) will increase or decrease the chance of seeing statistical significance.

	Increases the Chance of Statistical Significance	Decreases the Chance of Statistical Significance
Degree of change in consistency of change in urinary 6-β-hydroxycortisol/cortisol ratio D_m		
Consistency of change in urinary 6-β-hydroxycortisol/cortisol ratio SEM_d		
Subject number		

4. The reported p-value comparing posttreatment to baseline urinary 6-β-hydroxycortisol/cortisol ratios was $p = 0.003$. Explain what this means and whether you expected this statistical result or not.

5. In this study, did St. John's wort affect the urinary 6-β-hydroxycortisol/cortisol ratio, a measure of CYP3A4 activity?

6. A study published in *Pharmacotherapy* (20:622–628, 2000), "Gender Differences in Labetalol Kinetics: Importance of Determining Stereoisomer Kinetics for Racemic Drugs," compared the dose-corrected AUC (AUC/dose) in women ($n = 5$) and men ($n = 14$). The data is as follows:

Women ($n = 5$)   6.79 ± 2.11 (mean ± s)

Men ($n = 14$)   3.82 ± 1.37

Name the most appropriate statistical test to use to determine the probability that the following null hypothesis statement is true: "There is no difference in labetalol AUC/dose in men and women." Why?

7. For the data shown in question 6, are the variances equal in both groups?

8. Indicate the impact that each of the following factors has in determining whether the data in Question 6 is statistically significant.

    a. Difference in mean values

    b. Variance

    c. Subject number

9. The authors report a p-value of <0.05 for this data. Explain what this means and whether this is what was expected.

10. The disposition of nicotine was studied in 12 cigarette smokers using a within-subject crossover design to three treatments: (1) cigarette smoking, (2) inhalation of carbon monoxide, and (3) inhalation of air. Study, "Effects of Cigarette Smoking and Carbon Monoxide on nicotine and cotinine metabolism" was published in *Clinical Pharmacology and Therapeutics* (67:653–659, 2000). Data for nicotine clearance and renal clearance is as follows:

	Cigarette Smoking (CS)	Carbon Monoxide (CO)	Air (A)
Clearance, mL/min	1232 ± 242	1376 ± 297	1402 ± 302
Renal clearance, mL/min	58 ± 36	85 ± 90	84 ± 46

Which is the most appropriate statistical test to use to determine the probability that the clearance and renal clearance of nicotine is the same after cigarette smoking, carbon monoxide inhalation, and air inhalation? Why?

11. For renal clearance, are the within-group variances similar?

12. For both clearance and renal clearance, indicate the impact that each of the following factors may have on determining statistical significance.

SS_{bet}

SS_{wit}

Subject number

13. The p-value for nicotine clearance was reported as follows:

Clearance: $p < 0.01$ (CO, A > CS)

A Tukey posttest was used to determine CO, A > CS. Explain what kind of test this is.

14. The results for renal clearance were reported as not significant (NS). Explain why this result was not significant and the results for clearance were significant.

15. Explain when a multifactorial ANOVA would be used.

References

1. Ren S, Kalhorn TF, McDonald GB, et al: Pharmacokinetics of cyclophosphamide and its metabolites in bone marrow patients. Clin Pharmacol Ther 64:289–301, 1998.

2. Jann MW, ZumBrunneen TL, Tenjarla SN, et al: Relative bioavailability of odansetron 8-mg oral tablets versus two extemporaneous 16-mg suppositories: Formulation and gender differences. Pharmacotherapy 18(2):288–294, 1998.

3. Mitrovic V, Mudra H, Bonzel T et al: Hemodynamic and hormonal effects of quinilaprilat in patients with congestive heart failure. Clin Pharmacol Ther 59:686–698, 1996.

4. Harris RZ, Tsumoda SM, Mroczkowski P, et al: The effects of menopause and hormone replacement therapies on prednisolone and erythromycin pharmacokinetics. Clin Pharmacol Ther 59:429–435, 1996.

5. Leclercq I, Desager J-P, Horsmans Y: Inhibition of chlorzoxazone metabolism, a clinical probe for CYP2E1, by single ingestion of watercress. Clin Pharmacol Ther 64:144–149, 1998.

Chapter 9

Evaluating Statistical Results: Nonparametric Tests

Richard L. Slaughter

OUTLINE

Goals and Objectives

Chi-Square

   Special Cases

   Yates Correction Factor

   Fisher's Exact Test

   McNemar's Chi-Square

   Effect of Number on Chi-Square
     Statistic

Odds and Risk Ratios

   Risk Ratio

   Odds Ratio

Nonparametric Tests of Ordinal Data

Summary

Study Questions

References

KEY WORDS

Chi-square
Fisher's exact test
Kruskal-Wallis test
Mann-Whitney U test
McNemar's chi-square
Nominal

Nonparametric
Odds ratio
Ordinal
Risk ratio
Wilcoxan rank sum test
Yates correction factor

Goals and Objectives

The goal of this chapter is to discuss and demonstrate how common nonparametric tests are used and evaluated when reading primary drug literature sources.

The specific objectives are as follows:

1. To explain, based on study design considerations and study characteristics, when it is appropriate to use the following nonparametric tests for nominal data:

  a. Chi-square
  b. Chi-square with Yates correction factor
  c. Fisher's exact test
  d. McNemar's chi-square

2. To explain when it is appropriate to use the odds ratio (OR) and risk ratio (RR)

3. To explain the relationship between the two factors that influence nonparametric tests on nominal data and the outcome statistic (e.g., chi-square, odds ratio, etc.). These factors are:

  a. Observed differences in rates/proportions between groups
  b. Number of observations

4. To illustrate how to apply a nonparametric test on a parametric test

5. To introduce common tests used to analyze ordinal data

Introduction

Nonparametric tests are used to make statistical conclusions about data sets that are nominal or ordinal in nature. They are also used to make statistical conclusions concerning parametric data that does not follow a normal distribution. In this case the parametric data is converted to nominal or ordinal format, and as such will lose its parametric characteristics (e.g., mean and standard deviation). Data does not have to follow specific distributional characteristics for nonparametric tests to be used. This is an advantage of nonparametric tests. Different tests are used, however, based on the type of data being analyzed (nominal vs. ordinal). For example, nominal data can be compared using the chi-square test, Fisher's exact test, the odds ratio (OR), or the risk ratio (RR). Ordinal data is compared using the Mann-Whitney U, Wilcoxan rank sum test, or Kruskal-Wallis test. As with parametric tests, study design will influence which test is used. For example, for a crossover design (e.g., the data is paired), the McNemar test (a modification of a chi-square) is used on nominal data, and the Wilcoxan rank sum test on ordinal data. When a parallel design is employed (e.g., unpaired data), the chi-square or Fisher's exact test is used on nominal data and the Mann-Whitney U on ordinal data. This chapter provides an introduction to the basic nonparametric tests. As with Chap. 8, the focus is on when it is appropriate to use a specific test, and how to interpret and evaluate the results obtained from using nonparametric procedures. Tests used on nominal data are discussed first, followed by those tests used to evaluate data that is ordinal in nature.

Chi-Square

Data that is nominal in nature can be analyzed using a chi-square analysis. The distribution of nominal data among groups of subjects can be compared using a chi-square analysis. This analysis will determine the probability that the distribution of data is the same among the groups being compared. Data is presented in tabular format, as shown in Table 9-1. This data table is divided into rows and columns. By convention, the groups being compared are represented in rows and the outcomes in columns. In this example there are two groups (rows) of patients (A and B) that have two possible outcomes (A and B). A chi-square test will determine the probability that the outcomes (A and B) are the same in the two study groups (A and B). The chi-square will determine the expected result based upon the distribution of outcomes and the number of subjects in each group. It will then compare the expected value to the actual observed value. This procedure will provide the probability that the following null hypothesis statement is true:

The outcome of patients in Group A is the same as the outcome of patients in Group B.

The equation to calculate the chi-square statistic is:

$$\chi^2 = \Sigma \frac{(O - E)^2}{E} \tag{9-1}$$

where O is the observed value within a given cell (e.g., Cell A) and E is the expected observation. As is shown, the chi-square value is dependent on the difference between the observed and expected values $(O - E)$. The greater the difference, the larger the chi-square. Further, since this number is squared, as this difference increases the numerator in the equation becomes proportionally larger than just the raw difference. This phenomenon makes the chi-square statistic very dependent on the number of observations (note that there is a direct linear relationship between the chi-square statistic and the number of observations). Theoretically, very small differences can be detected if the sample size is large enough. The number of degrees of freedom v for a chi-square are determined from the number of rows and columns of data analyzed as follows:

$$v = (\text{no. rows} - 1) \cdot (\text{no. columns} - 1) \tag{9-2}$$

TABLE 9-1. **Example of a Data Table Used for Chi-Square Analysis**

Groups Compared	Outcomes Assessed		Totals
	Outcome A	Outcome B	
Group A	Cell A	Cell B	A + B
Group B	Cell C	Cell D	C + D
Totals	A + C	B + D	A + B + C + D

Two primary assumptions for using the chi-square are (1) that the groups being compared are independent from one another, and (2) that there are enough observations in each cell for the test to be accurate. By convention this is defined as 5 observations per cell for 20% or more of the cells in the chi-square table.

KEY CONCEPT

The chi-square tests for distributional differences between groups and is sensitive to the number of observations.

CASE STUDY

Consider the following data from an advertisement for Zosyn. In this advertisement the data shown in Table 9-2 was used to substantiate the statement "Proven effective versus Timentin in patients with community-acquired pneumonia . . . requiring hospitalization, of moderate severity only, caused by piperacillin-resistant, Zosyn susceptible, B-lactamase-producing strains of *Haemophilus influenzae*." The null hypothesis that the chi-square analysis is testing states:

There is no difference in the incidence of patients who are cured, improved or failed when Zosyn is compared to Timentin.

Note that the data in this example is nominal in nature. That is, a patient would fall into only one of three discreet categories: cured, improved, or failed. Since the data is nominal and the groups compared are independent from one another (or unpaired in nature), a chi-square analysis can be used. Conceptually, the chi-square test is very simple to analyze. When evaluating data that is analyzed by a chi-square, it is useful to realize that only two factors influence the chi-square statistic:

1. How similar or dissimilar the distribution of data points are between the groups being compared

2. The number of observations

TABLE 9-2. **Patients Cured, Improved, or Failed on Zosyn or Timentin**

Drug	Cured	Improved	Failed	Total
Zosyn	51 (69%)	11 (15%)	12 (16%)	74
Timentin	26 (49%)	10 (19%)	17 (32%)	53

The chi-square test will provide the probability that the distribution between groups is the same, or in this example, that the incidence of patients that are either cured, improved, or failed is the same whether they received Zosyn or Timentin. If the test determines that there is less than a 5% chance that they are the same, then the null hypothesis statement is rejected and a conclusion is made that the distribution of observations between the groups is different. The interpretation of the p-value is identical to that used for parametric tests.

The ability of the chi-square test to determine whether a given distributional pattern between groups is different is solely dependent on the number of observations. Any difference, no matter how small, can be shown to be statistically significant, if enough subjects are enrolled. Remember that with parametric tests, statistical difference was influenced by the degree of difference in the observations, the amount of variability in the data, and the number of observations. For nonparametric tests, statistical difference is influenced only by the degree of difference between the groups compared and number of observations. As with parametric tests, it is important to assess whether the differences being tested appear to be clinically significant. Using the previous example, does a 69% cure rate with Zosyn provide for a clinical advantage over Timentin that had a cure rate of 49%? This clinical assessment should be done before you either perform the statistical test or evaluate the results of a statistical test.

In order to calculate the chi-square, the number of expected observations needs to be determined for each cell. In this example, a total of 127 patients were studied, with 77 (60.6%) of the patients cured, 26 (16.5%) improved, and 29 (22.8%) patients who failed therapy. The expected values are determined by multiplying the overall percent response by the number of subjects studied in that group. For example, to determine the expected number of patients who were cured on Zosyn therapy, one would multiply 74 (the number of patients who received Zosyn) by 0.606 (the fraction of patients overall who were cured), which is 44.9. Table 9-3 shows the expected value and $(O - E)^2$ for the data in Table 9-2. A good check on this calculation is to sum all of the expected values for each treatment group. This sum should be equal to the actual number of patients studied, which in this case is 74 in the Zosyn group and 53 in the Timentin group. The sum of all of the $(O - E)^2$ terms shows a χ^2 value of 5.72. The number of degrees of freedom (v) is 2. For 2 degrees of freedom, using the chi-square table in App. C, you should see that this calculated χ^2 is between 2.41 and 5.99, showing a probability that the distribution of cure rates is similar between the Zosyn and Timentin of between 5 and 10%. The null hypothesis statement should therefore be accepted that the cure rates for Zosyn and Timentin are similar. Thus, Zosyn therapy would be evaluated as equivalent to treatment with Timentin.

Special Cases

There are circumstances when it is not appropriate to use a chi-square analysis, or when a modification needs to be made to provide a more accurate result. Two situations will be discussed. These are: (1) when there are two outcomes compared

TABLE 9-3. Expected Values for Patients Cured, Improved, or Failed on Zosyn and Timentin Therapy

Drug	Parameter	Cured	Improved	Failed	Total
Zosyn	E	44.9	12.2	16.9	74
	$(O-E)^2$	37.6	1.5	24.0	
	$(O-E)^2/E$	0.84	0.12	1.42	
Timentin	E	32.1	8.8	12.1	53
	$(O-E)^2$	37.6	1.5	24	
	$(O-E)^2/E$	1.17	0.17	1.98	

between two groups, and (2) when there are a low number of observations in one or more cells.

Yates Correction Factor

When two groups are being compared and there is only one discreet category (outcome) being compared, and the data are formatted into a 2×2 table with only 1 degree of freedom, then the Yates correction factor is to be used. This provides for a better approximation of the chi-square value when there is only 1 degree of freedom. Also, when data is formatted in this manner, the odds ratio or risk ratio can be used to analyze data. This is discussed in more detail later. The χ^2 with Yates correction is calculated as follows:

$$\chi^2 = \frac{(|O-E| - .5)^2}{E} \qquad (9\text{-}3)$$

As illustrated, the chi-square determined using the Yates correction factor will always be lower than that calculated when not using this correction. This is important when values are close to being at the level of statistical significance. Specifically, not using the Yates correction factor can result in an inappropriate conclusion of statistical significance, because a higher χ^2 value will be calculated. Using the previous Zosyn example, the data can be formatted into two possible outcomes: (1) a favorable response that includes the cured and improved responses as one category, and (2) unfavorable outcomes that include data from the patients who failed. Table 9-4 depicts an example of a 2×2 table using the data from this advertisement. Under these circumstances it is appropriate to use the chi-square with the Yates correction factor. In this example, the χ^2 value was calculated to be 3.55, which showed a probability of greater than 5% but less than 10% that the outcomes of Zosyn therapy were the same as with Timentin (see App. C). The statistical conclusion would be that the therapies are the same. If, however, the Yates correction is not used, a higher chi-square value will be obtained (which in this case is 4.41), which shows a p-value of <0.05. Thus, a statistical conclusion would be reached that the therapies are different, with Zosyn therapy showing a higher percentage of patients with favorable responses. Different statistical conclusions can be reached depending on whether the Yates correction factor is used. When borderline results are obtained, as in this case, a statistical conclusion can be altered based on whether the Yates correction factor is used.

A final comment about the Yates correction factor involves the number of subjects. Since this factor is a subtraction of 0.5 from the difference $O - E$, as this difference gets large in number (i.e., the number of observations is large), the Yates correction factor will become insignificant. Therefore, with large sample sizes the Yates correction factor is not needed.

KEY CONCEPT

Statistical conclusions can be changed based upon whether the Yates correction factor is used. This correction factor always gives a lower χ^2 value!

Fisher's Exact Test

When data is formatted in a 2×2 table, or in situations when there are a small number of observations, the chi-square test should not be used. The definition of a small number of observations is arbitrary, being defined as a total number of observations of <20, or less then 5 observations in a given cell. In these circumstances, a Fisher's exact test is used. As the name of the test implies, Fisher's exact test gives an exact value for p. For this reason, when data are formatted into a 2×2 table, it is preferred and more accurate to use the Fisher's exact test as opposed to the chi-square test.

A quirk of the Fisher's exact test is that two separate tests are used for one-tailed and two-tailed analysis. Most computer programs perform only one-

TABLE 9-4. An Example of a 2 × 2 Contingency Table

Drug	Improved	Failed	Total
Zosyn	62 (84%)	12 (16%)	74
Timentin	36 (68%)	17 (32%)	53

$\chi^2 = 3.55$, $v = 1$, $p > 0.05$

tailed analysis. Further, most studies do not mention whether a one-tailed or two-tailed test was performed. This can lead to some ambiguity in evaluating the results of Fisher's exact test. This again would be of concern when p-values are close to the .05 range, where the difference between a one- and two-tailed test can result in differences in statistical interpretation.

> **KEY CONCEPT**
>
> Exceptions to using the chi-square test include cases where there is 1 degree of freedom and when the number of observations is small.

McNemar's Chi-Square

The nonparametric tests discussed so far require that the data analyzed be independent from one another. Often, however, data is obtained from crossover-designed trials that have nominal data from the same subject taken on different occasions. In this case, McNemar's chi-square is used. This is a modification of the chi-square that accounts for samples coming from the same subject. When this procedure is used, patients will have been exposed to one treatment and then crossed over to another treatment. McNemar's chi-square will ignore subjects that respond the same way to both treatments and will analyze those patients who change response. If all subjects respond in the same way to the two treatments, then the McNemar's chi-square value will be small, because the before- and after-treatment values will be very close to one another. If they respond differently, then the number of patients who change response is large, and the corresponding McNemar's chi-square value will be large. How each individual subject changes in response to a treatment effect determines whether McNemar's chi-square is significant.

Effect of Number on Chi-Square Statistic

As previously mentioned, the chi-square statistic is very sensitive to the number of observations. The relationship between observation number and the calculation of the chi-square statistic is shown in Fig. 9-1. Note the direct linear relationship between the calculated chi-square statistic and the number of observations, showing a strong dependency of the chi-square statistic on subject number. Also note the effect that the tested difference has on the needed N to determine a difference (note this example illustrates differences of 22, 50, and 85%). A practical way of looking at this effect is to go back and evaluate the Zosyn advertisement. If the favorable responses were 82% (Zosyn) and 70% (Timentin) (instead of 84 and 68%; or a 17% difference as opposed to a 24% difference), the chi-square statistic would have shown a p-value >0.10 and <0.2. This would indicate that there is a greater than 10 but less than 20% chance that the cure rates are similar, and the null hypothesis would be accepted, resulting in a different statistical conclusion being reached.

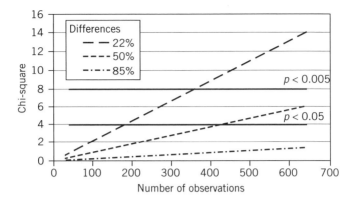

Figure 9-1. Effect of *N* and differences in distribution on chi-square.

This modest 2% directional change in response (84 to 82% effective), changed the statistical conclusions reached. Another way of showing this effect is to look at the number of subjects that would be required to determine a difference if the response rates showed an 82% cure rate for Zosyn and 70% for Timentin. As shown in Table 9-5, approximately 190 subjects would be needed—almost twice as many as required to detect a difference of 84 vs. 68%. When small changes in data can change statistical conclusions, be wary of the statistical conclusions reached! Under these circumstances, prior clinical knowledge and experience are important in evaluating data and assessing the relevance of the conclusions reached.

As another example see the data in Table 9-6, which is adapted from an advertisement for Activase. This advertisement showed 24-h, 30-day, and 1-year mortality data from patients with acute myocardial infarction who received either Activase, streptokinase/IV heparin, or streptokinase/SC heparin. Note that each group contained a very large number of patients (Activase 10,376; streptokinase/IV heparin 10,387; streptokinase/SC heparin 9814). This large subject number will allow for the detection of very small differences. The point of the advertisement is that there is a lower mortality rate with Activase as compared to streptokinase. This is true—

TABLE 9-5. **Effect of *N* on Chi-Square Analysis**

Parameter	Zosyn	Timentin	Critical N to Reach $p < 0.05$
Advertisement	84%	68%	~90
2% change from ad	82%	70%	~190
4% change from ad	80%	72%	~440

TABLE 9-6. Comparison of 30-Day Mortality in Patients after Receiving Activase and Streptokinase (SK)

Drug	N	% Mortality at 30 Days	p-Value
Activase	10,376	6.3%	$p < 0.003$ from SK/IV heparin $p < 0.007$ from SK/SC heparin
SK (IV heparin)	10,387	7.3%	
SK (SC heparin)	9,814	7.3%	

SOURCE: Adapted from an advertisement for Activase.

mortality rate is 1% lower (6.3 vs. 7.3%). This means that for every 100 patients treated with Activase, there will be 1 fewer deaths. The key to interpreting this result is whether a 1% difference in mortality can be detected at a given institution. Given all of the variables in managing acute myocardial patients within a health system, will the use of Activase in fact lower mortality by 1%—and is this difference detectable? Be careful about the extrapolation of small statistically significant results.

Two of the confusing aspects of nonparametric tests are the unusual names of tests and the exceptions that are applied to the use of these tests. The algorithm in Fig. 9-2 should help the reader determine the most appropriate test to use for nominal data based upon the type of study design and the exceptions that are to used. Hopefully this will help to demystify some aspects of nonparametric data analysis and interpretation.

Odds and Risk Ratios

The odds ratio or risk ratio will provide the odds or risks of an event occurring in one group as compared to another. The null hypothesis statement is as follows:

The odds or risks of an event occurring is the same in one group as compared to another.

Risk Ratio

A relative risk (RR) ratio is used when the risk of developing a specific outcome (e.g., mortality, disease occurrence) is desired within a specific category of patients (e.g., males, smokers, etc). A risk ratio is performed on data obtained from a prospective study when the outcome measure and the risk factor are nominal variables. Since there are two outcomes for the presence or absence of the risk factor, the data can be

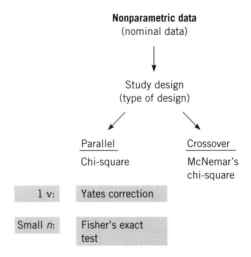

Figure 9-2. How to determine the most appropriate nonparametric test for nominal data based on study design. Exceptions shown in gray.

displayed in the format of a 2×2 contingency table. An example of a 2×2 table formatted for the risk ratio is shown in Table 9-7. The RR is determined from:

$$RR = \frac{a/(a+b)}{c/(c+d)} \qquad (9\text{-}4)$$

where a, b, c, and d are defined in Table 9-7. The confidence interval for RR is determined from:

$$100(1-\alpha)\%CI = RR^{1 \pm (z_\alpha/\sqrt{\chi^2})} \qquad (9\text{-}5)$$

where z_α is the two-sided z-value for the appropriate confidence interval. This value is 1.96 for a 95% CI. The χ^2 value is calculated as previously described. Eval-

TABLE 9-7. Example of Table Format Used for the Risk Ratio (RR)

	Outcome Measure		
Risk Factor	*Present*	*Absent*	*Total*
Present	a	b	$a+b$
Absent	c	d	$c+d$
Total	$a+c$	$b+d$	n

uation of Eq. (9-4) shows the RR compares the rate of occurrence of an outcome measure in a group of patients with a risk factor $[a/(a+b)]$ as compared to the rate of occurrence when the risk factor is absent $[c/(c+d)]$. If the rates of occurrence are same, the ratio will be 1.0. When the rates of occurrence are greater in the presence of a risk factor, the RR will be larger than 1.0. In contrast, when the rates of occurrence are smaller, then the RR value will be less than 1.0. Assessment of the RR is done by determining whether the value is different from 1.0. This is done by looking at the confidence interval. By convention, a 95% CI is used for statistical significance. If this interval includes 1.0, it is concluded that the RR is the same in the groups compared. If the interval excludes 1.0, then it is concluded that there is a higher (if RR > 1.0) or lower (if RR < 1.0) risk of occurrence of the outcome with the risk factor that is being evaluated. The value for RR is influenced only by the rates of occurrences of the outcome measure in the two groups being compared. The 95% CI interval is influenced by the number of observations n. This interval is inversely proportional to the number of observations. As this number increases, the confidence interval will get smaller. This allows smaller differences in the RR value from 1.0 to be statistically significant.

KEY CONCEPT

The risk ratio determines the risk of an event occurring in one group compared to another group. The ratio is compared to 1.0 using the 95% CI.

CASE STUDY

A study published in the *New England Journal of Medicine*[1] reported the results of a randomized, double-blind placebo-controlled trial that compared the effectiveness of digoxin to placebo on both mortality and hospitalization for heart failure in patients with heart failure who were in normal sinus rhythm. A total of 3397 patients were assigned to the digoxin group and 3403 to placebo. Patients were followed on average for 37 months. The study concluded that "digoxin did not reduce overall mortality, but it reduced the rate of hospitalization both overall and for worsening heart failure." Data from this study is shown in Table 9-8. The risk ratio is used because the study is prospective in nature and there are two possible outcomes (e.g., patients hospitalized for cardiovascular reasons or those hospitalized for other reasons) and two possible risk factors (receiving digoxin or placebo). In this case, the RR shows the risk that taking digoxin has on the incidence or occurrence of cardiovascular hospitalizations. The RR shows that there are lower hospitalizations for all cardiovascular reasons in patients on digoxin as compared to placebo [0.87 (95% CI: 0.81–0.93), $p < 0.001$]. This is statistically significant because the 95% CI does not include 1, ranging from 0.81 to 0.93. There is a higher RR for hospitalizations caused by digoxin toxicity [2.17, 95% CI (1.42–3.32), $p <$

0.001]. Note that the 95% CI does not include 1 (ranges from 1.42 to 3.32). In contrast, there was no difference between digoxin and placebo for hospitalizations caused by supraventricular arrhythmia or AV block arrhythmia/sinus bradycardia. Comparing the RR for hospitalizations for all cardiovascular reasons to those caused by supraventricular arrhythmias shows identical RR values (0.87), yet one is statistically significant (all cardiovascular reasons) and the other is not. The reason for this is that the CI for hospitalizations caused by all cardiovascular reasons is narrower (0.81–0.93) than the CI for hospitalizations caused by supraventricular arrhythmias (0.69–1.10). This is because there are more observations in the group of all cardiovascular reasons for hospitalization ($n = 3544$) than in the group hospitalized for supraventricular arrhythmias ($n = 287$), resulting in a narrower 95% CI. This example illustrates the impact that subject number has on the RR and how the statistical interpretation can change as a function of n.

KEY CONCEPT

The width of the 95% confidence interval for the risk ratio is inversely proportional to the number of observations.

Odds Ratio

The odds ratio (OR) is used when the odds of an event occurring in one group is compared to another when data is derived from a retrospective study. This test is similar to the risk ratio and is used when an outcome variable of nominal scale is compared between two groups, such that the data can be formatted into a 2×2

TABLE 9-8. **Reasons for Hospitalization in Patients Receiving Digoxin or Placebo**

Reason for Hospitalization	Digoxin, n = 3397	Placebo, n = 3403	Risk Ratio, 95% CI	p-Value
All cardiovascular reasons	1694 (49.9)	1850 (54.4)	0.87 (0.81–0.93)	<0.001
Supraventricular arrhythmia	133 (3.9)	152 (4.2)	0.87 (0.69–1.10)	NS
AV block arrhythmia, bradycardia	14 (0.4)	9 (0.3)	1.56 (0.68–3.61)	NS
Suspected digoxin toxicity	67 (2.0)	31 (0.9)	2.17 (1.42–3.32)	<0.001

SOURCE: Adapted from Table 3 in Digitalis Investigation Group (1).

table (see Table 9-7). The odds ratio compares event occurrence between two groups and is calculated from:

$$OR = \frac{ad}{bc} \qquad (9\text{-}6)$$

If the odds of event occurrence are the same in both groups, the odds ratio will be 1.0. The statistical procedures tests for differences from 1.0. The analysis is very similar to that described for the risk ratio. The odds ratio is always presented as the ratio and the 95% CI for that ratio. If the 95% CI encompasses the value 1.0, the null hypothesis is accepted. If the 95% CI does not encompass 1.0, the null hypothesis is rejected. The 95% CI for the OR is calculated as described in Eq. (9-4), except that the RR is replaced by the OR as defined in Eq. (9-6).

KEY CONCEPT

The odds ratio determines the odds of an event occurring from data obtained from a retrospective study. The OR is similar to the RR and is compared to 1.0 using the 95% CI.

CASE STUDY

An assessment of factors associated with participation in a pharmaceutical care program was published in the *Journal of the American Pharmaceutical Association*.[2] This paper surveyed HMO enrollees with chronic health conditions who were part of a study that evaluated the effectiveness of pharmaceutical care. They surveyed enrollees in the program ($n = 210$), refusers of the program ($n = 162$), and controls ($n = 368$) on the impact of pharmaceutical care on medication use awareness. They analyzed specific factors that predicted participation in the pharmaceutical care program. This data is shown in Table 9-9. A greater chance of participating in the pharmaceutical care program (comparing participants to refusers) was associated with the number of medications (OR = 1.27) and being employed part-time (OR = 2.21). This was because the OR was greater than 1.0 in both cases, and in both instances the 95% CI did not encompass the number 1 (see Table 9-8). In contrast, poor health (OR = 0.35) and living with a relative but not a spouse (OR = 0.21) were associated with a lower chance of participating in the pharmaceutical care program because the OR was less than 1.0. Look at the ORs for number of medications and being employed part-time. In the latter instance the OR is not quite twice that for number of medications (2.21 vs. 1.27), yet the *p*-value for number of medications is much lower than that for working part-time ($p = .0001$ vs. $p = .0428$). Also note that the range in the 95% CI is much different for these two observations, being 0.28 (1.42 − 1.14) for number of medications and 3.73 (4.76 − 1.03) for being employed part-time. The differences in *p*-values and ranges in the 95% CI can only be explained by differences in the number of observations between the two groups. There are fewer observations in the subgroups of patients working part-time, which accounts for a higher p-value and wider 95% CI, despite the OR being greater than in the number of medication group. This illustrates the effect that the number of observations can have on how the OR can be interpreted.

In summary, the odds ratio is influenced only by the incidence of occurrence of an event in a given group and by the number of observations in that group. The 95% CI is primarily influenced by the number of observations. As n increases, the 95% CI will get smaller. If the 95% CI includes 1.0, but the OR looks to be different from 1.0, check the subject number. If the number of subjects studied is small, then a Type II error could exist.

Nonparametric Tests of Ordinal Data

Only a brief introduction to the nonparametric tests that are used on ordinal data is provided here. Those wishing more in-depth discussion should review appropriate biostatistics textbooks. Unpaired ordinal data from two groups (e.g., data from a parallel-design trial) can be analyzed using the Mann-Whitney U test. This test rank orders all of the data from the lowest to the highest ranked value and compares the ranks between the two groups. Paired ordinal data from two groups (e.g., data from a crossover-design trial) can be compared using the Wilcoxan rank sum test. This test compares the directional change (plus or minus) as a result of the test procedure compared to control. The test also incorporates the magnitude of change observed. If there is no effect, then the directional change should be randomly positive and negative. In contrast, if there is an effect, the change will be in the direction of the effect (i.e., either positive or negative). As an example, the following data comes from a study that was designed to determine whether grapefruit juice affects the disposition of caffeine.[3] Note that this is being used as an illustration of how the Wilcoxan rank sum test can be used—not that it *is* the best test to

---

TABLE 9-9. **Factors That Predict Participation in Pharmaceutical Care Programs (Participants Compared to Refusers)**

Variable	OR	95% CI	p-*Value*
No. prescription medications	1.27	1.14–1.42	.0001
Employed part-time	2.21	1.03–4.75	.0428
Poor health 0.35	0.15–0.86	.0219	
Living with a relative (not a spouse)	0.21	0.07–0.63	.0056

SOURCE: Data adapted from Table 2 in Fisher et al., (2).

use on this data set. Table 9-10 provides caffeine AUC, $\mu g/(mL \cdot h)$, after administration with water and then grapefruit juice. The data is then ranked by absolute value from the lowest to the highest value and sorted by whether the change was in the positive or negative direction, as shown in Table 9-11. If grapefruit juice has no effect on caffeine disposition, one would expect that the distribution of rank order would be similar in the positive and negative columns. If there is an effect, then all or almost all of the change should occur in the appropriate column. For example, if grapefruit juice does increase caffeine AUC, then all of the ranks should be in the plus column. The Wilcoxon rank sum tests for movement from this case to the random, no-effect situation. Note that the test is on the distribution of ranks, and the actual change is converted to a rank and then tested. As with other nonparametric tests, this test is influenced by the distribution of the ranks and subject number. Comparing to the information used in parametric tests, as with the chi-square test, variance parameters (e.g., SEM as used in the paired t-test) are not used. This information is lost when nonparametric testing is performed.

In another example, a report compared the pharmacokinetics of phenytoin after oral and rectal administration.[4] The pharmacokinetic parameters obtained—C_{max} and AUC, which are parametric data—did not follow a normal distribution. For this reason, the data was reported as the median value and an interquartile range (25th to 75th percentile). For example, the median value and IQ for phenytoin AUC after oral administration was 36.2 (30.7–52.2) $\mu g/(mL \cdot h)$, and after rectal administration

TABLE 9-10. **Comparison of Caffeine AUC After Administration of Water and Grapefruit Juice, $\mu g/(mL \cdot h)$**

Pair	Water	Grapefruit Juice	Change
1	46.68	51.40	+2.72
2	48.52	49.51	+0.99
3	51.25	48.94	−2.31
4	47.60	59.78	+12.18
5	47.93	63.72	+15.79
6	46.68	60.13	+13.45
7	21.17	20.23	−0.94
8	49.05	72.48	+23.43
9	37.92	44.73	+6.81
10	47.41	29.93	−17.48

SOURCE: Data from Marsh et al., (3).

TABLE 9-11. **Rank Order of Differences in Caffeine AUC**

Pair	Difference, $\mu g/(mL \cdot h)$	Rank, +	Rank, −
8	+23.43	10	
10	−17.48		9
5	+15.79	8	
6	+13.45	7	
4	+12.18	6	
9	+6.81	5	
1	+2.72	4	
3	−2.31		3
2	+0.99	2	
7	−0.94		1

it was 5.4 (0.0–14.2) $\mu g/(mL \cdot h)$. Since this data was not normally distributed, it would be inappropriate to compare these values with a test such as a paired t-test. For this reason, the authors appropriately analyzed the data using a Wilcoxan signed rank test and found that the AUC values were different ($p = 0.046$).

Nonparametric tests used on ordinal data that have been discussed here have focused on two treatment groups and are analogous to the use of the paired and unpaired t-tests that are used on parametric data. The nonparametric test that is used when ordinal data is analyzed from more than three independent groups is the Kruskal-Wallis test. This is the nonparametric equivalent to analysis of variance (ANOVA) testing. An algorithm to assist the reader in determining which nonparametric test is appropriate to use on ordinal data, based on the design of the study employed, is shown in Fig. 9-3. In addition, these tests are compared to their parametric counterparts in Table 9-12.

KEY CONCEPT

Parametric data can be converted to nonparametric data and then analyzed with the appropriate test. This loses the input of variance, and as such a weaker statistical test is used.

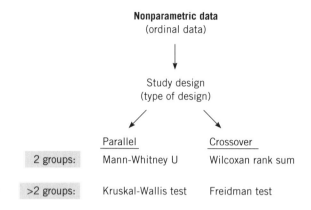

Figure 9-3. How to determine the most appropriate nonparametric test for ordinal data based on study design.

Summary

Nonparametric tests are used on data that is either nominal or ordinal in nature. A wide variety of nonparametric tests are used, based upon the study design and formatting of the data. These are summarized in Table 9-12. The large number of tests that can be utilized in some way adds to the complexity of understanding these procedures. In reality, nonparametric tests are fairly simple to understand. Independent of the specific test used, they will determine the probability that observations that are ordinal or nominal in nature come from the same population. These procedures are influenced by only two factors:

TABLE 9-12. Nonparametric Tests for Ordinal Data and Their Parametric Equivalent

Study Design	Nonparametric Test	Parametric Equivalent
Crossover design		
2 groups compared	Wilcoxan rank sum	Paired *t*-test
>2 groups compared	Freidman test	Repeated measures ANOVA
Parallel design		
2 groups compared	Mann-Whitney U	Unpaired *t*-test
>2 groups compared	Kruskal-Wallis test	ANOVA

1. The differences observed between the groups compared

2. The number of observations

If the observed differences are large and there is a reasonable number of observations, the chances are that the test will be significant. In contrast, if the differences are small and there are a small number of observations, the chances are that the test will not be significant. It should be realized that any difference can be determined to be statistically significant by increasing the number of subjects studied. The reader should be careful about extrapolating statistically significant but small differences. Always follow the statistical conclusions with your own clinical conclusion. Finally, be careful in how exceptions to the chi-square are used, as these can result in borderline values shifting in significance. One of the mysteries of nonparametric testing is the large number of tests that have unusual names. This should not be a barrier to understanding how these tests are used, as in reality the interpretation and use of these procedures are not difficult.

Study Questions

St. John's wort (250 mg hypericum extract ZE 117 twice daily) was compared to imipramine (75 mg twice daily) in a randomized, multicenter, double-blind, parallel group trial (H Woelk: Comparison of St. John's Wort and imipramine for treating depression: Randomized controlled trial, BMJ; 321:536–539, 2000). Adverse events by treatment group are as shown:

Adverse Event	Hypericum, n = 157	Imipramine, n = 167
Dry mouth	13	41
Headache	3	6
Sweating	2	13
Asthenia	2	11
Nausea	1	12
Dizziness	0	12

1. What is the most appropriate statistical test to use to determine the probability that the null hypothesis that adverse events are the same after hypericum as imipramine is true?

For the data in the previous question, describe the impact that the following factors would have on assessing statistical significance:

2. Differences in adverse events

3. Number of observations

4. The calculated χ^2 for the data in the first question is 51.12. What is the p-value? Is the null hypothesis statement accepted or rejected? Is there a difference in the occurrence of specific adverse events between hypericum and imipramine?

The number of patients who reported adverse events is as follows:

Hypericum ($n = 157$): 39%

Imipramine ($n = 157$): 63%

5. What is the most appropriate statistical test to provide the probability that the number of patients with adverse events is the same in patients exposed to hypericum as compared to imipramine?

6. The calculated χ^2 is 22.56; what is the p-value? In this example, do you think use of the Yates correction factor will result in a different statistical result as compared to the use of a chi-square without this correction factor?

The percentage of treatment withdrawals is as follows:

Hypericum ($n = 157$): 3%

Imipramine ($n = 157$): 16%

7. What is the most appropriate statistical test to determine the probability that the number of treatment withdrawals is the same in the hypericum group as compared to the imipramine group?

8. The effect of omeprazole treatment as compared to placebo was studied in patients after endoscopic treatment (JYW Lau, JJY Sung, KC Lee, et al: Effect of intravenous omeprazole on recurrent bleeding after endoscopic treatment of bleeding peptic ulcers, N Engl J Med, 343:310–316, 2000). Patients were randomized to receive omeprazole 80 mg followed by an infusion of 8 mg/h for 72 h or placebo. Data for recurrent bleeding is as follows:

	Omeprazole, n = 120	Placebo, n = 120
Number of patients with recurrent bleeding by day 7:	7	26
Ulcers within 30 days, no. patients/total no.:	5/56	17/62

Explain why the data just presented can be analyzed using a risk ratio.

9. For the data in the previous question, calculate the RR for placebo as compared to omeprazole.

The reported risk ratios were:

Recurrent bleeding by day 7: 3.71 (95% CI: 1.68–8.28)

Ulcers within 30 days: 3.85 (95% CI: 1.31–11.3)

10. Compare the range in 95% CI. Why is there a wider range in the ulcers within 30 days group as compared to the recurrent bleeding by day 7 group?

11. The effect of zinc lozenges in reducing cold symptoms was evaluated in 50 ambulatory patients presenting with cold symptoms (AS Prasad, JT Fitzgerald, B Bao, et al: Duration of symptoms and plasma cytokine levels in patients with the common cold treated with zinc acetate: A randomized, double-blind, placebo-controlled trial, Ann Intern Med 133:245–252, 2000). This was a randomized parallel designed trial comparing zinc lozenges to placebo. Participants graded cold symptoms as follows: 0 for none, 1 for mild, 2 for moderate, and 3 for severe.

What is the most appropriate test to determine if the probability of cold symptoms is the same in subjects who received zinc lozenges as compared to placebo? Why?

References

1. The Digitalis Investigation Group: The effect of digoxin on mortality and morbidity in patients with heart failure. N Engl J Med 336:525–533, 1997.

2. Fisher LR, Scott LM, Boonstra DM, et. al: Pharmaceutical care for patients with chronic conditions. J Am Pharm Assoc 40:174–180, 2000.

3. Marsh WA, Hampton EM, Whitsett TL, et al: Influence of grapefruit juice on caffeine pharmacokinetics and pharmacodynamics. Pharmacotherapy 16:1046–1052, 1996.

4. Burstein AH, Fisher KM, McPherson ML, Roby CA: Absorption of phenytoin from rectal suppositories formulated with a polyethylene glycol base. Pharmacotherapy 20:562–567, 2000.

Evaluating Statistical Results: Correlation, Regression, Survival, and Life Analysis

Richard L. Slaughter

OUTLINE

Goals and Objectives

Correlation Analysis

Types of Correlation Analysis

Regression Analysis

    Linear Regression Analysis

    Nonlinear Regression Analysis

Survival Life Analysis

Summary

Study Questions

References

KEY WORDS

Censored data
Correlation
Correlation coefficient
Coefficient of determination
Dependent variable
Independent variable
Nonparametric

Parametric
Pearson product-moment
  correlation
Regression analysis
Spearman rank correlation
Survival analysis

Goals and Objectives

The goal of this chapter is to discuss and demonstrate how correlation and regression analysis is used and evaluated when reading primary drug literature sources.

This chapter will introduce the reader to survival life analysis. After completing this chapter, readers should:

1. Understand concepts and terms used for correlation analysis. These include the correlation coefficient (r-value) and coefficient of determination (r^2-value).

2. Be able to assess the factors that will result in a statistically significant correlation.

3. Be able to describe when a statistically significant correlation may be clinically insignificant.

4. Be able to illustrate why it is important to visually evaluate correlation analysis.

5. Be able to describe and evaluate regression analysis.

6. Be able to differentiate between linear and nonlinear regression techniques.

7. Appreciate the limitations of regression analysis.

8. Be able to describe how survival analysis is used in primary drug literature.

9. Be able to define censored data.

Introduction

Very often, when data is obtained from clinical studies it is desirable to know if one variable is related to another. For example, is the systemic clearance of a drug such as an aminoglycoside antibiotic related to renal function or age? Correlation analysis will determine the statistical answer to this question. It will determine how strong the relationship is and whether the relationship is statistically significant. Sometimes it is useful to be able to predict one variable (e.g., drug clearance) from another variable (e.g., creatinine clearance) using an equation, such as that for a straight line. This procedure is referred to as *regression analysis.* This statistical test is often used to predict information about a drug that may be difficult to obtain routinely in the clinical setting, such as systemic clearance, from data that is easily obtainable, such as creatinine clearance or the patient's age. This is also the statistical test that is used to design dosing nomograms that are reliant on patient-specific information. As can be seen, this procedure is widely used. It is also a statistical procedure that can frequently overstate the significance of a relationship. It is one of the most used—and abused—procedures. As with all statistical tests, these tests require clinical and intuitive knowledge for appropriate interpretation. This chapter provides an overview of how these tests are performed, and focuses heavily on how to interpret the presentation of correlation and regression analysis.

Correlation Analysis

Correlation analysis, very simply, determines whether two or more variables are related to one another. This statistical procedure provides the probability that the null hypothesis statement "There is no relationship between a dependent and independent variable" is true. The results are typically displayed in a scattergram, with the y variable, by convention, being the dependent variable and the x variable the independent variable. In this case, the dependent variable should be related to (or dependent on) the independent variable. For example, systemic clearance for a drug that is renally eliminated would be expected to be dependent on a measurement of renal function, such as creatinine clearance. Systemic clearance would be the dependent variable. Factors that influence the independent variable should not be related to the dependent variable. In this case, factors that influence renal function are completely independent of drug clearance. That is, drug clearance does not influence renal function, whereas renal function may significantly influence drug clearance.

KEY CONCEPT

For correlation analysis, the dependent variable is placed on the x axis and the independent variable on the y axis.

- The dependent variable should have a clinical rationale for relating to the independent variable (systemic drug clearance may be expected to be related to or dependent on creatinine clearance).

- Factors that influence the independent variable should not be related to the dependent variable (factors that influence creatinine clearance, age, muscle mass, glomerular filtration, or factors not related to systemic drug clearance).

Correlation analysis may show a positive relationship, such that the values for the dependent variable increase in direct proportion to the values of the independent variable. A negative relationship may also exist such that the values of the dependent variable decrease in inverse proportion to those of the independent variable. The strength of this relationship is assessed from the correlation coefficient (r-value). The r-value can range from +1 to −1, where +1 is a perfect positive correlation (Fig. 10-1) and −1 is a perfect negative correlation (Fig. 10-2). Actual examples of positive and negative correlations are shown in Figs. 10-3 and 10-4. Figure 10-3 shows that ceftazidime total body clearance (dependent variable) is positively correlated ($r = 0.83$) with gestational age (independent variable) in preterm infants.[1] Figure 10-4 shows that the area under the curve (AUC; 0 to 72) value (dependent variable) for a drug metabolized by CYP2C9 P450 isozyme negatively correlates ($r^2 = 0.6778$; $r = 0.823$)

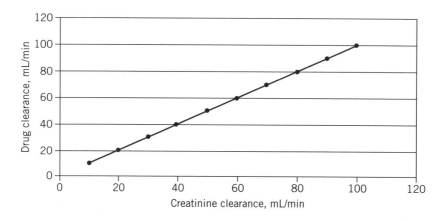

Figure 10-1. Hypothetical example of a perfect positive correlation.

with concentrations of serum albumin (independent variable) in patients who have liver cirrhosis.[2] An example of a very poor correlation is shown in Fig. 10-5. This figure shows the correlation between predicted peak and trough concentrations of tobramycin in premature infants. As shown, there is an unrelated scatter of data points, with no obvious correlation between the two variables.[3]

A linear regression model (this procedure is discussed in more detail later), where the two variables are related in a straight-line relationship, is used to show how the correlation coefficient is determined. Note that data points may be associated by a number of different types of mathematical relationships (e.g., exponential or quadratic); however, the linear model is most commonly used. When data is fitted to a linear model, the best-fit line is determined by the line that gives the smallest amount of deviation or variance of the data points from that line. This is determined by taking the difference of a data point from the fitted line and then squaring this difference. The sum of these squares is called the *sum of squared deviations from the regression line*. The r-value is determined from Eq. (10-1):

$$r = \sqrt{1 - \frac{SS_{reg}}{SS_{mean}}} \qquad (10\text{-}1)$$

where SS_{reg} is the sum of squared deviations of points from the regression line and SS_{mean} is the sum of squared deviations from the mean. One should be able to see that if the data points are very close to the regression line, the value for SS_{reg} will be small because the difference between the data points and the line will be small. The ratio SS_{reg}/SS_{mean} will approach 0 and the r-value will be close to 1. If the data points vary significantly from the regression line, SS_{reg} will be very large, because the square of the difference of the data point and the line will be large, and the ratio SS_{reg}/SS_{mean} will be large and the r-value very small. The r-value provides an indication of how strong the relationship is. A guide for relating a given r-value to the strength of a relationship is given in Table 10-1. This will provide an overall assessment of the

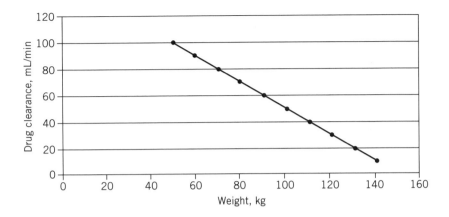

Figure 10-2. Hypothetical example of a perfect negative correlation.

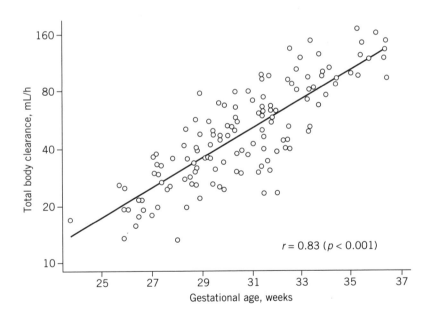

$r = 0.83 \ (p < 0.001)$

Figure 10-3. Linear regression analysis of total body clearance of ceftazidime versus gestational age in 136 preterm infants on day 3 after birth. Note logarithmically transformed vertical axis. *[From van den Anker et al. (1). Reproduced from Clin Pharmacol Ther 58:650–659, 1995, with permission from Mosby, Inc.]*

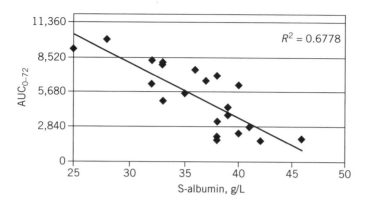

Figure 10-4. Individual AUC_{0-72} values for Drug A versus serum albumin levels in subjects with liver cirrhosis. *[From Bergquist et al. (2). Reproduced from Clin Pharmacol Ther 66:201–204, 1999, with permission from Mosby, Inc.]*

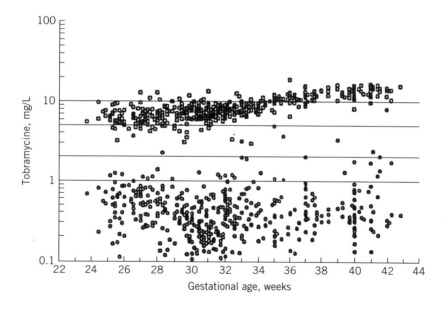

Figure 10-5. Predicted tobramycin peak (■) and trough (○) levels with revised dosing recommendation. *[From de Hoog et al. (3). Reproduced from Clin Pharmacol Ther 62:392–399, 1997, with permission from Mosby, Inc.]*

strength of a relationship but will not provide a statistical answer to the null hypothesis statement. This is done by calculating the t-statistic from Eq. (10-2):

$$t = r \sqrt{\frac{n-2}{1-r^2}} \qquad (10\text{-}2)$$

where n is the total number of observations and the number of degrees of freedom is determined from $n - 2$. Once the t-value is calculated, the p-value is obtained from the t-table in App. B, just as was done for a t-test. This will provide the probability that there is no correlation between the two variables evaluated. If the p-value is <0.05, the null hypothesis statement is rejected and it is concluded that there is a statistical correlation between the two variables. Inspection of Eq. (10-2) shows that only two factors influence the calculation of the t-statistic—the r-value and the number of observations—with the t-statistic being directly related to both. An important point to realize is that statistical significance can be achieved with very low r-values if there are enough observations. A correlation may be statistically significant while having almost no clinical utility. For this reason, visual inspection of the actual scattergram is a very important evaluative component when analyzing a correlation analysis. Do not rely on just the statistical report.

KEY CONCEPT

A correlation analysis may be statistically significant while the r-value is low and the relationship does not look clinically significant. Do not rely solely on the statistical output from a correlation analysis for interpretation.

TABLE 10-1. **Correlation of *r*-Value to Strength of Relationship**

r-*Value*	*Quality of Correlation*
0.9–1.0	Excellent correlation, relationship is probably predictive
0.7–0.9	Very good correlation, relationship may be predictive
0.6–0.7	Good correlation, but probability not predictive
0.5–0.6	Moderate correlation, not predictive
<0.5	Weak to no correlation

Another term frequently used in correlation analysis is the *coefficient of determination* or r^2-value. This value is the square of the correlation coefficient and is determined from Eq. (10-3):

$$r^2 = 1 - \frac{SS_{reg}}{SS_{mean}} \qquad (10\text{-}3)$$

This value is a function of how much deviation or variance there is in the data points from the regression line SS_{reg} as compared to the total variance of the sample SS_{mean}. Another way of looking at the r^2-value is that it explains the amount of variability in the dependent y-variable that is explained by the independent x-variable. For example, Fig. 10-3 shows the correlation between ceftazidime clearance and gestational age. The reported correlation coefficient (r-value) is 0.83, so the coefficient of determination (r^2-value) is 0.69. In this study the mean $\pm s$ for ceftazidime clearance is 55.7 $\pm$ 34.4 mL/h. Ceftazidime clearance shows a fair degree of variability in preterm infants with a coefficient of variation (CV; s/mean) of 62%. A large amount of this variability (about 69%, the r^2-value) can be explained by gestational age of infants. As one can readily see by inspecting Fig. 10-3, ceftazidime clearance does increase in a direct linear fashion across the age range of 25 to 37 weeks, so that older infants have larger clearance values than younger infants.

KEY CONCEPT

The coefficient of determination (r^2-value) indicates the amount of variability in the dependent variable that is explained by the independent variable. Do not confuse this with the correlation coefficient. The r^2-value will always be a smaller number.

Types of Correlation Analysis

There are special types of correlation analysis, based on the type of data that is analyzed. The data being related may be either parametric (as in the above examples) or nonparametric (ordinal or nominal data types). Also, parametric data may not be normally distributed. As with other statistical tests, there are parametric and nonparametric tests that are performed on the appropriate data set for correlation and regression analysis. For example, the Pearson product-moment correlation is performed on data that is parametric in nature, using the procedures previously described. The Pearson product-moment correlation also depends on data following a normal distribution. When data is ordinal in nature or does not follow a normal distribution, a Spearman rank correlation is used. The interpretation of the statistical result is the same as for the Pearson product-moment correlation; however, the calculation of the correlation coefficient is different and is designated as r_s:

$$r_s = 1 - \frac{6 \sum d^2}{n^3 - n} \qquad (10\text{-}4)$$

where d is the difference in ranks of the two ranks for a given point and n is the number of observations. If there is a strong correlation between the dependent x-variable and independent y-variable, the ranks of these values should be similar to one another. In this case, the numerator in Eq. (10-4) approaches 0, and the r_s value will approach 1. If there is no correlation between the two variables, then the rank values will be dissimilar; the numerator will be large and the r_s value small.

KEY CONCEPT

A Pearson product-moment correlation is performed on parametric data that is normally distributed, and a Spearman rank correlation is used on nonparametric data or parametric data that is not normally distributed.

CASE STUDIES

The study by Miettinen et al.[4] determined the effects of a margarine containing the plant sterol sitostanol on reducing serum cholesterol. This study compared the effects of 2.6 g/day of margarine containing sitostanol ester on 102 subjects to those on 51 patients who consumed plain margarine. One of the goals of the study was to see if reductions in serum cholesterol would be related to changes in serum campesterol concentrations. The absorption of campesterol, a dietary plant sterol not synthesized in the body, is reflective of intestinal absorption of cholesterol. Changes in campesterol concentrations may then reflect changes in intestinal absorption of cholesterol. The null hypothesis statement would be as follows:

> There is no correlation between campesterol concentrations and cholesterol concentrations

The relationship is shown in Fig. 10-6. The p-value determined was <0.001, indicating that there is a less than 0.1% chance that there is no correlation. The null hypothesis statement is therefore rejected, and this relationship is assessed as statistically significant ($p < 0.001$). This does not necessarily mean that the relationship is clinically important. The r-value for this relationship is 0.57, which in accord with Table 10-1 would be a moderate, but not predictive, relationship. This is what is shown in Fig. 10-6.

Cholesterol concentrations change as a function of campesterol concentrations, but they could not be accurately predicted from campesterol concentrations.

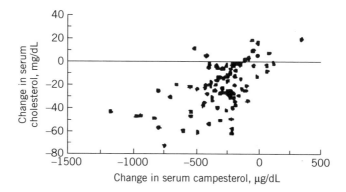

Figure 10-6. Correlation of changes in the total cholesterol concentration with those in the campesterol concentration after consumption of 2.6 g of sitostanol ester margarine per day for 6 months (*r* = .57, *p* < 0.001). *[From Miettinen et al. (4). Reproduced from N Engl J Med 333:1308–1312, 1995, with permission from the Massachusetts Medical Society.]*

Note that only 32% (the *r*-value squared, 0.57^2) of the variability in the change seen in serum cholesterol concentrations is accounted for by the change in serum campesterol. Finally, note that while this is not a strong relationship, it does show that these two variables are related to one another (see Fig. 10-6).

Figures 10-7 and 10-8 are from a study that compared the pharmacokinetics and pharmacologic effects of omeprazole in white and Chinese subjects.[5] One of the purposes of this study was to see whether the pharmacokinetics of omeprazole are related to the urinary enantiomeric ratio (S/R ratio) of mephenytoin, which would indicate that its metabolism is dependent on the CYP2C19 cytochrome P450 isozyme. Another purpose was to relate the pharmacologic effect of omeprazole as measured by plasma gastrin plasma concentrations of omeprazole to omeprazole AUC. The correlation between urinary S/R mephenytoin ratio and omeprazole AUC is shown in Fig. 10-7. This is a statistically significant relationship (*p* < 0.001) with an *r*-value of 0.82, indicating a very good and possibly predictive correlation. One might make this interpretation without looking at the figure. However, Fig. 10-7 actually shows a nonpredictive correlation that is heavily reliant on two outlying data points. Visually remove the two points in the upper right-hand part of the graph and then see if there is a relationship between the two variables. There is not. Also note that there is a noticeable gap in the data points between urinary S/R mephenytoin ratios of 0.4 and 0.8. It is not known what omeprazole AUC values would be in this range of mephenytoin ratios. A line drawn through this area, as has been done, can in some ways be misleading by drawing the reader's attention to areas in the correlation where there are no data points.

KEY CONCEPT

Always visually inspect correlation analyses for outlying data points that will change the characteristics of the correlation if removed from the analysis. Also watch for gaps that might exist in data sets.

Now look at Fig. 10-8, which shows the relationship between gastrin AUC and omeprazole AUC. This has the same p- and r-values as the previous example ($p < 0.001$ and $r = 0.82$), showing a statistically significant correlation that is very good and may be predictive. In contrast with the previous example, all of the data points are scattered fairly close to the regression line over the omeprazole AUC ranges given. Note that the data point in the far upper right-hand corner may be evaluated as an outlier. However, removal of this point would not change the interpretation of this correlation analysis. In contrast with the previous example, it can be readily concluded that these two variables (gastrin and omeprazole AUC) are related to one another.

Note the difference in the interpretation of two data sets with identical r-values and the same number of observations. The only difference is in how the data is scattered in the two graphs. In order to interpret correlation analyses one must be able to look at the data.

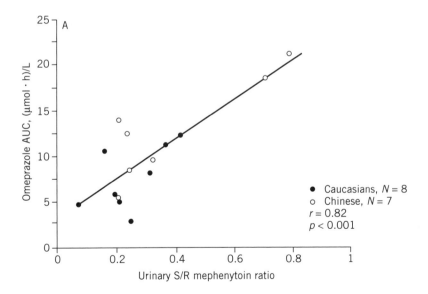

Figure 10-7. Correlation between mephenytoin S/R ratio and omeprazole AUC. *[From Caraco et al. (5). Reproduced from Clin Pharmacol Ther 60:163, 1996, with permission from Mosby, Inc.]*

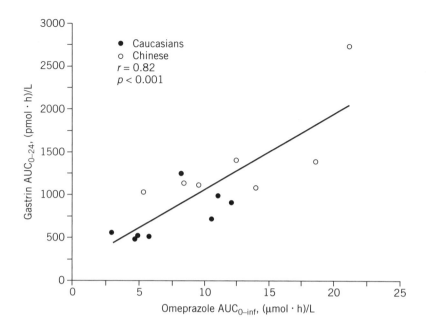

Figure 10-8. Correlation between omeprazole AUC and 24-h plasma gastrin AUC. *[From Caraco et al. (5). Reproduced from Clin Pharmacol Ther 60:157–167, 1996, with permission from Mosby, Inc.]*

KEY CONCEPT

Always visually inspect correlation analyses before making any conclusions.

Regression Analysis

Very often it is desirable to be able to predict one variable from another. This can be very helpful in determining pharmacokinetic parameters from patient information such as weight, age, or measurements of renal or hepatic function. Regression analysis can also be used to test the ability of model equations (such as the Hill equation, which relates pharmacologic effect to drug concentration) to predict a dependent variable from another independent variable. Regression analysis is commonly done to predict drug clearance from creatinine clearance and then use this information to develop dosing nomograms that can be used in patients with renal dysfunction. As an example, Table 10-2 shows a nomogram for dosing aminoglycoside antibiotics in patients with renal failure that was published in the *AHFS Drug Information 2000* text by the American Society of Health-System

Pharmacists. This is a very widely used nomogram that was developed from the correlation between aminoglycoside half-life and creatinine clearance.

Linear Regression Analysis

When regression analysis is based on a straight-line relationship, it is referred to as *linear regression analysis;* when the relationship is not a straight line (e.g., exponential or quadratic), it is referred to as *nonlinear regression analysis.* In both cases, the process is the same. The data is fitted to an equation that best describes the relationship. In most cases, this equation is that of a straight line:

$$y = mx + b \qquad\qquad (10\text{-}5)$$

where m is the slope of the line and b is the intercept value on the y axis. Regression analysis will obtain the best values for m and b that are described by the x, y data points. Typically, the output of regression analysis will be estimates for the values of m and b that describe the regression line and the correlation parameters, r-value, and p-value as described previously.

CASE STUDY

A study evaluated the disposition of piperacillin and tazobactam in 42 patients with varying degrees of stable renal failure, 5 patients on hemodialysis, 5 patients on chronic ambulatory peritoneal dialysis, and 8 health volunteers.[6] The total body clearance and renal clearance of these antibiotics were compared to creatinine clearance, a measure of renal function. Figure 10-9 shows this relationship for tazobactam. Both total body clearance and renal clearance of tazobactam correlate very well with creatinine clearance over creatinine clearance values ranging from 10 to 150 mL/min, with good representation of data throughout this range. Note that both total body clearance ($r^2 = 0.845$; $r = 0.919$) and renal clearance ($r^2 = 0.872$; $r = 0.934$) are highly correlated with creatinine clearance, showing that about 85 to 90% of the variance of tazobactam total and renal clearance is explained by creatinine clearance. The regression line for total body clearance Cl and creatinine clearance Cl_{cr} is as follows:

$$Cl, mL/min = 1.292 \times Cl_{cr} + 66.7$$

Thus, for any creatinine clearance value, a Cl value for tazobactam can be calculated.

Look at Fig. 10-9 and see the possible ranges of Cl that can occur for any given Cl_{cr} value. For most creatinine clearance values there is almost a twofold possible range of tazobactam clearance. For example, at a creatinine clearance of 50 mL/min, tazobactam Cl can range from about 75 to 150 mL/min. This might be acceptable for a drug with a fairly wide therapeutic range, such as this irreversible inhibitor of β-lactamase. It may not be for drugs with narrower therapeutic indexes, such as aminoglycoside antibiotics. This is why one should always visually inspect regression analyses, even those with fairly high r- and r^2-values.

TABLE 10-2. **Aminoglycoside Dosing for Adults with Renal Impairment**

Do not use in hemodialysis or peritoneal dialysis patients or in children.

Select loading dose in mg/kg (based on estimated ideal body weight) to provide peak serum concentrations in range listed for desired aminoglycoside.

Aminoglycoside	Usual Loading Dose, mg/kg	Expected Peak Serum Concentration, μg/mL
Tobramycin gentamicin	1–2	4–10
Amikacin kanamycin	5.0–7.5	15–30

Select maintenance dose (as percentage of chosen loading dose) to continue peak serum concentration indicated above according to desired dosing interval and the patient's corrected (for a 70-kg ideal body weight) creatinine clearance Cl_{cr}.

$$Cl_{cr} \text{ male} = \frac{(140 - \text{age})}{\text{serum creatinine}}$$

$$Cl_{cr} \text{ female} = 0.85 \times Cl_{cr} \text{ male}$$

Cl_{cr}, mL/min	Half-life,* h	8 h	12 h	24 h
90	3.1	84%	—	—
80	3.4	80	91%	—
70	3.9	76	88	—
60	4.5	71	84	—
50	5.3	65	79	—
40	6.5	57	72	92%
30	8.4	48	63	86
25	9.9	43	57	81
20	11.9	37	50	75
17	13.6	33	46	70
15	15.1	31	42	67
12	17.9	27	37	61
10†	20.4	24	34	56
7	25.9	19	28	47
5	31.5	16	23	41
2	46.8	11	16	30
0	69.3	8	11	21

*Alternatively, one-half of the chosen loading dose may be given at an interval approximately equal to the estimated half-life.

†Dosing for patients with $Cl_{cr} \leq 10$ mL/min should be assisted by measured serum concentrations.

SOURCE: From GK McEvoy (ed): *AHFS Drug Information 2000*. American Society of Health-System Pharmacists, 2000. [Reproduced with permission from the American College of Physicians–American Society of Internal Medicine, who is not responsible for the accuracy of the translation, and the American Society of Health-System Pharmacists.]

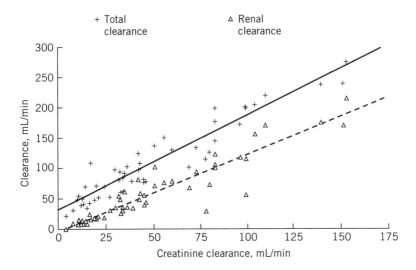

Figure 10-9. Tazobactam total body clearance versus creatinine clearance (predialysis patients): $y = 27.9 + 1.572x$; $r^2 = 0.845$; $p < 0.001$. Tazobactam renal clearance versus creatinine clearance (predialysis patients): $y = -3.2 + 1.27x$; $r^2 = 0.872$; $p < 0.001$. *[From Johnson et al. (6). Reproduced from Clin Pharmacol Ther 51:32–41, 1992, with permission from Mosby, Inc.]*

A study by Lande et al. analyzed the effect of dofetilide, a Class III antiarrhythmic drug, on QT interval prolongation in healthy male volunteers.[7] Figure 10-10 shows the relationship between the RRs and QTs interval during the baseline period and after exposure to dofetilide. Note the very high correlation value in both cases ($r = 0.99$), with each data point occurring on the regression line. The QTs interval can be accurately predicted from the RRs interval in this subject. Note that the two regression lines are as follows:

$$\text{QTs, ms} = 0.102 \text{ RRs} + 289 \qquad \text{Baseline}$$

$$\text{QTs, ms} = 0.144 \text{ RRs} + 303 \qquad \text{Dofetilide}$$

The QTs interval is prolonged by dofetilide, as indicated by a higher intercept value (303 vs. 289 ms). A steeper slope is also seen during dofetilide therapy (0.144 vs. 0.102), so that during dofetilide therapy a greater change in the QTs interval is seen for a given change in the RRs interval. This illustrates how regression analysis can be used to determine the effects that a drug may have on a physiologic parameter such as ventricular repolarization.

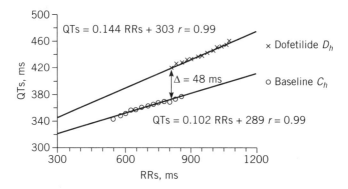

Figure 10-10. Correlation of QTs interval versus RRs interval at baseline and during dofetilide therapy in one volunteer. *[From Lande et al. (7). Reproduced from Clin Pharmacol Ther 64:312–321, 1998, with permission from Mosby, Inc.]*

Nonlinear Regression Analysis

When data can be fitted to an equation that is not a straight-line equation, nonlinear regression analysis is used. This procedure will provide estimates for the parameters in the equation that best describes the mathematical relationship between the x and y variables. This can be any equation that describes a relationship between two variables, and that equation can have more than two parameters that can be estimated using nonlinear regression. For example, a large number of drugs follow a two-compartment pharmacokinetic behavior such that the relationship between concentration C and time t can be described as follows:

$$C = A^{-\alpha t} + B^{-\beta t} \tag{10-6}$$

where A and B are intercept values and α and β are slope values. Nonlinear regression analysis will provide the best values for A, α, B, and β that describe how drug concentration behaves in time after an intravenous dose of a drug.

CASE STUDY

A study by Kichimoto et al. determined the effect of increasing doses of propofol in the topographic electroencephalogram (EEG) in normal volunteers.[8] A total of 10 volunteers received intravenous doses of propofol over targeted plasma concentration ranges of 0 to 1200 ng/mL. The EEG was recorded and then compared to propofol concentrations using the following equation:

$$\text{EEG} = \frac{E_{\max}C^n}{ED_{50} + C^n} \tag{10-7}$$

where $E_{\max}$ is the maximal effect, ED_{50} is the concentration at 50% of maximum effect, C is propofol concentration, and n is the slope of this curve. The relationship

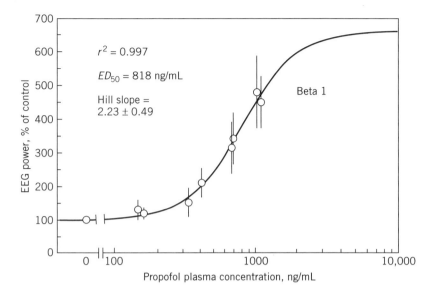

Figure 10-11. Correlation between EEG power and plasma propofol concentrations. *[From Kichimoto et al. (8). Reproduced from Clin Pharmacol Ther 58:666–674, 1995, with permission from Mosby, Inc.]*

between EEG and propofol concentration is shown in Fig. 10-11. Note that this is not a linear relationship, so a nonlinear regression analysis will be used. The three parameters that will be estimated are n, E_{max}, and the ED_{50} value. In this example, they reported a value of 2.23 for n (Hill slope), and 818 ng/mL as the ED_{50} value. A very strong relationship was found ($r^2 = 0.997$) when correlating EEG power to propofol concentration. As with all regression analyses, it needs to be kept in mind that estimates of parameters are obtained. When these data are obtained, the parameters provided by the regression analysis are given with an estimate of variance (usually a sum of squares value) that will provide the researcher with an idea of how reliable the estimates are. In most cases, variance estimates for regression analysis are not provided in manuscripts. One needs to use one's knowledge in the area in which one is reading coupled with how the data actually appear when interpreting data from regression analyses.

KEY CONCEPT

Regression analysis provides estimates for parameters such as slope and intercept. These are best guesses for what the true values may be. They should be interpreted as such—as a good guess.

Survival Analysis

Only a very brief description of survival analysis is presented here. This is sometimes referred to as *time series analysis*. The purpose of this procedure is to look at how an outcome variable may change over time. The variable does not have to be survival, but it does have to be a one-time event. The data used for survival analysis is nominal in nature—the event either occurred or it did not occur.

Outcomes such as mortality or the occurrence of events such as acute myocardial infarction, onset of breast cancer, or discharge from an intensive care unit can all be analyzed using survival analysis. Very often the effectiveness of drug regimens in reducing mortality or increasing survival are compared.

There are two methods for determining a survival curve. One is an actuarial method that divides the x axis into regular time intervals (days, months, years) and then calculates the survival data for that appropriate interval. A more common approach is the Kaplan-Meier method. As opposed to calculating survival within predefined intervals, the Kaplan-Meier method recalculates survival each time there is a change in event occurrence (e.g., each time a patient dies). This is a fairly straightforward approach; however, it is much more tedious than the actuarial analysis. Examples of how survival analysis is shown in literature articles are given, with the purpose of introducing the reader to this topic.

A study published by the Global Use of Strategies to Open Occluded Coronary Arteries in Acute Coronary Syndromes (GUSTO IIb) Angioplasty Substudy Investigators compared treatment with angioplasty to accelerated thrombolytic therapy with tissue plasminogen activator (tPA) in patients who presented within 12 hours of an acute myocardial infarction.[9] The endpoint of the study was a composite outcome of death, nonfatal reinfarction, and nonfatal disabling stroke at 30 days. The incidence of the composite endpoint was 9.6% in the angioplasty group and 13.7% in the tPA group (OR-0.67; 95%, CI, 0.47 to 0.97; see Chap. 9 for a discussion of odds ratio). The composite events were statistically significant while individually they were not: 5.7% of the angioplasty patients died, as compared to 7.0 percent of the tPA patients ($p = 0.37$); the incidence of reinfarction was 4.5 and 6.5% ($p = 0.13$), respectively; and the incidence of disabling stroke was 0.2 and 0.9% ($p = 0.11$). The survival analysis curve comparing overall survival over 30 days is shown in Fig. 10-12. Note that the y axis in this curve starts at 90, so the differences in survival between the angioplasty and tPA group will be exaggerated. Shortening the axis will always magnify the results displayed. Even with this exaggeration there is no strong apparent difference in survival between these groups compared over the 30-day evaluation period. The survival analysis curve for freedom from composite events is shown in Fig. 10-13. Again note that the y axis starts at 0.86, which again will exaggerate the differences between the treatment groups. Also note that freedom from composite event occurrence is very similar between the two groups through about 5 days, at which point the curves for the two treatments diverge, with higher freedom from event occurrence being evident with the angioplasty group.

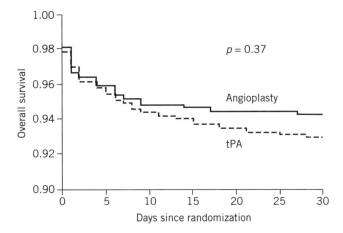

Figure 10-12. Kaplan-Meier curves for survival in the study patients within the 30 days after randomization, according to treatment group. *[From GUSTO IIb (9). Reproduced from N Engl J Med 336(23):1621–1628, 1997, with permission from the Massachusetts Medical Society.]*

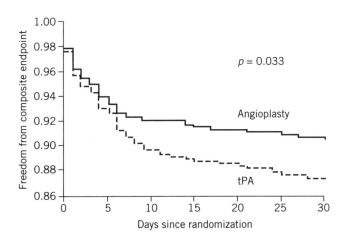

Figure 10-13. Kaplan-Meier curves for freedom from the composite endpoint of death. *[From GUSTO IIb (9). Reproduced from N Engl J Med 336(23):1621–1628, 1997, with permission from the Massachusetts Medical Society.]*

A study published by the Bypass Angioplasty Revascularization Investigation (BARI) Investigators compared the outcomes of patients with multivessel coronary artery disease who were treated with coronary artery bypass grafting (CABG; $n = 914$) to those who were treated with percutaneous transluminal coronary angioplasty (PTCA; $n = 915$).[10] Overall survival and survival free from Q-wave myocardial infarction are shown in Fig. 10-14. Very often with survival life analysis, a large number of patients are included at the start of the study, but very few are followed through the entire duration. This is referred to as *censored survival data,* since not all of the patients who enter the study are analyzed, and their data therefore cannot be used for analysis. In this sense the data is considered to be censored. This is particularly true for studies that have long follow-up periods (e.g., 5 or 10 years). This is illustrated in Fig. 10-14. At time 0 in this study, 914 patients were in the CABG group and 915 were in the PTCA group. At 3 years, there were 857 and 840 in the overall survival category in each respective group. By 5 years, the numbers had decreased to 542 and 537, respectively. The reasons why the numbers of patients evaluated toward the end of survival analysis studies are lower than at the beginning are as follows:

1. Patients are enrolled in the study who have not met the endpoint outcome (i.e., they are alive, but they have not been followed over the entire time frame used for the survival analysis).

2. Patients drop out of the study.

When evaluating survival analyses, always look to see that the data are reasonably comparable between the groups being compared over the entire duration of the survival curve. In particular, dropout rates should be similar between compared groups.

KEY CONCEPT

When comparing censored data between two or more groups using survival analysis techniques, evaluate the dropout rates between the compared groups.

Survival analysis is an often-used statistical procedure. The purpose of this section is to introduce the reader to how data is displayed by authors who use this procedure. Graphical manipulation is common when presenting survival curves. This will magnify the y axis and exaggerate differences, so always be aware of the scale used on the y axis. Always be careful about interpreting the data toward the end of survival curves that display data over a long period (5 to 10 years). The number of patients evaluated at the end of the evaluation period could be very dif-

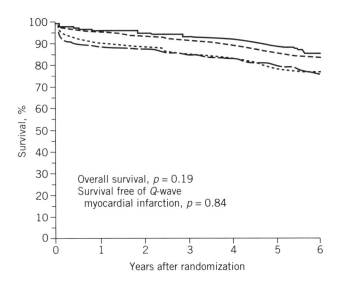

Overall Survival			
CABG	914	857	542
PTCA	915	840	537

Survival Free of Infarction			
CABG	914	782	485
PTCA	915	780	487

Figure 10-14. Overall survival (heavy lines) and survival free from Q-wave myocardial infarction (light lines) after study entry. Patients assigned to CABG are indicated by solid lines, and patients assigned to PTCA by dashed lines. The numbers of patients at risk are shown below the graph at baseline, 3 years, and 5 years. *[From BARI (10). Reproduced from N Engl J Med 335(4):217–225, 1996, with permission from the Massachusetts Medical Society.]*

ferent from that evaluated at the beginning. The number of observations between groups could also be different because of differences in dropout rates.

Summary

Correlation and regression analysis are frequently used statistical procedures. They determine whether two variables are related to one another. Caution must be used in interpreting the results of correlation analyses. Remember that a statistically significant relationship often may not be clinically important. You must always visualize the relationship, and match your visual interpretation with the statistical conclusions drawn. Keep in mind the following key points:

1. Look to see if the two variables are correlated with one another.

2. Data presented should cover the entire range of x, y data points, with no large gaps identified.

3. Be careful regarding how outlying data points influence the correlation.

When evaluating regression analyses, again visually inspect the relationship. Look closely and see what the possible ranges in x values may be for any given y value. This will give you an idea of the error that could be made using the regression equations. If this is an acceptable range of error in prediction, then the relationship can be used. If the range is unacceptable for the drug involved, be cautious about overinterpreting the exactness of the results. Remember to use your experience and common sense when interpreting data from correlation and regression analyses. Never accept results without looking at the scattergram of the data.

Study Questions

1. The pharmacokinetics and pharmacodynamics of tamsulosin, a selective α_1-adrenergic receptor antagonist activity, was evaluated in nine healthy normotensive men with an age range of 21 to 38 years.[11] Figure 10-15 shows the correlation between systolic blood pressure (SBP) and diastolic blood pressure (DBP) and tamsulosin concentrations.

   a. Which is the dependent variable? Why?

   b. Which is the independent variable? Why?

   c. Is this an example of a positive or negative correlation analysis? How would you describe the strength of these analyses?

   d. Approximately what percent of the variability in the change in SBP and the change in DBF is explained by tamsulosin concentrations?

2. The statistical results showed a p-value of 0.08 relating the change in SBP to tamsulosin concentrations and $p = 0.11$ for change in DBP.

   a. What is the statistical conclusion?

   b. What factors influence the statistical result of a correlation analysis?

   c. Which of these factors had the primary influence on this statistical result? Why?

3. The following statement occurs in this paper in reference to Fig. 10-15:

   Although statistically insignificant, negative correlations were observed between plasma tamsulosin concentrations and the changes in systolic blood pressure ($r = -0.42$; $p = 0.08$) and diastolic blood pressure ($r = -0.36$; $p = 0.11$) caused by standing up.

Comment on the accuracy and intent of this statement. Does it reflect the data in the figures?

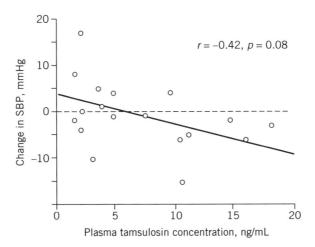

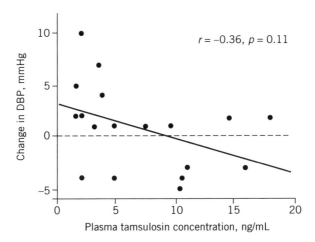

Figure 10-15. Correlation between (*a*) systolic blood pressure (SBP) and (*b*) diastolic blood pressure (DBP) and tamsulosin concentrations. *[From Harada et al. (11). Reproduced from Clin Pharmacol Ther 67:405–412, 2000, with permission from Mosby, Inc.]*

4. The pharmacokinetics and pharmacodynamics of argatroban, a small-molecule synthetic thrombin inhibitor, were studied in healthy volunteers ($n = 52$), patients with hepatic dysfunction ($n = 5$), and patients with varying degrees of renal dysfunction ($n = 24$).[12] Figure 10-16 shows a scattergram of ACT, (Fig. 10-16a) and a PTT, (Fig. 10-16b) versus predicted argatroban plasma concentrations.

   a. What are the dependent and independent variables? Why?

   b. This is an example of what type of statistical procedure?

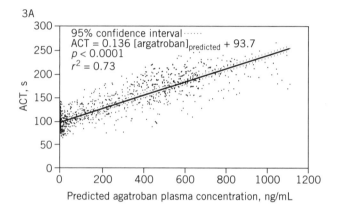

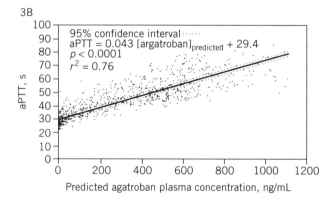

Figure 10-16. (*a*) ACT and (*b*) aPTT versus predicted argatroban concentration for all subjects. Equations represent regression parameters calculated from pooled data. *[From Swan and Hursting (12). Reproduced from Pharmacotherapy 20:318–329, 2000, with permission from Pharmacotherapy Publications, Inc.]*

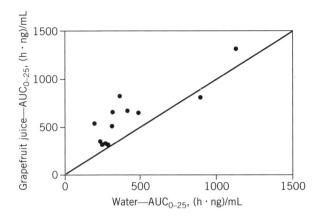

Figure 10-17. Relationship between cisapride area under the plasma concentration–time curve from 0 to 25 hours [AUC_{0-25}; (h · ng)/mL] after ingestion with water or grapefruit juice ($r_s = 0.747$; $p = .003$; $n = 13$). The line of unity is shown. *[From Gross et al. (13). Reproduced from Clin Pharmacol Ther 65:395–401, 1999, with permission from Mosby, Inc.]*

c. What is the correlation coefficient? How strong is this correlation?

d. Can response (ACT or aPTT) be predicted from argatropin concentrations? How much variance can be seen in response for a given argatropin concentration?

5. The effect of grapefruit juice on the pharmacokinetics of cisapride was studied in 14 normal healthy volunteers.[13] Figure 10-17 shows the relationship between cisapride area under the plasma concentration–time curve (AUC) after ingestion with water (*x* axis) or grapefruit juice (*y* axis). The line shown is the unity line.

a. Why was a Spearman rank correlation used to analyze this relationship?

b. What impact do outliers have on the interpretation of this relationship?

6. Methotrexate at a weekly dose of 25 mg intramuscularly was compared to placebo in patients with active Crohn's disease.[14] Figure 10-18 shows remission rates weeks since randomization.

a. What type of statistical test would be used to compare remission rates over time between the methotrexate group and placebo?

b. Compare the number of patients in each group at the beginning and the end of the study. Are the numbers the same or different?

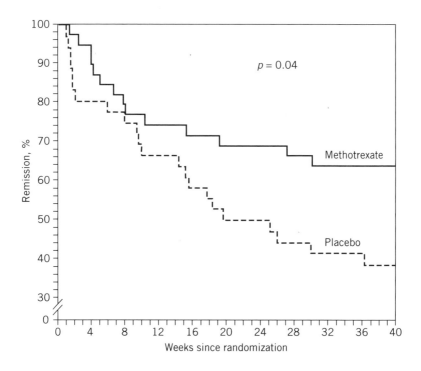

Group	No. at Risk										
Methotrexate	40	36	30	29	28	27	27	26	25	24	19
Placebo	36	29	28	24	21	18	18	15	15	15	12

Figure 10-18. Methotrexate versus placebo in patients with active Crohn's disease. *[From Feagan et al. (14). Reproduced from N Engl J Med 342:1627–1632, 2000, with permission from the Massachusetts Medical Society.]*

References

1. van den Anker JN, Schoemaker RC, Hop WCJ, et al: Ceftazidime pharmacokinetics in preterm infants: Effects of renal function and gestational age. Clin Pharmacol Ther 58:650–659, 1995.

2. Bergquist C, Lindegard J, Salmonson T: Dosing recommendations in liver disease (letter to the editor). Clin Pharmacol Ther 66:201–204, 1999.

3. de Hoog M, Schoemaker RC, Mouton JW, van den Anker, JN: Tobramycin pharmacokinetics in neonates. Clin Pharmacol Ther 62:392–399, 1997.

4. Miettinen TA, Puska P, Gylling H, et al: Reduction of serum cholesterol with sitostanol-ester margarine in a mildly hypercholesterolemic population. N Engl J Med 333:1308–1312, 1995.

5. Caraco Y, Lagerstrom P-O, Wood AJJ: Ethnic and genetic determinants of omeprazole disposition and effect. Clin Pharmacol Ther 60:157–167, 1996.

6. Johnson CA, Halstenson CE, Kelloway JS, et al: Single-dose pharmacokinetics of piperacillin and tazobactam in patients with renal disease. Clin Pharmacol Ther 51:32–41, 1992.

7. Lande G, Maison-Blanche P, Fayn J, et al: Dynamic analysis of dofetilide-induced changes in ventricular repolarization. Clin Pharmacol Ther 64:312–321, 1998.

8. Kichimoto T, Kadoya C, Sneyd R, et al: Topographic electroencephalogram of propofol-induced conscious sedation. Clin Pharmacol Ther 58:666–674, 1995.

9. The Global Use of Strategies to Open Occluded Coronary Arteries in Acute Coronary Syndromes (GUSTO IIb) Angioplasty Substudy Investigators: A clinical trial comparing primary coronary angioplasty with tissue plasminogen activator for acute myocardial infarction. N Engl J Med; 336(23):1621–1628, 1997.

10. The Bypass Angioplasty Revascularization Investigation (BARI) Investigators: Comparison of coronary bypass surgery with angioplasty in patients with multivessel disease. N Engl J Med 335(4):217–225, 1996.

11. Harada K, Kawaguchi A, Ohmori M, Fujimura A: Antagonistic activity of tamulosin against human vascular α_1-adrenergic receptors. Clin Pharmacol Ther 67:405–412, 2000.

12. Swan SK, Hursting MJ: The pharmacokinetics and pharmacodynamics of argatroban: Effects of age, gender and hepatic or renal dysfunction. Pharmacotherapy 20:318–329, 2000.

13. Gross AS, Goh YD, Addison RS, Shenfield GM: Influence of grapefruit juice on cisapride pharmacokinetics. Clin Pharmacol Ther 65:395–401, 1999.

14. Feagan BG, Fedorak RN, Irvine J, et al: A comparison of methotrexate with placebo for the maintenance of remission in Crohn's disease. N Engl J Med 342:1627–1632, 2000.

Critical Appraisal of Meta-analyses

John Devlin

OUTLINE

Goals and Objectives

Clinical Scenario

Introduction

Role of Meta-analysis in Evidence-Based Medicine

Advantages of Meta-analyses

The Focused Clinical Question

Criteria to Select Articles for Inclusion

Identifying Relevant Studies for Inclusion into the Meta-analysis

Appraising the Validity of Included Studies

Identifying Heterogeneity

Combining Studies

Interpreting the Results

Applying the Results to Patient Care

Study Questions

References

KEY WORDS

Meta-analysis	Cochrane collaboration
Systematic reviews	Medical literature
Heterogeneity	Critical appraisal
Evidence-based medicine	Statistics

Goals and Objectives

After reading this chapter, the reader should be able to:

1. Describe what a *meta-analysis* is, as well as the indications and contraindications for its use.

2. Discuss the role of the meta-analysis when providing evidence-based medicine to patients.

3. Understand the key methodological steps that must be completed in a well-designed meta-analysis.

4. Define *heterogeneity* and list common methods that are used to detect and minimize it.

5. Differentiate between the traditional and random-effects statistical models that are used to combine primary studies in a meta-analysis.

6. Discuss methodological factors that may affect meta-analysis quality.

7. Identify factors that may limit the meta-analysis as a replacement for the large randomized, controlled trial.

8. Be able to interpret the results of a meta-analysis and apply these results to the care of patients.

Clinical Scenario

A 55-year-old female is admitted to the medical ward at your hospital with pre-sumed pyelonephritis and started on 80 mg intravenous gentamicin every 8 h and 2 g intravenous ampicillin every 6 h. On patient rounds, the medical resident asks you, the clinical pharmacist, if this patient's gentamicin should be changed to a once-daily dosing regimen because he heard that it is associated with better efficacy and decreased toxicity. A Medline search identifies 26 studies that compare once-daily aminoglycoside dosing to traditional dosing. Study results appear equivocal. Some of the studies conclude that once-daily aminoglycoside dosing is superior, whereas others find traditional dosing to be the preferred dosing strategy. In addi-tion, not all of the studies measured aminoglycoside-related nephrotoxity as an endpoint, and the types of patients and the infections these patients had varied con-siderably between studies. As you start to search further, one of your pharmacist colleagues enters the library. After you explain this therapeutic dilemma to her, she suggests looking for a meta-analysis of trials comparing traditional to once-daily aminoglycoside dosing. Further Medline searching locates such a meta-analysis, re-cently published in *Annals of Internal Medicine,* and you sit down to review it.[1]

Introduction

The pharmacy clinician is faced with an ever expanding pharmacotherapy litera-ture.[2] State-of-the-art reviews of a particular drug therapy or disease state, which include recent and pertinent studies, are published to aid practitioners in making informed therapeutic decisions. Until recently, most therapeutic reviews were nar-rative in nature and were authored by a recognized expert in the field. These re-views usually included a qualitative summary of studies that were felt by the author to be important to the topic at hand. The review usually ended with a series of conclusions based on the evidence presented. Narrative reviews, however, have inherent weaknesses that compromise validity, including author bias in relation to the choice of studies included in the review and the conclusions that are drawn.[3]

Authors frequently include only those studies that support their own viewpoint or that are published by thought leaders in prestigious journals.[2-5]

In narrative reviews, clinicians frequently compare the number of positive studies supporting a particular therapy with those studies showing negative results.[4] With this "vote-counting" exercise, large and small studies are given equal weights. In addition, studies with potentially nonsignificant (but potentially clinically important) results are counted as negative. Moreover, a reader cannot tell anything about the magnitude of the clinical effect using vote counting, even when studies are appropriately classified into those demonstrating a positive or negative therapeutic trend.

To avoid the subjectivity and poor construct validity of narrative reviews, the concept of systematic overviews was developed in the 1970s.[6] Systematic reviews assemble, critically appraise, and synthesize the results of primary investigations addressing a specific topic or problem. The explicit methods by which they are completed limit bias and random error. Meta-analyses, a quantitative synthesis, using statistical techniques, of two or more studies of the same outcome, are the most robust type of systematic overview. Systematic reviewers, in general, will set out trying to complete a meta-analysis of the primary literature for the clinical question being asked. In many cases, however, a meta-analysis may not be able to be completed because of a lack of studies or excessive methodological disparity between studies. A best-evidence synthesis is produced instead.[5-7]

Role of Meta-analysis in Evidence-Based Medicine

Evidence-based medicine, incorporating timely, pertinent evidence from the medical literature into clinical practice, should be an integral component of clinical decision making for every health practitioner. Many clinicians, however, lack the time, motivation, and basic skills needed to find, critically appraise, and synthesize individual primary studies into practice. Meta-analyses are increasingly being used in practice not only to make therapeutic decisions for individual patients but to summarize evidence when developing practice guidelines and completing pharmacoeconomic analyses.[4] In addition, systematic reviews such as meta-analyses can be a useful decision-making tool for health care consumers and policymakers by objectively summarizing large amounts of information, identifying gaps in medical research, and identifying beneficial or harmful interventions.[4]

More than 1000 meta-analyses have been published up to 1999 with countless more available from other sources such as the Internet.[2] More recently, a worldwide network of clinicians, epidemiologists, and other health professionals has been established.[8] The Cochrane Collaboration promotes the preparation, maintenance, and dissemination of systematic reviews of the effects of health care. Currently, the Collaboration has over 15 international sites, each concomitantly working on hundreds of systematic overview projects. Another important objective of the Cochrane Collaboration, through the Internet, is to continuously update all systematic overviews and meta-analyses as new clinical trial evidence becomes available.[9,10]

Meta-analysis has several advantages, as detailed in Table 11-1.[3–5,7] It has the ability to combine findings from smaller studies to generate a more precise and robust conclusion. For example, eight small, randomized studies individually were underpowered to show a reduction in mortality when streptokinase was administered to patients with acute myocardial infarction. When these studies were pooled, however, they showed a significant decrease in mortality associated with streptokinase therapy that was later confirmed in a larger randomized, controlled trial.[11] A meta-analysis can help arbitrate between studies that generate different conclusions. Finally, it can inform clinicians about efficacy and toxicity-related endpoints that are not studied in the primary clinical trial. Although meta-analyses have many advantages and strengths over traditional therapeutic reviews, they may result in false conclusions, like any statistical manipulation, if completed incorrectly.[12,13] Meta-analyses are most useful for summarizing clinical trial evidence and identifying sources of heterogeneity. Their value in definitively assessing the efficacy of a clinical intervention still remains somewhat controversial. In addition, controversy surrounds the validity of the conclusions that can be made from meta-analyses and whether the meta-analysis is a replacement for the large, randomized controlled study.[11,14–16]

This chapter, in the context of the clinical decision presented, will review the components of a good meta-analysis, specifically highlighting the common methodological pitfalls that may lead to false conclusions and/or discordant results.[2,3,17] The science of meta-analysis is imperfect; clinical pharmacists must always scrutinize meta-analyses involving pharmacological interventions before adopting their conclusions into clinical practice.

KEY CONCEPTS

Systematic overviews assemble, critically appraise, and synthesize the results of primary investigations addressing a specific topic or problem.

Qualitative systematic reviews contain a summary of primary studies that are not statistically combined; a *quantitative* review (meta-analysis) results when two or more studies are statistically combined.

Meta-analyses should be planned like any other research project, by preparing a detailed written protocol before starting.

Meta-analyses of rigorously completed studies provide the best tool for practicing evidence-based medicine.

TABLE 11-1. Strengths and Weaknesses of Meta-analysis

Strengths

1. Provides preliminary data for calculation of sample size for a definitive large trial

2. Provides preliminary data for hypotheses to be tested in definitive large trial

3. Reduces possibility of Type II error when small studies show no treatment effect

4. Provides most reliable treatment recommendation in absence of definitive trial

5. Presents an assembly of trial information in a digestible format

Weaknesses

1. Biases and flaws of individual studies are incorporated.

2. New sources of bias may be introduced.

   a. Publication bias (favoring positive findings)

   b. Selection of studies (particular random-effects model) influences results

   i. Small studies tend toward extreme findings.

   ii. Prematurely terminated studies tend toward extreme findings.

3. Heterogeneity between studies may not be addressed adequately.

   a. Study design differences may exist or may not be fully recognized.

   b. Patient populations differ as a function of therapeutic advances over time.

   c. Risk or harm may not be fully recognized, because side effects are less uniformly assessed than primary endpoints.

   d. Statistical techniques testing for (fixed-effects model) or accounting for (random-effects model) heterogeneity are not a substitute for large-scale randomization.

4. Clinically relevant secondary outcomes and adverse effects of treatment may not be fully addressed.

SOURCE: Adapted from Borzak and Ridker (11). Reproduced from Ann Intern Med 123:873–877, 1995, with permission from the American College of Physicians–American Society of Internal Medicine, who is not responsible for the accuracy of the translation.

The Focused Clinical Question

Unless the meta-analysis clearly defines the clinical question it seeks to address, the clinician will have a difficult time determining whether the article is pertinent to the care of his or her patient. The clinical question to be addressed in the meta-analysis should have four basic components: (1) the type of person involved, (2) the type of exposure that the person experiences (e.g., intervention, risk factor, diagnostic test, etc.), (3) the type of control with which the exposure is being compared (e.g., another therapy versus placebo), and (4) the outcome(s) to be measured.[2,3,18] The outcomes to be evaluated should be clinically relevant to the patient. Indirect or surrogate outcome measures, such as laboratory or radiologic results, should be avoided or interpreted with extreme caution because they rarely predict clinically important outcomes accurately.[19] Finally, systematic reviews of therapy should measure not only clinical benefits but also any observed adverse effects.

Meta-analysis should always strive to use the best (i.e., least biased) literature available. Generally, this should be reports of randomized, controlled trials—particularly those having a well-concealed method of treatment allocation.[5] The clinical question to be addressed must not be too general. A broad topic will increase bias and heterogeneity in the analysis and limit the ability to accurately apply the results of the meta-analysis to specific patient populations. Inclusion criteria, however, should not be too narrow, as this may limit the amount of data that is available to include in the review and, thereby, increases the risk for false-positive and false-negative results. If the main question is not clear from the article's title or abstract, it is probably best to seek further articles to answer your question.[12,18]

After reviewing the once-daily aminoglycoside meta-analysis that you have extracted from the literature, you discover the authors have formulated a well-thought-out clinical question: to compare the efficacy, nephrotoxicity, and ototoxicity of once-daily aminoglycoside dosing with those of traditional aminoglycoside dosing regimens in immunocompetent adults.[1]

Criteria to Select Articles for Inclusion

Inclusion and exclusion criteria should be established a priori for each meta-analysis.[17] These should describe a specific methodological design (e.g., randomized, double-blinded), patient study population, and a particular outcome(s). It is important to find the appropriate balance between developing criteria that are not too restrictive (and limiting study inclusion) but not too loose (and thus compromising meta-analysis completion because methodological differences between the studies that are to be combined are excessive).[18,20]

The once-daily aminoglycoside meta-analysis you identified has the following inclusion and exclusion criteria:

1. It has a randomized, controlled study.
2. It compares an intravenous once-daily aminoglycoside regimen with a standard aminoglycoside regimen.
3. It comprises infected, immunocompetent adult patients (excludes surgical prophylaxis).
4. It uses any of the following outcome measures:
   a. Bacteriologic or clinical cure
   b. Mortality
   c. Nephrotoxicity
   d. Ototoxicity

5. It has a patient sample in which fewer than 50% of the patients had a lower urinary tract infection. (Optimal bactericidal levels of aminoglycoside in patients with lower urinary tract infections are achieved regardless of the dosing regimen because the entire daily dose is excreted unchanged into the urine.)[1]

Identifying Relevant Studies for Inclusion into the Meta-analysis

Flaws in data collection may invalidate the results of a systematic review; therefore, as many relevant primary studies as possible must be collected to minimize random error and bias.[18] It is important to use a Medline search strategy that is both sensitive (i.e., identifies all important articles) and specific (i.e., avoids identifying articles that do not fit the established inclusion and exclusion criteria). Mesh headings that correlate with each of the major inclusion and exclusion criteria developed that have been established [e.g., patient group(s), drug intervention, and outcomes of interest should be used]. Other databases such as Embase are sometimes used. See Chap. 2 for information on how to perform a search.

Only 32 to 91% of randomized, controlled trials published in journals indexed by Medline will be identified with a Medline search.[21] This is in large part due to both inadequate indexing and the use of incorrect keywords when the search is completed. Reviewers must take the time to plan their search systematically and obtain help from persons with database expertise. Medline only indexes 4000 of the approximately 16,000 journals available and does not index articles before 1966.[18] Currently, the Cochrane Collaboration is coordinating the manual searching of journals to identify all available randomized, controlled trials and has become one of the best sources of randomized, controlled trials.[22] Reference lists for each study retrieved through Medline should be checked to see if they meet the identified inclusion and exclusion criteria. Other sources of completed, but unpublished, studies include conference proceedings and communication with recognized experts in a particular therapeutic field.[3,18]

For practical reasons, many meta-analyses restrict articles to the English language. This practice is hard to justify, however, as the quality of research does not generally vary by publication language and the exclusion of non-English language studies has been shown to alter overall study results.[23] Unpublished studies should be included in the analysis. Fewer than half of the studies published as abstracts or conference proceedings go on to full publication—many because negative or nonsignificant results were initially reported. Meta-analysts risk introducing publication bias into the analysis, and overestimating the treatment effect, if they overlook studies with inconclusive or negative results (often not published).[21,24] Meta-analysts should account for the presence of publication bias in their overview. It has been shown that overviews of a small number of small studies with weakly positive effects are the most susceptible to publication bias.

Statistical techniques, such as funnel plots and the fail-safe N method, may be used to identify publication bias. Funnel plots are produced by plotting the summarized effect size for the outcome of interest versus the inverse of the variance of the individual study effect sizes. If no publication bias is present, the points produce a funnel shape, with the points centered around the true value of the effect size and the degree of scatter narrowing as variance decreases. The fail-safe N method calculates the number of studies with a z-statistic equal to zero (i.e., no significant result) that would need to exist in order for the combined z-score to become nonsignificant.[25]

After reviewing the meta-analysis, you note that the authors followed many of the methodological steps outlined previously.[1] Specific Medline search criteria were followed. Two reviewers independently completed the search. This technique has been shown to be more effective at retrieving studies than using a single reviewer.[26,27] In addition, interreviewer concordance (i.e., reliability) can be established using this technique. The references of all identified studies were manually searched by the authors, in addition to select infectious disease journals.

Appraising the Validity of Included Studies

Unfortunately, the original peer review process does not guarantee the validity of published research. Differences in study methods might explain important differences among results. For example, less rigorous studies tend to overestimate the effectiveness of therapeutic and preventative interventions.[28] The conclusions drawn from a meta-analysis can only be as valid as the quality of the individual studies that were incorporated into it.

The quality of the individual studies included in each meta-analysis should be appraised before being incorporated into the analysis.[3,12,17] Methods for assessing quality must be reliable (the results do not change if the procedure is repeated), impartial (not influenced by the study results), and explicit (unambiguous). Study quality should be approached with three objectives in mind:

1. To understand the validity of the study

2. To uncover reasons for differences among study results other than chance

3. To provide readers with sufficient information with which to judge for themselves the applicability of the systematic review to their clinical practice[3]

Important quality criteria include the following:

• Were patients randomly assigned to treatment?

• Was follow-up sufficiently thorough and were all of the patients accounted for?

• Were patients analyzed according to the groups to which they were randomly assigned?

• Did proper concealment and blinding occur between control and experimental groups?

Although there is no one correct way to assess quality, it is common to utilize scoring systems or checklists to complete this process. Although quality scoring does not completely eliminate the possibility of bias and does not address an individual study's external validity or statistical quality, it does make the reader aware that the authors went to great lengths to identify weak studies and to decrease their influence on the overall meta-analytic result.

In the aminoglycoside meta-analysis that you are reviewing, the authors used a quality scoring system similar to many others.[29] The total possible score for each article was 12 points: two points each for randomization, follow-up, and blinding, and one point for the remaining six criteria (Table 11-2). When methodological data was missing in the published study that was needed to properly assess quality, the primary author of the study was contacted to obtain the missing information.

Authors of meta-analyses must decide on the clinical studies to include in the analysis, the validity of the studies, and how to accurately extract data from them. Despite following predeveloped inclusion and exclusion criteria, it is challenging to decide which studies and articles should be included in the meta-analysis; thus, each of these decisions is subject to mistakes (random errors) and bias (systematic errors). Having two or more people participate in each decision guards against errors. The use of only one reviewer may introduce bias and distort the results. Degree of agreement between reviewers for study inclusion can be estimated using a kappa test. Good agreement between reviewers ($\kappa > 0.7$) allows the reader to be more confident in the overall results of the overview. It is suggested that reviewers (i.e., data extractors) be blinded to a study's author(s), institution, journal, and date of publication to further minimize extraction bias.[4,12]

KEY CONCEPTS

The clinical question should be developed a priori and should include four major components: (1) people, (2) exposure, (3) control group, and (4) outcome.

Publication bias results when all completed studies are not identified and included in the meta-analysis (e.g., nonpublished, non-English, nonsignificant results).

The presence of bias should be assessed by completing a sensitivity analysis, a funnel plot, or by using the fail-safe N method.

Unpublished, non-peer-reviewed data should not generally be included, particularly if the source of this data is an interested party (e.g., pharmaceutical manufacturer).

A predefined quality score should be used to evaluate the methodological quality (bias), likelihood of random errors (precision), and external validity (applicability to target population group).

TABLE 11-2. Methodological Quality Score

Study (Reference)	Randomization[a]	Follow-up[b]	Blinding of Outcome Assessor[c]	Intention-to-Treat Analysis[d]	Inclusion and Exclusion Criteria Specified	Cointervention[e]	Compliance[f]	Blinding of Patients	Defined Outcome Measures	Methodological Quality Score[g]
Hollender et al.	1	2	2	1	1	1	1	1	1	0.92
Maller et al.	2	2	1	1	1	1	0	0	1	0.75
Maller et al.	2	2	0	1	1	0	1	0	1	0.67
Marik et al.	2	2	0	1	1	1	1	0	1	0.75
Prins et al.	1	0	1	0	1	1	1	0	1	0.50
Sturm	2	2	0	1	1	1	1	0	1	0.75
ter Braak et al.	2	2	0	1	1	1	1	0	1	0.75
Mauracher et al.	1	2	0	1	1	1	1	0	1	0.67
de Vries	2	2	0	0	1	1	1	0	1	0.67
Vanhaeverbeek et al.	2	2	0	1	1	1	1	0	1	0.75
Gonzalez et al.	1	2	0	1	1	0	1	0	1	0.58
Tulkens	0	2	0	1	0	1	1	0	1	0.50
Vreede	2	2	0	1	1	1	1	0	1	0.75

[a]Two points were given for complete concealment of randomization, one point was given for partial concealment, and zero points were given if randomization technique was clearly manipulable or not stated.

[b]Two points were given if more than 50% of randomly assigned patients were accounted for in any of the outcome assessments; zero points were given if fewer than 80% were accounted for.

[c]Two points were given if the assessors were blinded for all outcome assessments; one point was given if the assessors were blinded for some outcome assessments; and zero points were given if the assessors were not blinded.

[d]One point was given for all other quality criteria.

[e]Assessment of whether cointervention antibiotic agents were equally distributed between both intervention groups.

[f]Assessment of whether length of treatment was recorded.

[g]Assessment of trial's methodological quality, obtained by dividing the sum score by the maximum attainable score (12).

SOURCE: From Hatala et al. (1). Reproduced from Ann Intern Med 124:721, 1996, with permission from the American College of Physicians–American Society of Internal Medicine, who is not responsible for the accuracy of the translation.

Identifying Heterogeneity

Despite the use of restrictive inclusion and exclusion criteria when completing a meta-analysis, differences in patients, treatment exposure, outcome measures, and research methods may vary significantly. It should be determined whether any of these identified factors are so different that it no longer makes sense to combine the study results in a meta-analysis. Statistical integration of heterogeneous studies can be misleading and can lead to a pooled estimate that does not apply to the population of interest.[27]

It is important to ascertain whether the studies being combined seem to be measuring the underlying magnitude of effect. Using homogeneity testing, investigators can test the extent to which differences among the results of individual studies are greater than one would expect if all studies were measuring the same underlying effect and the observed differences were due only to chance. The more significant the test of homogeneity [usually a chi-square (χ^2) test], the less likely the observed differences in the size of the effect observed is due to chance alone and that heterogeneity exists between studies. Both the average effect and the confidence interval around the average effect need to be interpreted cautiously because differences in patients, drug exposure and treatment, outcome, or study design may influence the overall study treatment effects observed. It must be noted, however, that heterogeneity testing is notorious for its lack of statistical power and that reviewers must still use caution in interpreting clinically important differences between study results, despite a nonsignificant test of homogeneity.[30]

Readers can also check for heterogeneity in a meta-analysis by visually inspecting the 95% confidence intervals (95% CIs) of the individual studies contained in the Peto diagram (see Fig. 11-1).[31] In a Peto diagram, each horizontal line represents an individual trial; the squares in the middle represent the single best estimate of the odds ratio (OR) of the effect (the larger the square, the larger the sample size in the study); and the width of the horizontal line represents the 95% CI around the estimate. The large vertical line that passes through the horizontal lines at 1.0 is called the *line of no effect*. When the 95% CI of a study crosses the line of no effect, one of two conclusions can be drawn: (1) There was no difference between the treatment and the placebo, or (2) the sample to detect this difference was not large enough. The triangle at the top is the pooled estimate from all the trials (point estimate) and usually has a narrower 95% CI (because of the larger combined sample size). If it does not cross the line of no effect, one can be more confident in inferring that a drug therapy is truly beneficial.

Combining Studies

There are two common methods by which to combine study results when completing a meta-analysis: (1) the traditional model (Mantel-Haenszel test) and (2) the random-effects model (DerSimonian-and-Laird method).[3,7] In general, the Mantel-Haenszel test is the preferred instrument by which to combine studies as randomization is preserved and the proportional size of both the within-study

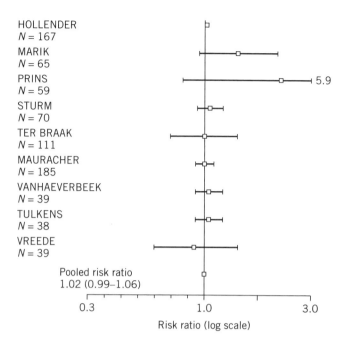

HOLLENDER
N = 167
MARIK
N = 65
PRINS
N = 59   5.9
STURM
N = 70
TER BRAAK
N = 111
MAURACHER
N = 185
VANHAEVERBEEK
N = 39
TULKENS
N = 38
VREEDE
N = 39

Pooled risk ratio
1.02 (0.99–1.06)

0.3   1.0   3.0

Risk ratio (log scale)

Figure 11-1. Peto diagram for bacteriologic cure: once-daily compared with standard aminoglycoside dosing. Individual study and pooled risk ratios for bacteriologic cure, with 95% CIs. Risk ratios to the left of 1.0 favor standard aminoglycoside dosing; those to the right favor once-daily aminoglycoside dosing. *N* = the total individual study sample for the outcome of bacteriologic cure. Test for heterogeneity: *p* > 0.2. Data is from sources cited in Hatala et al. *[From Hatala et al. (1). Reproduced from Ann Intern Med 124:717–725, 1996, with permission from the American College of Physicians–American Society of Internal Medicine, who is not responsible for the accuracy of the translation.]*

population as well as the variance of the study OR is taken into account. In addition, in the absence of statistically significant heterogeneity, the random-effects model may be preferable to the fixed-effects model since it yields a more conservative assessment of overall efficacy and the results can be more easily extrapolated into clinical practice. Moreover, given the generally poor power of heterogeneity testing and the fact that statistical homogeneity does not demonstrate clinical homogeneity, the random-effects model is the preferred statistical method for combining studies.[27]

In the presence of statistically significant heterogeneity, a single summary measure, even if the random-effects model is used, does not usually adequately describe the data. In such settings, the primary objective should be to explore the reasons for the observed heterogeneity.[15] Differences between these two study methodologies are highlighted in Table 11-3. In the once-daily aminoglycoside meta-analysis that you are examining, the authors calculated a pooled risk ratio for each study outcome using a random-effects model (i.e., DerSimonian-and-Laird method) as significant between-study heterogeneity was identified. Heterogeneity was most noticeable as it related to the microbiologic diagnosis of infection and each study's specific definition of bacteriologic and clinical cure.

Sensitivity analysis is a final evaluative step that should be completed at completion of the meta-analysis. Reviewers, by repeating the analysis after excluding one or more of the studies, can identify sources of heterogeneity, studies having the greatest effect on the overall effect size, and elucidate future research hypotheses.

TABLE 11-3. **Comparison Between Traditional and Random-Effects Models**

Traditional Model	*Random-Effects Model*
Mantel-Haenszel test.	DerSimonian-and-Laird method.
To combine OR* or RR* across studies using a weighted average of within-study results.	Used when heterogeneity among study results is suspected, but exploratory analyses have failed to identify the source of the heterogeneity.
ORs are combined across studies with weights that are proportional to the inverse of the variance of the within-study OR.	Incorporates hidden or unmeasured sources of heterogeneity into the weighting scheme when computing a weighted average summary estimate.
Randomization is preserved as comparisons are made within a study prior to combination across studies.	Randomization is not preserved.
More weight is assigned to larger studies than smaller studies (larger studies are more precise).	Assigns higher weights to smaller studies than traditional methods.
Underlying treatment effect that each study is estimating is assumed to be the same for all studies (i.e., any variation is assumed to be random).	Allows for the possibility that the underlying true treatment effect that each study is estimating may not be the same for all studies, even when examining studies with similar designs, protocols, and patient populations.

*OR, odds ratio; RR, relative risk.

> ## KEY CONCEPTS
>
> Results from individual studies should be displayed on a common scale (e.g., Peto diagram) and visually inspected for evidence of heterogeneity.
>
> Methodological features shown empirically to be most associated with heterogeneity in clinical trials include: patient characteristics, dose, randomization, blinding, and the methodology used for outcome assessment.
>
> Showing statistical heterogeneity is a mathematical exercise (e.g., use of χ^2 for homogeneity); explaining heterogeneity (just as important an exercise) requires intuition and clinical and research experience in the field.
>
> While traditional models are usually preferred over random-effects models when combining data because randomization is preserved, the traditional model often cannot be used due to excessive heterogeneity.

Interpreting the Results

Once a clinician is confident that the methodology behind the results of a particular meta-analysis are strong and that the authors were conscientious in minimizing bias, it is time to decide how the results can be applied to patients.[32]

The magnitude of the benefit or harm associated with a given pharmacologic intervention can be presented as relative risk reduction (RRR) or relative risk (RR). Relative risk is the ratio of the risk in the treatment group to that in the control group, and the RRR is simply 1 − RR. The disadvantage of the RRR is that it may falsely magnify the perception of benefit with a specific therapy since it is independent of different baseline risks. A more meaningful way to represent the magnitude of benefit is to calculate the absolute risk reduction (ARR). This is done by subtracting the risk in the treatment group from the risk in the control group (baseline risk) or by multiplying baseline risk by the RRR. A more practical application is to calculate the reciprocal of the ARR, which is referred to as the number necessary to treat (NNT) or the number of patients required to treat or prevent one harmful outcome.[33,34] For example, if only 10/20 (50%) of patients treated with Drug A survive but 15/20 (75%) survive who receive Drug B, then the RRR = 1.5, the ARR = 0.25, and the NNT is 4.

Occasionally, outcome measures that are used in studies are similar but not exactly the same. If the patients and the interventions are reasonably similar, it is possible to estimate the average effect of the intervention on the outcome being studied. One way of doing this is to summarize the results of each study as an "effect size."[35] The effect size is the difference in outcomes between the intervention and control groups divided by the standard deviation(s). The effect size summarizes the results of each study in terms of the number of standard deviations of difference between the intervention and control groups. Investigators can then calculate a weighted average of the effect sizes from studies that measured an outcome in different ways. While it is generally desirable to have a quantitative summary of the results of a structured overview, it is not always appropriate. In some instances, unexplained heterogeneity is excessive or the individual studies are of such poor quality that the overall results would be uninterpretable.

In the aminoglycoside meta-analysis, the authors estimated the pooled risk ratio for the bacteriologic cure endpoint to be 1.02 (95% CI, 0.99–1.05), indicating that the standard and once-daily aminoglycoside dosing regimens are equivalent.[1] For clinical cure, individual trial results were found to be too heterogeneous to combine. Four separate sensitivity analyses, wherein studies were stratified according to the four identified sources of heterogeneity (methodological quality, the specific aminoglycoside used, the cointervention antibiotic used, and the site of infection), still demonstrated significant heterogeneity, and thus individual study results were not pooled to obtain a common risk ratio. The pooled risk ratio for nephrotoxicity was 0.87 (95% CI, 0.35–1.28), corresponding to an RRR of 13% with the once-daily regimen. Given a 10% baseline risk for nephrotoxicity, 77 patients would need to be treated with the once-daily regimen.

Applying the Results to Patient Care

A major advantage of overviews, such as meta-analyses, are that since they include many studies, the results come from a very diverse range of patients.[34] If the results are consistent across studies, they apply to this wide variety of patients. Clinicians need to consider whether their patients fit the demographics of the patients considered in the studies and that the drug therapy that is being considered is exactly what was studied in the meta-analysis. In an effort to measure the effect of drug therapy in a subset of study patients (for example, the elderly), subgroup meta-analyses may be completed. One must view conclusions that are drawn based on between-study subgroup comparisons with some skepticism, however.[20]

Factors increasing the credibility of subgroup analyses include:

- A big difference in the treatment effect
- A highly statistically significant difference in the treatment effect (the lower the p-value, the more credible the difference)
- A hypothesis that was made before the study began and was one of the only hypotheses tested
- Consistency across studies
- Indirect evidence in support of the difference (biologic plausibility)

If these criteria are not met, the results of the subgroup analysis are less likely to be trustworthy, and you should assume that the overall effect across all patients and all treatments, rather than the subgroup effect, applies to the patient at hand and to the treatment under consideration. In summary, meta-analytic subgroup analysis, like subgroup analysis within a clinical trial, is prone to bias and needs to be interpreted with caution.[20]

Does the completion of a meta-analysis preclude the completion of large randomized trials having adequate power to answer the clinical question? There are numerous examples, in a variety of clinical areas that would suggest no.[11,14–16] One review examined the role of thrombolytics, early beta-blocker therapy, nitroglycerin, and magnesium in the setting of acute myocardial infarction (MI).[16] For each of these four post-MI therapies, meta-analyses (combining small clinical trials) were published before the completion of a definitive, large clinical trial. For thrombolytics, the beneficial effects first demonstrated in a meta-analysis have been subsequently confirmed in large randomized, controlled trials. This is not the case, however, with the other three therapies. An early meta-analysis of post-MI beta-blocker therapy demonstrated no benefit; however, a subsequent clinical trial demonstrated a significant mortality benefit. The opposite trend occurred for the post-MI use of both nitroglycerin and magnesium. While initial meta-analyses

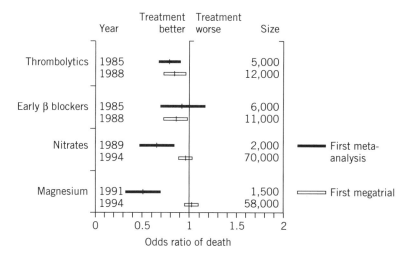

Figure 11-2. Concordance and discordance between meta-analyses and megatrials. Comparison of the ORs and 95% CIs for the given treatments. The first published meta-analysis is shown by the solid bars; the first published megatrial is shown by the open bars. Years of publication are given on the left; the numbers of patients included in each trial or meta-analysis are given on the right. Data is from sources cited in Borzak and Ridker. *[From Borzak and Ridker (11). Reproduced from Ann Intern Med 123:873–877, 1995, with permission from the American College of Physicians–American Society of Internal Medicine, who is not responsible for the accuracy of the translation.]*

suggested benefit, later, large randomized, controlled trials demonstrated no clinical benefit, and in the case of magnesium, suggested harm (Fig. 11-2).

Although the definitive clinical trial has yet to be completed comparing once-daily aminoglycoside therapy with standard dosing, the meta-analysis you have reviewed suggests that standard and once-daily dosing regimens are equivalent with regard to bacteriologic cure, and once-daily dosing shows a trend toward reduced mortality and toxicity. The outcome that the medical resident is most interested in knowing about, however, clinical cure, was not able to be assessed in this meta-analysis because of excessive heterogeneity.

Meta-analysis is now a common statistical method to systematically quantify the vast, ever-increasing amount of clinical trial data. There are numerous methodological pitfalls, however, that can affect the robustness of any conclusions that can be made.[2,12,17] Pharmacists should use a systematic process to scrutinize the methodological quality of meta-analysis before adapting the results of any analysis into clinical practice (Table 11-4).

TABLE 11-4. **Key Points to Consider When Critically Appraising a Meta-analysis**

---

1. Was an important, well-focused question described that includes people, exposure, control group, and outcomes?

2. Were the inclusion and exclusion criteria clear and logical?

3. Was the search strategy sensible, thorough, and clearly reported?

4. Did the authors retrieve data from more than just Medline?

5. Did all of the studies that were selected for inclusion in the meta-analysis undergo the same rigorous critical appraisal process that focused on the rigor of the studies, the sources of heterogeneity between the studies, and did they provide the reader with sufficient detail with which to judge the applicability of the review to their clinical practice.

6. Results from individual studies should be graphically displayed using a common scale to allow for visual examination of heterogeneity.

7. A fixed-effects model is generally preferable to a random-effects model for combining data, unless significant heterogeneity is detected as the fixed-effects model preserves randomization.

8. A thorough sensitivity analysis is essential to assess the robustness of combined estimates to different assumptions and inclusion criteria.

SOURCE: Adapted from Lau et al. (12). Reproduced from Ann Intern Med 127:820–826, 1997, with permission from the American College of Physicians–American Society of Internal Medicine, who is not responsible for the accuracy of the translation.

> ## KEY CONCEPTS
>
> Sensitivity analysis is essential to assess robustness of the results over different assumptions and inclusion criteria.
>
> A comprehensive approach to evaluating systematic reviews is important before their results are applied. Important steps include: assessing the exhaustiveness of the search, selection criteria, quality of the included studies, and whether study designs and results are similar across studies.
>
> Results from a meta-analysis can help ground clinical decisions in research evidence, although they never obviate the need for sound clinical reasoning when caring for patients.

Study Questions

1. Differentiate between a narrative review and a systematic review (e.g., meta-analysis) using the following features:

   a. Clinical question

   b. Search strategy and source(s) for literature

   c. Selection of studies

   d. Appraisal of studies

   e. Synthesis of studies

   f. Confidence in using results for patient care

2. One of your colleagues describes an 84-year-old patient with chronic atrial fibrillation and asks your opinion about whether anticoagulation would benefit this patient. Based on this scenario, develop a well-formulated clinical question that could be used in completing a systematic overview or meta-analysis.

3. A meta-analysis that includes 22 studies examining the effects of β-adrenergic blockers after myocardial infraction has a fail-safe N of 26. What is the fail-safe N method? Is a result of 26 likely to be of significance in this meta-analysis?

4. A meta-analysis of trials studying the effect of a new antiretroviral agent (CDD) on CD4+ T cell count was completed. In asymptomatic HIV patients, the OR was 0.96, and the 95% CI was 0.75 to 1.22. In patients with AIDS, the OR was 0.04, and the 95% CI was 0.01–0.33. Based on these results, in which patients would you recommend the use of CDD?

References

1. Hatala R, Dinh T, Cook D: Once-daily aminoglycoside dosing in immunocompetent adults: A meta-analysis. Ann Intern Med 124:717–725, 1996.

2. Etminan M, Levine M: Interpreting meta-analyses of pharmacologic interventions: The pitfalls and how to identify them. Pharmacotherapy 19:741–745, 1999.

3. Oxman AD, Cook DJ, Guyatt GH: User's guide to the medical literature. VI. How to use an overview. JAMA 272:1367–1371, 1994.

4. Cook DJ, Mulrow CD, Haynes RB: Systematic reviews: Synthesis of best evidence for clinical decisions. Ann Intern Med 126:376–380, 1997.

5. Sacks HS, Berries J, Reitman D, Arcona-Berk VA, Chalmers TC: Meta-analyses of randomized controlled trials. N Engl J Med 316:450–455, 1987.

6. Cooper RM, Rosenthal R: Statistical versus traditional procedures for summarizing research findings. Psychol Bull 87:442–449, 1980.

7. L'Abbe KA, Detsky AS, O'Rourke K: Meta-analysis in clinical research. Ann Intern Med 107:224–233, 1987.

8. *Cochrane Collaboration* (brochure). UK Cochrane Centre, National Health Service Research and Development Programme, Oxford, UK, 1984.

9. Huston P: Cochrane collaboration helping unravel tangled web woven by international research. Can Med Assoc J 154:1389–1392, 1996.

10. Jadad AR, Cook DJ, Jones A, Klassen TP, Tugwell P, Moher M, Moher D: Methodology and reports of systematic reviews and meta-analyses: A comparison of Cochrane reviews with articles published in paper-based journals. JAMA 280:278–280, 1998.

11. Borzak S, Ridker PM. Discordance between meta-analyses and large-scale randomized, controlled trials. Ann Intern Med 123:873–877, 1995.

12. Lau J, Ioannidis JPA, Schmid CH: Quantitative synthesis in systematic reviews. Ann Intern Med 127:820–826, 1997.

13. Eysenck HJ: Meta-analysis and its problems. BMJ 309:789–792, 1994.

14. Cappelleri JC, Ioannidis JPA, Schmid CH, de Ferranti SD, Aubert M, Chalmers TC, Lau J: Large trials vs meta-analysis of smaller trials: How do their results compare? JAMA 276:1332–1338, 1996.

15. DerSimonian R, Levine RJ: Resolving discrepancies between a meta-analysis and a subsequent large controlled trial. JAMA 282:664–670, 1999.

16. DeLorier J, Gregoire G, Benhaddad A, Lapierre J, Derderian F: Discrepancies between meta-analyses and subsequent large randomized controlled trials. N Engl J Med 337:537–542, 1997.

17. Cook DJ, Sackett DL, Spitzer WO: Methodological guidelines for systematic reviews of randomized controlled trials in health care from the Potsdam consultation on meta-analysis. J Clin Epidemiol 48:167–171, 1995.

18. Counsell C: Formulating questions and locating primary studies for inclusion in systematic reviews. Ann Intern Med 127:380–387, 1997.

19. Fleming TR, DeMets DL: Surrogate end points in clinical trials: are we being misled? Ann Intern Med 125:605–613, 1996.

20. Oxman AD, Guyatt GH: A consumer's guide to subgroup analysis. Ann Intern Med 116:78–84, 1992.

21. Dickerson K: The existence of publication bias and risk factors for its occurence. JAMA 263:1385–1389, 1990.

22. The Cochrane Controlled Trials Register, in *Cochrane Library. CD ROM and online. Cochrane Collaboration* (no. 2). Oxford, U.K., Update Software, 1999.

23. Gregoire G, Derderian F, DeLorier J: Selecting the language of the publications included in a meta-analysis: Is there a Tower of Babel bias? J Clin Epidemiol 48:159–163, 1995.

24. Easterbrook PJ, Berlin JA, Gopalan R, Mathews DR. Publication bias in clinical research. Lancet 337:867–872, 1991.

25. Begg CB, Berlin JA: Publication bias: A problem in interpreting medical data. J R Stat Soc 15:445–463, 1988.

26. Landis JR, Kock GG: The measurement of observer agreement for categorical data. Biometrics 33:159–174, 1977.

27. Mulrow C, Langhorne P, Grimshaw J: Integrating heterogenous pieces of evidence in systematic reviews. Ann Intern Med 127:989–995, 1997.

28. Detskey AS, Naylor CD, O'Rourke K, McGeer AJ, L'Abbe A: Incorporating variations in the quality of individual randomized trials into meta-analysis. J Clin Epidemiol 45:255–265, 1992.

29. Verhagen AP, de Vet HCW, de Bie RA, Kessels AG, Boers M, Bouter LM, Knipschild PG: The Delphi list: A criteria list for quality assessment of randomized clinical trials for conducting systematic reviews developed by Delphi consensus. J Clin Epidemiol 12:1235–41, 1998.

30. Lau J, Ioannidis JP, Schmid CH: Summing up evidence: One answer is not always enough. Lancet 351:123–127, 1998.

31. Peto R: Why do we need systematic overviews of randomized trials? Stat Med 6:223–230, 1987.

32. McQuay HJ, Moore RA: Using numerical results from systematic reviews in clinical practice. Ann Intern Med 126:712–720, 1997.

33. Laupacis A, Sackett DL, Roberts RS: As assessment of clinically useful measures of the consequences of treatment. N Engl J Med 318:1728–1733, 1988.

34. Hunt DL, McKibbon KA: Locating and appraising systematic reviews. Ann Intern Med 126:532–538, 1997.

35. Rosenthal R: *Meta-analytic Procedures for Social Research,* 2d ed, Sage, Newbury Park, CA, 1991.

Chapter 12

Evaluating Pharmacoeconomic Literature

Daniel R. Touchette

James G. Stevenson

OUTLINE

Goals and Objectives

Introduction

Types of Pharmacoeconomic Analyses

Comparing the Cost-Effectiveness of Two Therapies

Evaluating Pharmacoeconomic Literature

Currently Published Guidelines

Defining the Question

Measurement of Effectiveness or Consequences

Measurement of Relevant Costs

Decision Analysis As a Tool for Pharmacoeconomic Analysis

Simple Decision Trees

Markov Models

Evaluating the Validity of Conclusions

Study Questions

References

KEY WORDS

Pharmacoeconomics

Cost minimization

Cost-effectiveness

Cost-utility

Cost-benefit

Incremental cost-effectiveness

Perspective

Efficacy

Effectiveness

Utility

Fixed costs

Variable costs

Semifixed costs

Discounting

Opportunity cost

Decision analysis

Simple decision tree

Goals and Objectives

After reaching the end of this chapter, you should be able to:

1. List and describe the various types of pharmacoeconomic analyses

2. Define *perspective, efficacy, effectiveness,* and *utility*

3. Determine whether cost and effectiveness estimates were appropriate in a pharmacoeconomic analysis, based on its perspective

4. Interpret simple decision trees and calculate their expected values

5. Critique the conclusions of pharmacoeconomic analyses

Introduction

Pharmacoeconomics is a relatively new discipline that prior to the early 1980s few clinicians had even heard of. However, as the recognition that health care was becoming more costly than available funding could bear, the need for detailed, evidence-based analyses examining both costs and effectiveness became very apparent. Health care costs have been steadily increasing since the 1960s. Over the last 10 years, medical inflation has outpaced cost of living increases by almost 200% (Bureau of Labor Statistics *Consumer Price Index* for all goods versus medical goods, January 1990 to January 2000). During this time, the cost of medical care has increased by 64% and currently accounts for 13.5% of the nation's gross domestic product (HCFA, 1998 data), compared with only 12.1% in 1990.

These increases in health care spending occurred during a time when the entire medical system was undergoing an upheaval. Throughout the 1990s several important trends were adopted in health care in an attempt to reduce the overall cost of health care administration. For example, during this period a dramatic decline was observed in the number of inpatient admissions and in hospital length of stay, with a corresponding shift to outpatient therapy for many diseases. Managed care has flourished, replacing traditional insurance-based medicine as the primary method of insurance in some states.

Government insurance plans have also adopted a number of methods to manage costs. In many states, both Medicare and Medicaid benefits are now administered by managed care organizations. Throughout the United States reimbursement rates to hospitals by government programs have been dramatically reduced. The combination of reduced payments from third-party payers and the government, plus the increasing costs of providing medical care, have forced hospitals to carefully examine programs that they administer.

Despite the motivation for evidence-based analyses examining the costs and outcomes of therapy, the acceptance of pharmacoeconomic analyses into clinical and administrative decision making has been slow. The pharmacoeconomic literature is expanding rapidly, with analyses frequently appearing in clinical medicine and pharmacy journals, as well as in several newer journals catering specifically to pharmacoeconomic and health economic topics. Courses in pharmacoeconomics are becoming more common in pharmacy curricula. Hospital systems, managed care organizations, and government agencies highly value clinicians possessing the ability to read, interpret, and critique pharmacoeconomic analyses. This chapter focuses on helping the reader develop these skills by introducing pharmaco-economic principles and terminology, modeling techniques, and critical evaluation of the pharmacoeconomic literature. The following chapter discusses the use of sensitivity analysis in pharmacoeconomics. *Sensitivity analysis* is a method of determining uncertainty in a pharmacoeconomic model, and is used in a similar manner to statistical analysis in traditional research.

Types of Pharmacoeconomic Analyses

Pharmacoeconomic studies are typically categorized into one of several categories of analysis. Included among these are *cost-minimization, cost-effectiveness, cost-utility,* and *cost-benefit analyses.* Unfortunately, the term "cost-effectiveness" is often used inappropriately to describe a variety of situations. Each of the four primary types of pharmacoeconomic analyses is appropriate for specific situations, as described in the following paragraphs:

1. *Cost-minimization analysis* is a technique that is used when the outcomes of two or more alternatives are considered to be equivalent, but when costs may vary. Since the outcomes are considered equivalent, the "effectiveness" component of the analysis can be omitted. It becomes a cost comparison of alternatives to achieve this outcome. This is one of the simplest forms of pharmacoeconomic analysis to perform. However, it is critical when conducting cost minimization studies that the outcomes of the alternatives in fact be equivalent, and that all valid costs are identified and considered appropriately in the analysis.

2. *Cost-effectiveness analysis* is used when the options being considered have a common outcome parameter (e.g., life years saved, mmHg reduced, etc.) but when the degree of effectiveness is variable between the alternatives. The numerator is typically expressed in dollars while the denominator is expressed in some measure of clinical effectiveness.

3. *Cost-utility analysis* is a type of cost-effectiveness analysis, but it also incorporates a humanistic component. The costs of alternatives are measured as in cost-effectiveness analysis. However, the outcomes that are described are modified by health state preference or utility scores. For example, a cost-effectiveness study of two chemotherapeutic regimens for breast cancer may be expressed in terms of dollars per life year saved. A cost-utility analysis of the same scenario would incorporate the impact on the patients' quality of life in addition to the years of life saved. In this case the analysis might be expressed in dollars per quality-adjusted life year (QALY) saved.

4. *Cost-benefit analysis* is a technique that is used when comparing the potential value of two or more alternatives that are not related by having the same outcomes measure. In this type of analysis, the outcomes of each of the alternatives are expressed purely in economic terms. This is a difficult task in many cases. However, in the example of a person attempting to determine whether to invest funds in an immunization effort versus a lipid control program, a cost-benefit analysis may be used to help guide the decision.

KEY CONCEPT

Pharmacoeconomic analyses can be categorized into cost-minimization, cost-effectiveness, cost-utility, and cost-benefit analyses depending on how the costs and outcomes are expressed.

Table 12-1 compares the four basic types of pharmacoeconomic analyses that are commonly used in the literature.

Comparing the Cost-Effectiveness of Two Therapies

Often we are faced with situations where a new treatment or service is more effective but also more expensive than the current standard practice. Decision makers are faced with a value judgment of determining whether the new treatment should be adopted in practice. *Incremental cost-effectiveness analysis* is often used in this situa-

TABLE 12-1. **Four Basic Types of Pharmacoeconomic Analyses**

Type of Analysis	Measure of Cost	Measure of Outcomes	Comments
Cost minimization	Dollars	None	Outcomes assumed to be equivalent.
Cost-effectiveness	Dollars	Same measure of effectiveness between alternatives	Examples include life years saved, mmHg reduced, LDL cholesterol reduced.
Cost-utility	Dollars	Same measure of effectiveness between alternatives, but preferences or utilities are included	Example of outcome measure is quality-adjusted life years (QALY) saved.
Cost-benefit	Dollars	Dollars	Used to evaluate alternatives that have different outcomes or benefits.

tion to help guide the decision. Incremental cost-effectiveness quantifies the additional expenses that will be borne for an incremental improvement in outcomes by subtracting the cost of one therapy from the other and then dividing by the difference in the effectiveness measure (see Table 12-2). Decision makers must then determine whether there is sufficient value in the outcome improvement for the cost increase. This is commonly accomplished by comparing the incremental cost-effectiveness of the more effective agent with other commonly accepted therapies.

KEY CONCEPT

Incremental cost-effectiveness analysis is the preferred method of comparing two therapies. It quantifies the additional expenses that will be incurred for an incremental improvement in the outcome measure (e.g., cost per additional year of life saved).

Evaluating Pharmacoeconomic Literature

Currently Published Guidelines

There are several published guidelines that aid in reviewing pharmacoeconomic analyses. These guidelines summarize the most important aspects involved in conducting and interpreting pharmacoeconomic analyses. Some are written specifically to guide pharmacoeconomic research,[1,2] while others focus on interpretation of analyses.[3,4] Following these guidelines helps the clinician to determine the validity of that analysis. These guidelines are not all-inclusive, but serve as a good reference point of what should be covered in a pharmacoeconomic analysis or study.

TABLE 12-2. **Costs, Effectiveness (Utility), and Incremental Cost-Effectiveness (Cost-Utility)**

Prophylaxis	Cost	QALYs	Incremental Cost per QALY Saved	
			Warfarin vs. Aspirin	*Warfarin vs. No Therapy*
Warfarin	$9000	6.70		
Aspirin	5400	6.67		
No therapy	6300	6.51		
Cost-effectiveness			$360,000	$14,000

Defining the Question

A key component in any study is the definition of a clear and relevant question. The question should clearly identify those alternatives that are being considered and that are clinically appropriate. For example, a study that evaluates two antibiotic regimens for the treatment of pneumonia but which compares a clinically inferior dosing regimen for one of the alternatives must be suspect when results indicate that "Drug A is more cost-effective in the treatment of pneumonia than Drug B."

The question also needs to identify the *perspective* from which the analysis is being taken. For example, is the problem being addressed from the perspective of the patient, the provider, the payer, the health care system, the employer, society, or other? The perspective is a key component in any analysis since it will determine which costs and consequences will be included in the evaluation. An analysis of the benefits of two treatments from the perspective of a hospital will not include components such as the cost to the patient's employer of lost work, or the transportation costs and out-of-pocket expenses of the patient. It will be focused on those costs that accrue to the hospital alone. Therefore, when examining pharmacoeconomic literature, a fundamental step is to determine the perspective of the analysis and decide whether the relevant costs and consequences from that perspective have been included in the analysis.

Measurement of Effectiveness or Consequences

Just as with clinical studies, pharmacoeconomic analyses should include an assessment of the effectiveness of the regimens being compared. It is essential that the consequences of therapy be evaluated prior to embarking on a pharmacoeconomic analysis so as to ensure that decisions are not made on cost alone. How these outcomes are measured depend on the question being asked and how the information will be used.

An important aspect of clinical outcomes utilized in pharmacoeconomic analyses is the quality of the evidence used in the analysis. As when evaluating clinical studies, comparative prospective studies are generally preferred. However, it is important to understand that studies that control for bias using randomization and blinding are not always optimal when comparing two therapies for use in medical practice. Clinical trials often introduce abnormal practices in order to minimize the bias. Practices such as randomization and blinding and restricting patient enrollment to certain age groups or patients with certain conditions make direct application of the results to the general population inaccurate. Clinical studies that control for bias and minimize outside influences evaluate the *efficacy* of medications or programs. Studies that evaluate medications or programs in actual practice evaluate their *effectiveness.* Effectiveness studies usually consider patient noncompliance and inefficiencies that exist in the delivery of care, such as delayed or missed patient visits or drug level monitoring. As a result, medications tend to be less effective and are occasionally more toxic when evaluated in effectiveness trials. Effectiveness trials are generally preferred when determining the cost-effectiveness of medications or programs in a managed care plan. However, the U.S. Food and Drug Administration recommends efficacy trials for evaluation of cost-effectiveness and approval of medications.

Also, the effectiveness measure used to compare therapies should make sense. Where possible, effectiveness should be measured using a method that allows comparisons with other therapies, potentially for other disease states. Two commonly used effectiveness endpoints are life expectancy expressed as life years saved (LYS) and utility-adjusted life expectancy expressed as quality-adjusted life years saved (QALYs). Other intermediate effectiveness endpoints, such as reduction in blood pressure in mmHg or adverse events avoided, are occasionally used when effects on quality of life (utility) or life expectancy are unknown or very small. The use of intermediate clinical endpoints is very practical in situations when a comparison is being made between the only two available therapies for a disease and those therapies do not need to be compared to other therapies for the purpose of policy decision making. The results can still be difficult to interpret and misleading if the clinical outcome is not consistent and cannot be translated into monetary terms or compared with other commonly accepted standards. For example, in an analysis that compares the adverse event rates of two otherwise similar antibiotics (i.e., the antibiotics have similar cure rates or effectiveness, but differ in their adverse event profiles), one could theoretically use a cost-effectiveness study design using cost per adverse event (AE) avoided as the outcome parameters. If comparison of these agents with other treatments that have differing effectiveness were not necessary, this would be a reasonable approach. However, the difficulty comes in interpreting the results of the analysis. Suppose that the AEs avoided using one therapy included seizures, coma, and a minor rash. Using a combination of AEs makes the measure ambiguous and impossible to quantify. As a reviewer, it is difficult to place a value on such a measure. Even when the clinical outcome is not ambiguous, it may be very difficult to place a monetary value or even a preference on the benefits of the therapy. An example of such an intermediate measure would be the improvement in FEV_1 seen with asthma therapies.

KEY CONCEPT

Outcomes used in cost-effectiveness analyses should be comparable to other therapies and make clinical sense. Whenever possible, intermediate outcomes should be avoided in favor of final and more economically quantifiable outcomes.

In summary, the ultimate pharmacoeconomic trial would use clinical endpoints that make sense and are economically quantifiable. It would also use prospective, comparative trials that account for irregularities in practice and patient noncompliance with therapy. Ultimately, the clinical outcomes used would allow comparisons not only between medications or programs that are similar, but also between programs that are very different.

Measurement of Relevant Costs

There are many costs that can be identified in clinical economics. As mentioned earlier, those costs that are included in a pharmacoeconomic analysis are largely influenced by the perspective of the evaluation. There are many components that would be considered a cost from one perspective but not from another.

The source of the cost estimates must be examined for relevance. For example, what costs are being used in the analysis? Are drug costs expressed as contract costs at a particular institution or as average wholesale price? How generalizable are these costs to other health providers?

For the first question, only those costs that would be expected to vary when a program is implemented should be included in the analysis. The *variable costs* of care are those that vary when a program is implemented or two treatments are being compared. Examples of variable costs include medication costs, costs of treating adverse events, and hospital "hotel" costs, which usually include laundry and food costs.

The *fixed costs* include costs such as hospital building maintenance, heating, and lighting, and should not be included in most analyses. These costs do not change even if a patient receives a new medication that reduces hospital length of stay. The building must still be maintained, lit, and heated regardless of whether a patient occupies a hospital bed.

A third category of costs that is more difficult to assign encompasses what are termed *semifixed costs*. These costs are those that do not typically vary with treatment, but that may change if enough patients are involved or if enough time is saved to impact them. The typical representative of semifixed costs is labor costs. For example, nursing time may be reduced by the administration of an intramuscular drug as compared with an intravenous drug. However, the nurse would still be on the patient care unit and would be paid by the hospital even if the intramuscular drug was administered, resulting in similar costs from the hospital perspective. If a program was implemented that all patients would receive intramuscular injections of this drug, and there were many patients receiving this drug, it is conceivable that eventually one less nurse might be required on the unit, resulting in a lower cost. Whether labor costs should be included in an analysis will depend on the impact of the therapies being compared. For most situations, labor costs should not be included in the analysis.

KEY CONCEPT

Variable costs should be used when determining the cost-impact of a therapy or program. Fixed and semifixed costs should be incorporated only when these costs are actually affected by the therapy or program.

There is considerable regional variation in costs, with items costing more in some areas as compared with others. Also, the size of an institution or system will influence its buying power and result in variations in costs between institutions or systems of different sizes. It is generally recommended that pharmacoeconomic analyses use generalizable costs such as national averages for hospital costs and physician services. Average wholesale cost or a percentage of this cost is recommended for valuing medications. Institutions and health care systems usually have a good idea of how their costs compare with national averages and can make more informed decisions than if they had to compare their costs with an unknown institution.

It is important that the time basis of the costs is also expressed, since comparing costs over time will need to consider the impact of inflation. All costs should be inflation-adjusted to a given year, usually the year the study was performed. This is best accomplished by applying the medical inflation rate to costs that have been derived from data from previous years.

Another important consideration is whether future costs incurred with the treatments being compared have been discounted. *Discounting* is the concept that a given sum of money ($10, for example) is worth more today than it will at some future time (e.g., 5 years from now). The *opportunity cost* is the earning potential of that $10 over the 5-year period, if it was invested and produced interest in the best alternative manner. The discount rate is usually based on the opportunity cost of that $10. While different discount rates may be used, the rate usually falls between the cost of inflation (approximately 2% per year) and an upper end of 10% per year. A commonly used discount rate is 5%.

KEY CONCEPT

Costs incurred over a period of several years should be inflation-adjusted to a given year (usually the year the analysis is performed). Costs predicted to be incurred in the future should be discounted using an appropriate rate of discount.

Decision Analysis as a Tool for Pharmacoeconomic Analysis

Pharmacoeconomic analysis is frequently used to aid in decision making. For example, a new and effective, but costly, medication released onto the market must be evaluated for admission onto a hospital formulary. The value of a new outpatient hyperlipidemia clinic must be weighed against existing methods of delivering similar care. The need for immediate information cannot always wait for a prospective research study. In the past, these decisions were typically made by internalizing as much information as possible to derive a conclusion. The decision making processes behind these conclusions were not always apparent and had a great potential for bias. It is often difficult to secure rational evidence-based decisions due to political agendas, personal preferences and experience, difficulty in incorporating available facts, and difficulty in interpreting the relative importance of economic and outcome-related goals.

Decision analysis improves on traditional decision making methods in two ways. When compared with prospective research trials, it allows us to evaluate a program quickly and inexpensively. It also provides a method of explicitly stating assumptions and organizing information into "variables" so that others may see and critique the decision making process. Decision analysis does not make decisions for us, but it is a tool that provides us with more information to help in the process. It also allows us to predict costs and events that would otherwise be too difficult or costly to determine.

Simple Decision Trees

There are two types of decision models—(1) *simple decision trees,* and (2) *recursive decision trees.* Simple decision trees are well-suited to modeling outcomes that occur in the short-term and have a definite conclusion, such as acute illness. Recursive decision trees are cyclical in nature and are therefore well-suited to modeling chronic illnesses. An example of a recursive decision tree is the *Markov model.*

Tree Structure.   A simple decision tree appears in a research report by Brown[5] (Fig. 12-1). This analysis examines the question of adding either metformin or insulin to oral sulfonylureas in patients with type-2 diabetes. The decision tree starts on the left with the question, "If patients fail therapy with oral sulfonylureas, would it be preferable (more cost-effective) to add metformin or insulin?" To the right of the starting point, labeled "Oral sulfonylurea failed," is the first branch in the tree. The two branches are separated by a square symbol termed the *decision node.* Theoretically, the options shown in a decision tree should represent all available possibilities, although it is more typical to see a comparison of two products in published analyses. The two options in this analysis are "Add metformin" and "Add insulin," which are appropriate to the question being asked. More branches could have been added that identified other therapy options such as "No additional therapy" and "Replace sulfonylurea with insulin."

To the right of each of the options is a circle separating another branch in the decision tree. This symbol is called a *chance node.* It separates two events that occur with a certain probability. In this analysis, these events are "Success" and "Failure." The probabilities with which they occur are usually indicated below each of the chance events. The probability of a successful outcome if metformin is added to sulfonylurea therapy in this analysis is 0.44 or 44%. The chance events to the right of a decision node should always be mutually exclusive and should add up to 1.0 (100%). In this analysis, a patient treated with metformin could not be classified as being a success and a failure, so they are mutually exclusive. A quick addition of the probabilities (success = 0.44 and failure = 0.56) shows that they do indeed add up to 100%. Chance nodes should only have two chance events branching off of them. Trees with more than two chance nodes will still be functional, but may not work properly when performing *sensitivity analyses.*

Simple decision trees should be symmetrical, meaning that chance events that occur for one treatment option occur for the other option also. However, the probabilities of these chance events may differ by treatment option. In this analysis, the probability of success with insulin is different from that of metformin (44% and 33% respectively).

It is possible to model more complex decisions than what are shown in this tree, by adding more chance nodes to the right of existing chance events, leading to a tree that grows exponentially in size.

To the right of the chance events are placed the *terminal nodes.* These nodes are represented by triangles. The terminal nodes indicate the end of the tree, where no further chance events can occur. To the right of the terminal nodes are the *payoffs.* These are typically the costs or outcomes associated with that branch of the decision tree. In Fig. 12-1, the cost (payoff) for the branch where metformin has been successful when added to sulfonylurea therapy has been calculated to be $99.13. In other words, patients who have a successful outcome when metformin is added typically cost that amount as calculated by the author using cost data from the VA Medical Center. Similarly, patients who failed on metformin therapy cost $111.12 on average.

Using Variables in Place of Payoffs and Probabilities.   It is always important to remember that each of the probabilities and payoffs in our tree carries some degree of uncertainty and/or variability. It is for this reason that we use variables in their place. This allows us to design the tree giving each probability and payoff a different name that can then be made to equal a value derived from the literature

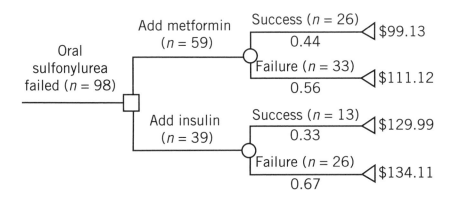

Figure 12-1. Decision tree used in the cost-effectiveness analysis. *[From Brown (5). Reproduced from Am J Health-System Pharm 55:524–527, 1998, with permission from the American Society of Health-System Pharmacists.]*

or from a database. In fact, many probabilities and payoffs are derived from several variables. In Fig. 12-1, the payoff for the cost of therapy failure while on metformin was likely made up of several variables, including the cost of metformin, the cost of sulfonylurea therapy, additional clinic visits, laboratory tests to assess fasting blood glucose and glycosylated hemoglobin, and other treatment costs to maintain fasting blood glucose levels with another agent. Each of these variables may carry a different cost based on the structure and billing system of the medical center, the geographical location of the center, and the demographics of the patient population. By using variables, we can quickly evaluate different scenarios by changing the value of the variable based on data obtained from another source. Using variables also allows us to perform sensitivity analyses on the model.

Rolling Back the Tree.   Once a decision tree has been constructed and all the probabilities and costs have been determined, it is time to see the results of our labors. Determining which option is the least costly, most effective, or produces the highest return is called *rolling back the tree.* The calculation is essentially a weighted average of each of the possible branches of the tree based on the probability of that branch occurring. The result of rolling back the tree is the *expected value* for each option. These expected values can then be compared to each other and the optimal option determined.

KEY CONCEPT

The expected value of a treatment option in a decision tree is a weighted average of all the potential costs that may be incurred by people receiving that therapy.

The expected value for each option is calculated by multiplying the payoff at the right of each branch by the probabilities of that payoff occurring and adding them to the subsequent calculations of all weighted payoffs for the option. In the example previously given, we would calculate the payoff (cost) of metformin therapy by multiplying the payoff by the probability of successful treatment with metformin occurring ($99.13 × 0.44) and adding it to the payoff and probability of failing metformin therapy ($111.12 × 0.56). This gives us an expected value of $105.84. Similarly, the expected value for insulin therapy is: $129.99 × 0.33 + $134.11 × 0.67 = $132.75. Since we are modeling the costs of therapy, the preferred option would be the one with the lower cost, which in this case is metformin therapy.

For a larger decision tree with more payoffs at the end, each payoff would be multiplied by the probabilities leading up to that payoff and then added to all the other similar payoff calculations for that option.

Markov Models

Markov models are recursive decision trees well suited to modeling chronic conditions. The principles behind Markov models are fairly simple; however, the calculations and design of the models can become complex. A discussion on developing Markov models is beyond the scope of this chapter. Interested readers are referred to an article by Sonnenberg[6] for a more detailed explanation of building and interpreting Markov models.

Evaluating the Validity of Conclusions

Evaluating pharmacoeconomic literature typically demands those skills needed to interpret clinical literature and a thorough understanding of pharmacoeconomic principles, cost data, and decision modeling. Pharmacoeconomic literature differs from a clinical trial in several ways. Unlike most clinical data, economic data changes considerably over time, affecting the decisions made regarding available choices and occasionally forcing us to use different methods to compare the options being tested. For example, a study was published in 1999 that compared immediate-release glipizide to delayed-release glipizide tablets. The analysis, using brand name cost data, recommended that delayed-release glipizide was the most cost-effective agent available.[7] However, glipizide became available as a generic product around this time—altering the costs for patients treated with this option and changing the conclusions of the analysis.

The cost of therapy tends to increase over time, and the value of preventative measures decreases if the benefits are to be realized in the distant future as compared with the more immediate future (see the explanation on *discounting* earlier in this chapter). Both of these conditions commonly affect pharmacoeconomic analyses that assess treatments for chronic conditions or preventative efforts. Handling these difficult situations often requires us to use techniques other than statistical analyses, such as predictive decision models, to compare treatment options.

Decision analysis has a number of limitations that must be carefully evaluated. Since it is a retrospective modeling process, the potential for bias is high. As mentioned previously, comparative trials are by far the preferred method of comparing efficacy or effectiveness estimates. The sources of all data should be described in detail, as this data may contain considerable bias. In addition, the model design and inputs should be very easy to follow and understand (i.e., "transparent"). These will help to make interpretation of the results easier and make any potential biases (intended or unintended) more apparent. Overly complex models with hidden or difficult-to-comprehend inputs should be avoided, as the interpretation of these models and ultimate believability are compromised.

CASE STUDY

Application of guidelines evaluating a pharmacoeconomic analysis. We have developed guidelines for evaluating the validity and interpretability of pharmacoeconomic analyses in a practical setting. These guidelines are outlined in Table 12-3.

Here we apply these guidelines in critically evaluating a recent pharmacoeconomic analysis by Reddy et al.[8] that examines the cost-effectiveness of amiodarone for atrial fibrillation (AF) prophylaxis after coronary artery bypass graft (CABG).

In this analysis, the authors developed a cost-effectiveness model comparing amiodarone to no therapy in the prophylaxis of atrial fibrillation in patients undergoing cardiac surgery. Efficacy data was obtained from two comparative clinical trials of amiodarone versus no therapy.[9,10] Cost data was obtained from hospital-specific databases. The costs were inflation-adjusted, but not discounted. Assumptions regarding length of stay were made for each therapy based on hospital-specific data. One-way sensitivity analyses were performed on all variables, and a Monte Carlo analysis was performed.

The base-case analysis showed that amiodarone was the preferred option, with a net savings of $1676. This decision was relatively stable during most one-way sensitivity analyses. The Monte Carlo analysis demonstrated 95% confidence intervals that did not overlap.

Note that the numbered entries in the following discussion of Reddy et al. relate to the corresponding guidelines in Table 12-3.

TABLE 12-3. **Guidelines for Evaluating Pharmacoeconomic Literature**

---

1. What is the perspective of the model?

2. Does the model make clinical sense?

   a. Are all available treatment options included?

   b. Are all important clinical outcomes included in the model? If not, are reasonable explanations given as to why they were omitted?

   c. Does the clinical outcome make sense when combined with costs (e.g., LYS vs. FEV1)?

   d. Are assumptions explicitly stated? Are the assumptions believable? What are the results of the assumptions? Are they conservative (favoring the less effective agent)?

   e. Were clinical or outcome-based trials used in populating the model? Were the trials used for estimating important parameters such as treatment effect comparative? Was compliance with therapy included in the model?

   f. Were all available trials evaluated? Were any important trials left out (studies that may have reported a different finding)?

   g. Were other methods of estimating clinical model parameters used (nonvalidated databases, expert opinion, or other), and if so, how might these methods affect the model's results?

   h. Do the clinical outcomes included follow the perspective?

3. Do economic variables make sense?

   a. Are appropriate costs used for the perspective?

   b. Does the paper describe from where the economic variables were obtained? Were fixed costs excluded; were cost-charge ratios used, administrative database used, etc.?

c. Are the economic variables institution-specific or from a more global database?

d. Are the cost values believable?

e. Are costs inflation adjusted? Are costs appropriately discounted?

4. Is the model transparent?

a. Is the structure of the model presented? Are all branches labeled?

b. Is the flow of the model easy to comprehend and well marked? Can you easily follow the path of a simulated patient through the model and determine where it would go and what the probability would be?

5. Are the results presented appropriately?

a. Are the cost and effectiveness estimates presented independently?

b. Are the costs and effectiveness estimations combined in an appropriate way? Do all comparisons use incremental cost-effectiveness ratios?

6. Were sensitivity analyses used to explore the uncertainty?

a. Were all variables included in one-way sensitivity analyses?

b. Were the parameters used in the sensitivity analyses appropriate to the variability in that estimate and in the method of estimating it?

c. Were multiway sensitivity analyses used to assess combined variability of significant or unknown variables?

d. Were Monte Carlo simulations necessary, and were they performed?

7. Are the conclusions consistent with the results?

a. Are statements consistent with results of the model and sensitivity analyses?

b. Are assumptions and their impact on the model discussed?

c. Are limitations in the analysis discussed?

d. Is the applicability of the results to similar and other practice settings discussed?

---

1. The perspective is explicitly stated as being that of the hospital.

2a. Next, we must look at the alternatives that are compared. The competing therapies included in the analysis are well described. The omission of beta blockers and digoxin as possible therapies[11] limit the conclusions of this analysis. The authors do explain that they omitted these agents because of their own doubts as to the agents' effectiveness.

2b. The model includes the most relevant clinical outcomes. Successful conversion from AF to normal sinus rhythm can be accomplished through spontaneous conversion, electrical cardioversion, or electrical cardioversion plus sotalol. In addition, the possibility of controlling AF rate instead of cardioverting patients is also considered in the model. The adverse events of amiodarone and sotalol are not included in the model. The authors justify the omission of amiodarone's adverse events from the model, but do not justify the omission for sotalol. However, this omission would likely have a small to negligible effect on the conclusions of the model, given the small percentage of patients who would receive sotalol.

2c. The efficacy measure used in this analysis is AF event avoided. Although this is an appropriate unit, it is difficult to place a monetary value on this event or even compare it with other therapies. A more appropriate unit would have been a quality-of-life (utility) measure or life expectancy expressed as life years saved (if this therapy had been shown to increase life expectancy). The costs included in this analysis are appropriate for the hospital perspective and are well described. The inclusion of labor costs for preparing and administering the infusions is not appropriate, since the labor costs to the hospital do not change, but would benefit the no-therapy group and is therefore conservative.

2d. The assumptions are explicitly stated in the methodology section and are believable. Assumptions were made with regard to ICU, step-down unit, and hospital length of stay and for when AF developed in this analysis. If the length of stay due to AF were erroneously high, the placebo group would cost more in the model than in clinical practice.

2e. Evaluating the evidence supporting the regimens in the trial is the next important step. In this analysis, the effectiveness results were obtained from several comparative trials. The main studies from which efficacy data was obtained were randomized and double-blinded.[9, 10] Although these trials may not exactly reflect what is actually done in clinical practice, they are a very close reflection of standard care for patients undergoing cardiac surgery. Ideally, we would prefer to have the results of several clinical trials to ensure that the efficacy estimates are consistent and similar, but this is rarely possible. Compliance with therapy was not evaluated, but that factor is unlikely to make a difference in the results since therapy is of short duration, in-hospital, and not much different from care given in the studies used for the effectiveness estimates.

2f. Most of the published trials evaluating amiodarone for AF prophylaxis are included. One important omission demonstrated no benefits to prophylaxis with amiodarone or other agents,[12] but had small numbers. Other studies that have become available since this study was published show similar benefits with amiodarone, although statistical significance was not achieved in all trials.[9, 13]

2g. Observational studies were used to populate some parameters in the model. Less reliable methods (such as expert opinion) were not used.

2h. Clinical outcomes used do reflect the hospital perspective.

3a. The costs included are those for hospital stays, drug acquisition and administration, cardioversion, and monitoring costs. Where costs were not available, cost-charge ratios are used to determine hospital costs from hospital charge data. These costs are appropriate for the hospital perspective.

3b. The costs are valued using true hospital cost data, where available, and hospital charge data with cost-charge ratios for all other data. Although cost-charge ratios are not the most accurate method of determining costs, they are an appropriate method if cost data is not available. The data used to determine hospital length-of-stay costs is not well described and may have included fixed costs. Inclusion of fixed costs would lead to a much higher estimate for each additional day spent in hospital and would favor the amiodarone treatment arm.

3c. The use of hospital-specific cost data may result in costs that are considerably different from costs incurred by other institutions, depending on geographical location and hospital size. The use of standardized costs, when available, would have made interpretation of the cost data easier.

3d. Cost data used is presented in a table, but is not clearly defined. Hospital cost data was combined for the entire length of stay in each ward. One day in an ICU costs approximately $1400, and a day in the SDU costs $1100. These costs are reasonable estimates for daily costs in each of these types of units when compared with cost data from other sources. Since these estimates were derived from hospital-specific data, it is more difficult to compare with other hospitals' costs than if a more standard cost had been used. Other cost data appears to be reasonable when compared with appropriate cost sources, such as average wholesale price for the medications and reimbursement data for services such as physician consults for electrical cardioversion.

3e. The costs are inflation-adjusted to 1998 U.S. dollars. Discounting is not necessary due to the short time horizon.

4a. The model structure is presented and the branches are labeled.

4b. The model is easy to interpret and is straightforward. There appear to be no hidden branches. The model does have one chance node from which three chance events can occur. This could complicate sensitivity analyses.

5a. The final cost and effectiveness estimates from the model are not presented independently. It is therefore difficult to determine how different the two options were for cost and effectiveness. Fortunately, these estimates can be calculated directly from the decision tree as the inputs have been included.

5b. The average cost-effectiveness of each treatment is presented. Since the amiodarone arm was more effective and less costly than usual care, an incremental analysis was not necessary (i.e., there is no increase in cost to achieve a higher level of effectiveness).

6a. One-way sensitivity analyses were performed on most cost data, but not on all variables independently. Any variables that impacted cost by 5% or greater were included in the one-way sensitivity analyses. The ICU length of stay and cost per day were not altered directly, but were indirectly altered through adjusting the cost of hospitalization. Separating out each of these variables would have been preferable.

6b. These variables were altered until a change in the decision was induced, which is appropriate. It is left to the reader to determine whether the value at which the decision changes is an attainable value.

6c. Multiway sensitivity analyses were not employed.

6d. Monte Carlo simulations were performed and provided considerably more insight into the problem.

7a. This analysis is generally well done, but does not sufficiently examine the uncertainty in the decision. The model generally supports statements made in the discussion, although there are some inconsistencies. For example, an important omission is the cost-effectiveness of other alternatives that are believed to be effective. Incremental analysis should always be performed so as to evaluate all possible regimens. It is entirely possible that beta blockers are more effective and less expensive than amiodarone; or that they are less effective, but amiodarone is much more costly, resulting in a high incremental cost-effectiveness. The authors do explain again why beta blockers were not included in the analysis; however, their view is not shared by all clinicians.[11]

7b. Assumptions and their impact on the model are not included in the discussion, although they had been previously stated and it is easy to evaluate their impact due to the transparency of the model.

7c. The limitations of the analysis are well described in the discussion section.

7d. The omission of all possible therapies for prophylaxis of AF in heart surgery limits the usefulness of the analysis in developing practice guidelines. The use of hospital-specific cost data and incomplete sensitivity analyses may also affect the generalizability of these results. The model is well designed and very clear, making it possible for decision makers to input their own data with relative ease, but this does not overcome the possibility that beta blockers may be the medication of choice in this situation.

Study Questions

1. Which of the following statements is false?
   a. Cost-minimization analyses assume that outcomes between two therapy options are clinically identical
   b. Cost-benefit analyses are useful for comparing programs with different outcome measures
   c. Cost-effectiveness analyses measure both costs and outcomes in monetary terms only
   d. Cost-utility analyses express effectiveness in terms of quality of life, willingness to pay, or preference

2. Which of the following costs would not be considered if using a managed care perspective for a pharmacoeconomic study?
   a. Cost of hospitalization(s)
   b. Cost of lost patient productivity
   c. Physician treatment costs
   d. Cost of home care

3. What is the expected value for Antibiotic A?

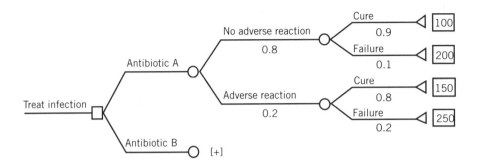

a. $34
b. $122
c. $88
d. $38
e. $161

4. Which of the following statements is false?

a. Semifixed costs should not be included in most pharmacoeconomic analyses
b. "Hotel" costs are an example of fixed costs
c. The opportunity cost represents the foregone earnings or interest of the best alternative investment
d. Perspective can influence which costs are included in an analysis

References

1. Jolicoeur LM, Jones-Grizzle AJ, Boyer JG: Guidelines for performing a pharmacoeconomic analysis. Am J Hosp Pharm 49:1741–1747, 1992.

2. Halpern M, Luce B, Brown R, Geneste B: Health and economic outcomes modeling practices: A suggested framework. Value in Health 1:131–147, 1998.

3. Richardson WS, Detsky AS: Users' guides to the medical literature. VII. How to use a clinical decision analysis. A. Are the results of the study valid? Evidence-Based Medicine Working Group. JAMA 273:1292–1295, 1995.

4. Richardson WS, Detsky AS: Users' guides to the medical literature. VII. How to use a clinical decision analysis. B. What are the results and will they help me in caring for my patients? Evidence-Based Medicine Working Group. JAMA 273:1610–1613, 1995.

5. Brown RR: Cost-effectiveness and clinical outcomes of metformin or insulin add-on therapy in adults with type 2 diabetes. Am J Health-Syst Pharm 55:S24–S27, 1998.

6. Sonnenberg FA, Beck JR: Markov models in medical decision making: A practical guide. Med Decis Making 13:322–338, 1993.

7. Leaf E, King JO: Patient outcomes after formulary conversion from immediate-release to extended-release glipizide tablets. Am J Health-Syst Pharm 56:454–456, 1999.

8. Reddy P, Richerson M, Freeman-Bosco L, Dunn A, White CM, Chow MS: Cost-effectiveness of amiodarone for prophylaxis of atrial fibrillation in coronary artery bypass surgery. Am J Health-Syst Pharm 56:2211–2217, 1999.

9. Redle JD, Khurana S, Marzan R, et al: Prophylactic oral amiodarone compared with placebo for prevention of atrial fibrillation after coronary artery bypass surgery. Am Heart J 138:144–150, 1999.

10. Daoud EG, Strickberger SA, Man KC, et al: Preoperative amiodarone as prophylaxis against atrial fibrillation after heart surgery [see comments]. N Engl J Med 337:1785–1791, 1997.

11. Bharucha DB, Kowey PR: Management and prevention of atrial fibrillation after cardiovascular surgery. Am J Cardiol 85:20D–24D, 2000.

12. Yilmaz AT, Demirkilic U, Kuralay E, et al: Long-term prevention of atrial fibrillation after coronary artery surgery. Panminerva Med 39:103–105, 1997.

13. Katariya K, DeMarchena E, Bolooki H: Oral amiodarone reduces incidence of postoperative atrial fibrillation. Ann Thorac Surg 68:1599–1603, 1999.

Managing Uncertainty in Decision Analysis with Sensitivity Analysis

Daniel R. Touchette

Muhammad M. Mamdani

R. Michael Massanari

James G. Stevenson

OUTLINE

Goals and Objectives

Introduction

   What Is Decision Analysis?

   Uncertainty Associated with Decision Analyses

Sensitivity Analysis

   Simple Sensitivity Analysis

   Scenario Analysis

   Probabilistic Sensitivity Analysis

How Is Sensitivity Analysis Performed?

General Guidelines

Calculation of Sensitivity Analyses

   One-Way Sensitivity Analysis

   Two-Way Sensitivity Analysis

Discussion

Study Questions

References

KEY WORDS

Decision analysis

Base case

One-way

Two-way

Multi-way

Sensitivity analysis

Monte Carlo simulation

Threshold analysis

Scenario analysis

Analysis of extremes

Confidence intervals

Goals and Objectives

At the end of this chapter, readers should be able to:

1. List and describe the types of sensitivity analyses used in pharmacoeconomic studies.

2. Interpret the results of sensitivity analyses presented in pharmacoeconomic studies.

3. Critique sensitivity analyses used in pharmacoeconomic studies for appropriateness and omissions.

4. Conduct a simple one- or two-way sensitivity analysis, given a decision tree and range, for the uncertain variable

Introduction

What Is Decision Analysis?

The clinician is often faced with difficult diagnostic and therapeutic decisions in caring for patients when several alternative approaches to therapy may be appropriate. In making a responsible decision regarding a health practice, numerous variables must be considered before a solution can be proposed. The clinical outcomes, economic implications, and effects on patient quality of life (i.e., utility) may be considerably different between the various options being considered. Given the complexity of modern medicine and the unprecedented access to vast amounts of medical information, assimilating all pertinent information and arriving at an optimal solution may be overwhelming. Decision analysis provides an orderly analytical approach to assist decision makers in weighing the consequences of each possible intervention.[1] It is characterized by a systematic analysis of evidence to identify viable alternatives and their consequences or outcomes. It forces the analyst to explicitly state these alternatives and their outcomes by assigning probability, economic, and qualitative values to each outcome. The average expected value is then determined for each alternative. The reader is referred to Chap. 12 and to other appropriate textbooks for a more detailed discussion on decision analysis.[2–4]

Uncertainty Associated with Decision Analyses

In a clinical decision analysis there must be a reasonable fit between the question being addressed, the structure of the model, and the data available.[1] When building decision models, assumptions may be made to compensate for limitations of the available data, and to simplify otherwise complex models.[5] These simplifications, rather than representing shortcomings of the model, may be necessary and useful compromises that facilitate the analyses. When applying the model to a real-world situation, however, notable discrepancies may exist between the analysis and the actual patient problem being addressed as a result of the compromises. These disparities can include study design characteristics such as the perspective of the analysis and the time horizon studied. As in clinical trials, careful attention must be paid to patient- and disease-specific characteristics examined in the analysis to ensure consistency with that of the actual clinical problem. Finally, the availability and accessibility of the diagnostic and therapeutic resources outlined in the analysis may result in unwanted compromises. The reviewer must be satisfied that the decision model sufficiently reflects the actual problem being addressed. When considering the structure of the model, the analysis should address all of the relevant strategies in a consistent, comprehensive, and unbiased manner. Structural characteristics of decision models are discussed in greater detail in other sources.[1, 3, 4]

After considering threats to external validity, the reviewer must now tackle the remaining sources of variability. A reality of medical decision making is that the outcome probability, cost, and utility data that are incorporated in a decision analysis are often imprecise. Furthermore, many sources of data are used in a decision model, including published and unpublished clinical trials, population studies,[6] meta-analyses,[7, 8] expert opinion,[9] registries,[10] clinical records,[11] institution-specific cost-accounting systems, national cost estimates from Medicare diagnostic related group (DRG) weights,[12] average wholesale drug prices,[13] and utility assessment methods.[1] Available data may be considered too inconsistent, insufficient, or of poor quality to build an ideal decision model.[5] These difficulties create a degree of uncertainty with the results of the decision analysis. This discrepancy may occur because of differences in patient selection criteria, regional differences, and normal variation within samples selected from the population. Other sources of variability include study size, design, and duration, as well as definitions, clinical or surrogate endpoints used, and attrition rate.

Further complicating the situation are clinicians who often wish to estimate the performance of a drug in the actual practice environment (effectiveness) rather than in the strict confines of a clinical trial (efficacy). However, the only efficacy and safety data that may be available are from controlled clinical trials in which patients were carefully selected, monitored, and in whom factors such as medication compliance was strictly controlled. These controlled conditions cannot be duplicated in the setting of routine medical practice. Although controlled clinical trials are recognized as the best source of data on the efficacy of health care interventions,[14] the circumstances of controlled clinical trials are so atypical that it may be difficult to extrapolate data on resource use obtained during the trial.[15] Another concern regarding data that is used in decision models deals with the extrapolation of intermediate endpoints from clinical trials to long-term consequences. The use of intermediate endpoints introduces an additional degree of uncertainty in a decision as to which option results in optimal outcome.

With all of these potential concerns regarding the data incorporated into a decision analysis, how confident can one be with the results?

Sensitivity Analysis

Sensitivity analysis is commonly used to assess the effects of uncertainty and, therefore, lends validity to the information from a decision analysis.[4, 16, 17] In a decision analysis model, the *best* estimate of the value for each variable is utilized in the *base-case,* or initial, analysis. To account for the uncertainty of the best point estimate, a range of plausible values may be used to estimate the value of interest. Sensitivity analyses test whether varying each of the estimates through the range of plausible values changes the decision.

> ## KEY CONCEPT
>
> The *best* estimate of the value for each variable is utilized in the *base-case,* or initial, analysis. Sensitivity analyses test whether varying each of the estimates through the range of plausible values changes the decision.

Several factors are taken into consideration when establishing the ranges of plausible values for each of the estimates. The range of values will depend on the nature and quality of the data and the perspective of the analysis.[16] Estimates from high-quality randomized studies reporting similar incidence rates (i.e., those with small variances) may result in the ability to use a narrow range of plausible values. On the other hand, when studies of variable quality or small sample size with large differences in clinical outcomes (i.e., those with large variances) must be used, wider ranges should be employed. Similarly, probability estimates based solely on expert opinion or very limited data may necessitate the use of a wide range. The reviewer should be satisfied that ranges applied are adequately defined and encompass values from all significant studies.

Depending on the perspective of the study, cost estimates used in the decision model can vary significantly. For example, a hospital may pay much less for a medication, diagnostic test, or procedure than a patient or provider would be charged. Therefore, a drug cost estimate from an institutional perspective may be quite different from that of the patient or payer. Furthermore, cost estimates may vary greatly from one institution to another and even from one geographic locale to another.[18]

The estimation of a utility value for a particular outcome state often involves a degree of uncertainty due to the patient-specific nature of reporting utilities. If large numbers of patients or knowledgeable and representative members of the general public gave similar ratings to the outcome states, a narrow range for the particular utility estimate may be sufficient.[16] A wider range of utility values may be necessary when the ratings were gathered from a small group of patients, or if individuals varied widely in their preferences. Since the uncertainty involved in assigning these estimates can be substantial, it is in these situations that sensitivity analysis can be particularly useful in assessing the applicability of the decision model to a given population.

Sensitivity analysis is a collection of approaches to better manage the uncertainty involved in assigning probabilities, costs, and utilities to the various options and outcomes considered in a decision model. Typically, all uncertain component estimates (probabilities, costs, utilities) are expressed as variables rather than fixed values. In sensitivity analysis, the decision model is reworked using different assumptions or values for items of uncertainty, and the impact of varying these assumptions on the optimal decision is assessed.

Three general types of sensitivity analyses are commonly used: (1) simple sensitivity analysis, (2) scenario analysis, and (3) probabilistic sensitivity analysis. Each of these methods is suitable in selected circumstances to provide increased confidence in the results of the decision analysis model and thus to increase validity. We review these techniques and recommend when the different approaches are appropriate, based on the nature of the decision being considered. It should be stressed that these analytical techniques are only useful for evaluating the effect of variability for the data used in the model. These methods do not provide any additional insight into the validity of the model structure itself.

Simple Sensitivity Analysis

Perhaps the most common form of testing for validity in decision analysis is through simple sensitivity analysis in which one or more parameters are varied across a plausible range.[17] Simple sensitivity analysis can take the form of a *one-way* or a *multiway* sensitivity analysis, depending on the number of variables that are simultaneously tested.

One-Way Sensitivity Analysis.   A one-way sensitivity analysis establishes the separate, isolated effect of a single variable on the results of the analysis.[17] The question assessed with a one-way sensitivity analysis is: Would the results of the model change if the value of a specific variable was different? In this type of analysis, the variable in question is systematically allowed to assume a range of plausible values determined by the analyst while other values in the decision model are held constant at their base-case specifications (i.e., their original values). The expected value of the decision model is then recalculated for each value of the variable within this range. The results can then be plotted on a graph with the expected value on one axis (usually the y axis) and the variable value on the other (usually the x axis). (See Fig. 13-1.[19])

KEY CONCEPT

A one-way sensitivity analysis establishes the separate, isolated effect of a single variable on the results of the analysis.

The critical pieces of information that a one-way sensitivity analysis may identify are *decision threshold values*,[20] where the preferred option changes. A decision threshold value implies that the overall decision is sensitive to the specific variable

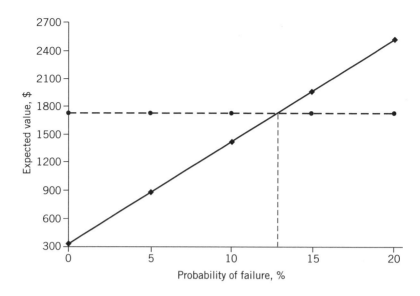

Figure 13-1. Graphical representation of a one-way sensitivity analysis. One-way sensitivity analysis was performed on the failure rate associated with cefoxitin, which varied from 0 to 20%. Results of the analysis show that the frequency of complications in the cefoxitin group would have to decrease to approximately 13% (dotted vertical line) before its cost would be lower than the cost associated with ampicillin-sulbactam in the treatment of intraabdominal infection. The values represent the cost of treatment with cefoxitin with an aggregate complication probability. ■ = cefoxitin; ● = ampicillin-sulbactam. *[From Messick et al. (19). Reproduced from Pharmacotherapy 18:175–183, 1998, with permission from Pharmacotherapy Publications, Inc.]*

and will change beyond the given threshold. An estimate containing a decision threshold value in its assigned range may be referred to as a *critical variable.*

Studies should report all uncertain estimates subjected to sensitivity analysis, the respective ranges over which these estimates were varied, any threshold values found for corresponding variables in the analysis, and the resulting change in the optimal decision if applicable. Ideally, all estimates used in a decision model should be tested using one-way sensitivity analysis.[16]

KEY CONCEPT

All estimates used in a decision model should be tested using one-way sensitivity analysis.

Threshold Analysis. A variation of a one-way sensitivity analysis that is concerned with identifying regions of decision threshold values of individual variables at which the optimal decision will change is a *threshold analysis.* A threshold analysis offers the ability to search for decision threshold values of a particular estimate beyond the defined plausible ranges assigned in a standard one-way sensitivity analysis. It is perhaps most useful when a parameter is indeterminate.[21]

Multiway Sensitivity Analysis: Two- and Three-Way Sensitivity Analysis.

It should be noted that if a sensitivity analysis performed on a particular estimate does not reveal any decision threshold values, the variability of the component within the given range will not independently affect the overall decision. This does not mean, however, that the combined variability of several estimates void of a decision threshold within their assigned ranges cannot potentially change the optimal decision. Therefore, limiting validity testing to one-way sensitivity analyses may be inadequate when analyzing the overall validity of the decision analysis model.

Multiway sensitivity analyses assess the effects of varying two or three variables simultaneously over the respective ranges of plausible values while other values in the decision model retain their original or base-case specifications. A two-way sensitivity analysis is typically displayed by graphing each of the variables on an axis. When displayed in this manner, the expected values for each of the options are not apparent on the graph as with a one-way sensitivity analysis. However, *regions of preference* are identified encompassing all combinations of the variables of interest for which an optimal decision is assigned. The observation of two distinct regions of preference implies that the combined effects of the two variables within their respective ranges can influence the optimal decision. The straight line separating the two distinct regions represents threshold values for various combinations of the estimates being examined. If, on the other hand, only one region of preference is observed, the combination of the two variables does not influence the optimal decision. (See Fig. 13-2.)

KEY CONCEPT

Multiway sensitivity analyses assess the effects of varying two or three variables simultaneously over the respective ranges of plausible values while other values in the decision model retain their original or base-case specifications.

CASE STUDIES

One-way and two-way sensitivity analysis.   Messick et al.[19] performed a pharmacoeconomic analysis of ampicillin-sulbactam compared with cefoxitin in the treatment of intraabdominal infections. In this analysis, the results of a clinical trial comparing these two antibiotics were used. Since detailed cost data was not avail-

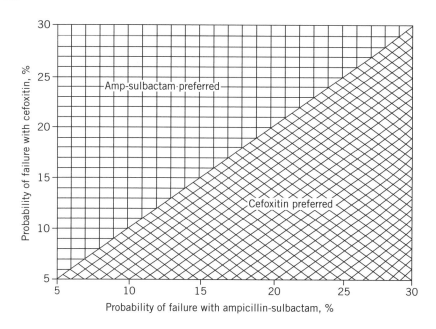

Figure 13-2. Graphical representation of a two-way sensitivity analysis. Two-way sensitivity analysis examining the relationship between ampicillin-sulbactam and cefoxitin with respect to failure rates when treating intraabdominal infections. Shaded areas represent regions of preference in which one option would be preferred over the other, given the combination of values chosen. For example, if the failure rate associated with ampicillin-sulbactam was 12% and that of cefoxitin was 18%, the combination of these values would lie in the region of preference corresponding to the use of ampicillin-sulbactam as opposed to cefoxitin with respect to costs. *[From Messick et al. (19). Reproduced from Pharmacotherapy 18:175–183, 1998, with permission from Pharmacotherapy Publications, Inc.]*

able from the trial, a decision analytic model was used to predict costs and outcomes associated with the use of either antibiotic. Economic data was approximated using submitted charges and the ratio of cost to charges for their institution. Costs were discounted at 3% annually.

The results of the analysis including all outcomes revealed ampicillin-sulbactam to cost $1732 per patient and cefoxitin $2622 per patient under the base-case assumptions. One-way sensitivity analyses were performed on all variables, identifying the frequency of failure with cefoxitin as the only variable to have a significant impact on the model. (See Figs 13-1 and 13-2.)

Another method of displaying a two-way sensitivity analysis places the expected value on the y axis and one of the variables on the x axis. A series of lines on the graph represents how the second variable impacts the expected value of the model, each line representing a different value of the second variable. (See Fig. 13-3.[22])

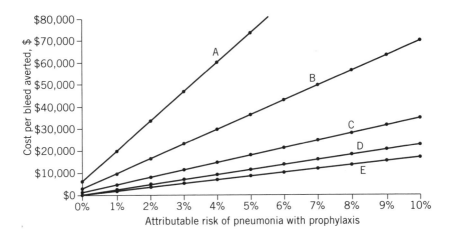

Figure 13-3. Graphical representation of a two-way sensitivity analysis displaying expected value on the *y* axis. Effect of nosocomial pneumonia on the cost per bleeding episode averted. Two-way sensitivity analysis of stress-related hemorrhage prophylaxis reflect the effects of the risk of nosocomial pneumonia and the risk of stress-related hemorrhage on the cost per bleeding episode averted. Risk reduction with prophylaxis is constant at 50%. Each plotted line represents a different risk of developing stress-related hemorrhage: *A,* 1.5%; *B,* 3%; *C,* 6%; *D,* 9%; *E,* 12%. *[From Ben-Menachem et al. (22). Reproduced from Crit Care Med 24:338–345, 1996, with permission from Lippincott Williams and Wilkins.]*

Two-way sensitivity analysis. In their analysis of prophylaxis for stress-related gastrointestinal hemorrhage, Ben-Menachem et al.[22] constructed a decision tree comparing *prophylaxis* to *no prophylaxis.* The marginal cost-effectiveness was calculated separately for prophylaxis with cimetidine or sucralfate. Data to complete the tree was abstracted from a literature search identifying all controlled clinical trials of stress-related hemorrhage prophylaxis published in the past 10 years from the study date. Cost data was based on the cost of medications and administration at the authors' institution.

With the base-case assumptions, the incremental cost-effectiveness of sucralfate was determined to be $1144 per bleeding episode averted as compared with a respective figure of $7538 for continuous-infusion cimetidine. Due to conflicting reports in the literature, the authors conducted a series of sensitivity analyses to further elucidate which variables most influenced the model. Both the risk of stress-related hemorrhage and the risk reduction afforded by prophylaxis significantly influenced the findings. A table from the paper demonstrates that using sucralfate becomes cost savings when the risk of stress-related hemorrhage exceeds 12% and the risk reduction afforded by sucralfate exceeds 75%. In contrast, the costs of using sucralfate become cost-prohibitive at lower values of these variables. (See Table 13-1.[22])

TABLE 13-1. **Representation of a Two-Way Sensitivity Analysis of Cost per Bleeding Episode Averted with Sucralfate Prophylaxis***

RRP[†] (%)	Risk of Stress-Related Hemorrhage					
	0.1%	*3%*	*6%*	*9%*	*12%*	*33%*
10	$521,005	$16,792	$8,098	$5,201	$3,752	$986
25	$208,045	$6,360	$2,882	$1,723	$1,144	$37
50	$103,725	$2,882	$1,144[‡]	$564	$274	($279)
75	$68,452	$1,723	$564	$178	($15)	($384)
90	$57,361	$1,337	$371	$49	($112)	($419)

*Two-way sensitivity analysis assuming different risks of stress-related hemorrhage, and different risk reductions due to prophylaxis (numbers in parentheses represent cost savings).

[†]RRP, risk reduction with prophylaxis.

[‡]Base-case estimates: 6% risk of stress-related hemorrhage and 50% risk reduction with prophylaxis.

SOURCE: From Ben-Menachem et al. (22). Reproduced from Crit Care Med 24:341, 1996, with permission from Lippincott Williams and Wilkins.

A two-way sensitivity analysis from the same study examines the impact of stress-related hemorrhage prophylaxis and the risk of nosocomial pneumonia (see Fig. 13-3). For this sensitivity analysis, the risk reduction with prophylaxis was held constant at 50% so that the cost per bleed avoided could still be displayed on the y axis.

When conducting a three-way sensitivity analysis, similar implications apply for the combined effects of three variables. Graphically, two of the variables are displayed on each of the axes. The impact of the third variable on the model is usually shown by a series of lines dividing zones of preference. Each line represents a new value for the third variable, allowing the zones to change size and possibly shape as the third variable is altered. (See Fig. 13-4.[23])

Multiway sensitivity analyses are typically limited to analyzing three or less variables simultaneously (i.e., a three-way sensitivity analysis) since the combined effects of more than three variables on the final decision are difficult to represent graphically and to comprehend.[24, 25] Therefore, limiting validity testing of the entire model to multiway sensitivity analyses when more than three variables contain decision threshold values in their respective ranges may be inadequate. Other methods such as scenario analysis and probabilistic sensitivity analysis may then be required to observe the impact of critical variables on the model.

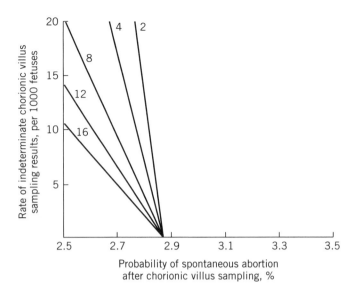

Figure 13-4. Graphical representation of a three-way analysis. Three-way sensitivity analysis of the probability of spontaneous abortion after chorionic villus sampling, the rate of indeterminate chorionic villus sampling results, and the probability of an abnormal amniocentesis after an indeterminate chorionic villus sampling. The numbers on the lines indicate the probability of an abnormal amniocentesis after an indeterminate chorionic villus sampling. For any line, the region to the right represents combinations of the probability of spontaneous abortion after chorionic villus sampling and the rate of indeterminate chorionic villus sampling results for which amniocentesis is the preferred strategy; the region to the left represents combinations for which chorionic villus sampling is preferred. (All other probabilities and utilities are assumed to remain constant at their baseline values.) *[From Heckerling and Verp (23). Reproduced from J Clin Epidemiol 44:657–670, 1991, with permission from Elsevier Science.]*

Scenario Analysis

Scenario analysis incorporates specific values for variables to generate scenarios.[17] The most common example is that of a best-case/worst-case scenario, which is often referred to as an *analysis of extremes.* An analysis of extremes should be performed by assigning worst-case extreme values of given ranges (i.e., high cost/low effectiveness) to the optimal decision as determined from the base-case analysis and best-case extreme values of given ranges (i.e., low cost/high effectiveness) to the nonoptimal strategies being compared. In this scenario, the extreme impacts of a decision on resource utilization can be calculated. (See Table 13-2.[26])

TABLE 13-2. **Best- and Worst-Case Scenarios for 12 Months of Interferon-α Treatment**

Variable	Best-Case Scenario	Base-Case Scenario	Worst-Case Scenario
Assumptions			
Monthly cost of interferon-α treatment, $	400	500	600
Annual cost of treatment for decompensated cirrhosis, $	30,000	20,000	10,000
Utility weight for chronic hepatitis C	0.85	0.95	1.0
Cure rate with interferon-α, %	25	17	5
Results (cost per quality-adjusted life-year), $			
30-year-old cohort	Net benefit	1,800	35,200
40-year-old cohort	Net benefit	3,700	48,300
50-year-old cohort	Net benefit	6,900	72,800
60-year-old cohort	1,400	12,800	122,500

SOURCE: From Kim et al. (26). Reproduced from Ann Intern Med 127:871, 1997, with permission from the American College of Physicians–American Society of Internal Medicine, who is not responsible for the accuracy of the translation.

KEY CONCEPT

An analysis of extremes is performed by assigning worst-case extreme values of given ranges (i.e., high cost/low effectiveness) to the optimal decision as determined from the base-case analysis and best-case extreme values of given ranges (i.e., low cost/high effectiveness) to the nonoptimal strategies being compared.

Scenario analysis is a particularly useful method for assessing the total range of values one can expect for each option being compared given the variability in the decision model. In addition to the range of values generated from an analysis of extremes, inferences can be made regarding the overall implications of the variability of the data used in the decision model. If the values of the reported ranges have considerable overlap, one cannot confidently conclude that any one option would consistently have a lower cost–to–quality-adjusted life year (QALY) ratio relative to the other given the large variability of the data in the decision model.

Scenario analysis alone will not identify critical variables, their threshold values, or corresponding regions of preference.

Probabilistic Sensitivity Analysis

Monte Carlo Simulation. Limitations exist with the use of one-way and multiway sensitivity analyses. While these analyses are essential for determining which variables contribute the most to the uncertainty in the decision, they do not demonstrate how multiple variables may affect a decision when there are greater than three variables adding some degree of uncertainty to the model. They also cannot provide reasonable confidence estimates around the expected value, since they exclude data from many of the variables.

A thorough test of validity and statistical significance can be accomplished through probabilistic sensitivity analysis.[24, 27, 28] Through this method, each probability, utility, and cost estimate in the decision model is represented by a distribution function from which estimates can be simultaneously selected in a random manner. A discussion on the selection of appropriate distributions to characterize estimates used in decision models for Monte Carlo simulation is beyond the scope of this chapter, and the interested reader is referred elsewhere for a more complete discussion.[29] The difference between two expected values is repeatedly calculated for a predetermined number of trials based on these random numbers, resulting in a different expected value for each trial. As a result, the difference between the two expected values of the decision model is itself a variable whose distribution function depends on those of the individual probabilities, utilities, and costs.

KEY CONCEPT

In a Monte Carlo analysis, each probability, utility, and cost estimate in the decision model is represented by a distribution function from which estimates can be simultaneously selected in a random manner.

The information provided at the end of the simulation is sufficient to calculate the confidence intervals (CIs)[30, 31] of the expected value of each of the options being compared in the decision analysis model and the frequency with which each option is optimal.[24, 27, 32] When examining the frequency with which each option is optimal, the reviewer of the decision analysis should be satisfied that the optimal strategy has the best expected value in at least a certain percentage of trials. This requirement may be different given the nature of the decision being made and the expectations of the reviewer. For example, in very important decisions one may require a particular strategy to have the optimal expected value in at least 95% of trials to be confident in the decision. For less important decisions, a minimal frequency of 80% may suffice. (See Figs. 13-5 and 13-6.[19, 33])

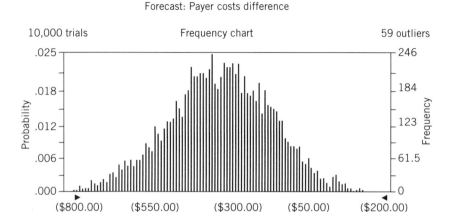

Figure 13-5. Monte Carlo simulation of the difference between two treatment options. *[From Doyle et al. (33). Reproduced from Semin Oncol 23:51–60, 1996, with permission from W. B. Saunders Co.]*

The Monte Carlo simulation is a means of managing uncertainty in decision analysis, especially when more than three critical variables are identified in the model. It is preferable, however, to conduct Monte Carlo simulations in all decision analyses, regardless of the number of critical variables to capture the combined effects of the variability of all the estimates on the overall decision. Unfortunately, Monte Carlo simulations alone will not identify critical variables in the decision model nor their threshold values or corresponding regions of preference.[34] The retrieval of such information necessitates the use of simple sensitivity analysis techniques.

Other Techniques for Estimating CIs for Cost-Effectiveness Analyses.   Other techniques have been developed and are continually being improved upon in an effort to minimize and properly characterize the variability seen with cost-effectiveness ratios.[2, 35, 36] At present, the most commonly used and accepted method for modeling cost-effectiveness ratios is bootstrapping. Monte Carlo analysis, although considered a type of bootstrap analysis, typically uses distributions selected by the investigator rather than distributions sampled from actual data. Bootstrap analysis in its purest form refers to analyses done on wholly stochastic data. In other words, efficacy and cost data must be sampled from the same patients in a study.[35] When this type of study is performed, it is then possible to develop CIs based on parametric and nonparametric bootstrap methods. These methods have the advantage over Monte Carlo simulation in that there is less possibility for manipulation by the investigator as sampled distributions are used instead of selected ones.[35] They are limited in that they are unable to take discount rates or other nonsampled, uncertain variables into account, as do Monte Carlo simulations. These methods are described in further detail elsewhere.[35, 37]

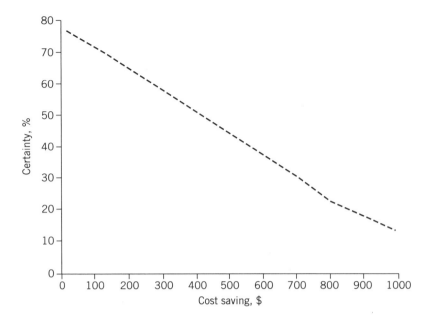

Figure 13-6. Monte Carlo simulation demonstrating the likelihood that one treatment option is preferred to another. Certainty estimation associated with Monte Carlo simulation. This graph represents the amount of certainty one can expect (vertical axis) in realizing certain amounts of specified savings (horizontal axis) when ampicillin-sulbactam is chosen over cefoxitin. *[From Messick et al. (19). Reproduced from Pharmacother 18:175–183, 1998, with permission from Pharmacotherapy Publications, Inc.]*

How Is Sensitivity Analysis Performed?

Conducting sensitivity analysis can impose substantial computational burdens. Over the past 2 decades, however, computer programs have been developed that facilitate exploration of decision tree models. Computer software specifically designed for the creation of decision models and their data validation using sophisticated sensitivity analysis techniques are available.[25, 38–41] For the experienced modeler, spreadsheet programs provide a flexible but more mathematically intense method of generating models and sensitivity analyses. Add-on programs for spreadsheets that specialize in certain types of sensitivity analysis such as Monte Carlo simulation[32] are also available.

General Guidelines

In determining whether proper testing of the results of a decision analysis model was conducted, a simple approach is proposed based on the number of critical variables in the model, as outlined in Table 13-2. The number of critical variables in the model can be determined by conducting a series of one-way sensitivity analyses on all of the estimates used in the model. Given a problem that contains two critical variables, a two-way sensitivity analysis with or without a Monte Carlo simulation and/or an analysis of extremes would be sufficient to test the validity of the decision model. Although a two-way sensitivity analysis would be the basic sensitivity method in this circumstance, Monte Carlo simulation and analysis of extremes may provide additional useful insight. Although these guidelines are by no means definitive, they may serve as a useful guide to assessing sensitivity testing of a decision analysis model. (See Table 13-3.)

Calculation of Sensitivity Analyses

One-Way Sensitivity Analysis

The calculations required for producing a one-way sensitivity analysis are no different than for calculating the expected value. The calculation for the expected value for the tree in Fig. 13-7 would be as follows:

$$EV_{Antibiotic\ A} = payoff1 * pcure * pnoAE + payoff2 * pfail * pnoAE + payoff3 \\ * pcure * pAE + payoff4 * pfail * pAE$$

$$EV_{Antibiotic\ B} = payoff5 * pcure2 * pnoAE2 + payoff6 * pfail2 * pnoAE2 + payoff7 \\ * pcure2 * pAE2 + payoff8 * pfail2 * pAE2$$

TABLE 13-3. **Suggested Approach to Validity Testing in Decision Analysis Models**

Number of Critical Variables	Optimal Sensitivity Analysis Method
0	Threshold analysis ± Monte Carlo simulation and/or analysis of extremes
1	One-way sensitivity analysis ± Monte Carlo simulation and/or analysis of extremes
2	Two-way sensitivity analysis ± Monte Carlo simulation and/or analysis of extremes
3	Three-way sensitivity analysis ± Monte Carlo simulation and/or analysis of extremes
>3	Monte Carlo simulation and/or analysis of extremes

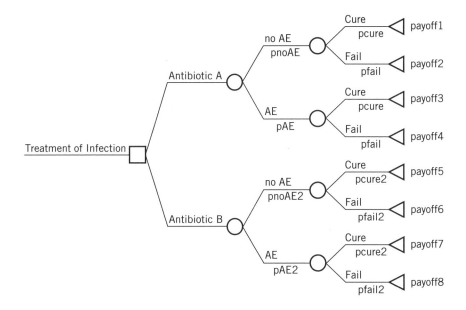

Figure 13-7. Simple decision model illustrating the choice of two different antibiotics in the treatment of infection. Chance events appear above branches, and the probabilities of those events occurring appear below branches as variables.

The one-way sensitivity analysis would graph the change in the expected value resulting from a change in one of the variables.

Two-Way Sensitivity Analysis

When performing the calculations for a two-way sensitivity analysis, the line that separates the zones of preference is where the expected values for the two treatment options are equal. The first step in determining this line is to set the two expected value equations equal to each other. We will pick pcure and pAE2 as the variables that we would like to perform a two-way sensitivity analysis on.

$$EV_{\text{Antibiotic A}} = EV_{\text{Antibiotic B}}$$

Therefore

$$payoff1 * pcure * pnoAE + payoff2 * pfail * pnoAE + payoff3 * pcure * pAE$$
$$+ payoff4 * pfail * pAE = payoff5 * pcure2 * pnoAE2 + payoff6 * pfail2$$
$$* pnoAE2 + payoff7 * pcure2 * pAE2 + payoff8 * pfail2 * pAE2$$

We would then collect the variable on the *y* axis (pcure) on the right-hand side of the equation and all others on the left-hand side, isolating the *x* axis (pAE2) variable:

1. Move payoff2 * pfail * pnoAE + payoff4 * pfail * pAE from the left-hand to the right-hand side of the equation.

payoff1 * pcure * pnoAE + payoff3 * pcure * pAE = payoff5 * pcure2
* pnoAE2 + payoff6 * pfail2 * pnoAE2 + payoff7 * pcure2 * pAE2
+ payoff8 * pfail2 * pAE2 − **payoff2** * **pfail** * **pnoAE**
− **payoff4** * **pfail** * **pAE**

2. Isolate pcure and pAE2.

pcure * (payoff1 * pnoAE + payoff3 * pAE) = **pAE2** * (payoff7 * pcure2
+ payoff8 * pfail2) + payoff5 * pcure2 * pnoAE2 + payoff6 * pfail2
* pnoAE2 − payoff2 * pfail * pnoAE − payoff4 * pfail * pAE

3. Divide both sides by payoff1 * pnoAE + payoff3 * pAE.

pcure = [pAE2 * (payoff7 * pcure2 * + payoff8 * pfail2) + payoff5
* pcure2 * pnoAE2 + payoff6 * pfail2 * pnoAE2 − payoff2 * pfail * pnoAE
− payoff4 * pfail * pAE] / (**payoff1** * **pnoAE** + **payoff3** * **pAE**)

4. Vary pAE2 and graph how pcure varies in response.

Discussion

By generating explicit structures for the decision problems, decision analysis can be a powerful tool, providing insight into real-world problems. The applicability and practicality of decision analysis have been demonstrated through several clinical trials demonstrating favorable results when applying decision analysis to actual practice.[42–46] Some degree of uncertainty in such models is, however, inevitable.[17] Although sensitivity analysis is useful for managing uncertainty arising from the data inputs in decision models, it should not be viewed as a substitution for good data. When data of uncertain quality is used in a decision model, it may lead to inaccurate, unreliable results.

Once the basic composition of the decision model is deemed acceptable, validity testing of the results should be performed using explicit, prespecified criteria such as those outlined in this article. The complete analysis of a decision model, however, requires not only explicit, prespecified criteria, but also judgment and scientific intuition. Essentially, the model must make clinical and economic sense. Although several guidelines are available to assess decision model structure and overall validity,[2, 16, 47, 48] the rationale behind all assumptions and outcomes considered must be assessed through clinical judgment and scientific knowledge. As with all clinical problems, logic, knowledge, and clinical judgment are essential components in making optimal patient care decisions.

Study Questions

1. Touchette and Rhoney[49] performed a cost-minimization analysis comparing fosphenytoin to phenytoin in the emergency department. The results of their decision analysis were tested using various sensitivity analyses. A two-way sensitivity analysis varied the cost of treating purple glove syndrome and the incidence of purple glove syndrome with phenytoin. The Monte Carlo simulation showed the expected difference in the two therapies when adverse event frequencies in the cost of purple glove syndrome are varied. These are shown in Figs. 13-8 and 13-9.

    a. Which agent is preferred when the cost of purple glove syndrome is estimated at $6000 per case and the incidence of purple glove syndrome is 2.5%?

    b. From the Monte Carlo simulation, estimate the mean cost savings expected with using phenytoin in the emergency department.

    c. Under the assumptions made by Touchette et al. in the Monte Carlo simulation, would fosphenytoin ever be a preferred agent?

2. Cagnoni et al.[50] compared liposomal amphotericin B with conventional amphotericin B in persistently febrile neutropenic patients. Figure 13-10 shows a one-way sensitivity analysis from this article.

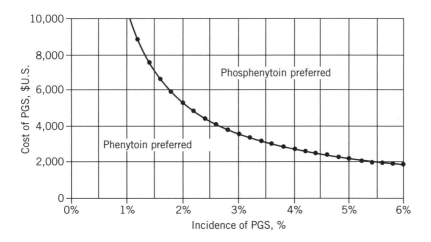

Figure 13-8. Two-way sensitivity analysis of the frequency of incidence and cost of treating purple glove syndrome (PGS). [From Touchette et al. (49). Reproduced from Pharmacother 20:913, 2000, with permission from Pharmacotherapy Publications, Inc.]

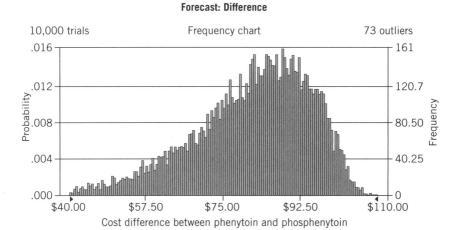

Figure 13-9. Monte Carlo analysis of the difference in costs of fosphenytoin and phenytoin therapies when frequency of adverse events and cost of treating purple glove syndrome (PGS) are varied. *[From Touchette et al. (49). Reproduced from Pharmacother 20:913, 2000, with permission from Pharmacotherapy Publications, Inc.]*

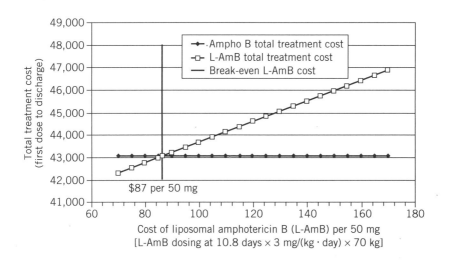

Figure 13-10. Sensitivity and break-even analysis of drug costs versus total hospital costs for all patients. Study drug costs for conventional therapy (Ampho B) are held constant at $5 per 50 mg; study drug costs for liposomal therapy (L-AmB) are varied. *[From Cagnoni et al. (50). Reproduced from J Clin Oncol 18(12):2481, 2000, with permission from Lippincott Williams and Wilkins.]*

    a. If the cost of liposomal amphotericin B is $120 per 50 mg, which agent is preferred?

    b. If the cost of liposomal amphotericin B is $120 per 50 mg, what is the approximate total treatment cost of conventional amphotericin B?

3. Table 13-4 shows univariate sensitivity analyses from Marra et al.[51] The base-case analysis favored imipenem/cilastatin with the mean cost difference of $979. Under the assumptions given for the base value and ranges of the variables in the table, answer the following questions as true or false.

TABLE 13-4. Univariate Sensitivity Analyses

Parameter	Base Value (Range)[a]	Cost Difference per Treatment Course, $CDN (Range P/T–I/C)
Probability of success with I/C	0.68 (0.48–0.88)[b]	−799 to 2756
Cost of I/C 500 mg, $	28.75 (14–42)	683 to 1308
Cost of hospitalization for success with I/C, $	9,136 (47–18,225)[c]	−5205 to 7159
Cost of hospitalization for failure with I/C, $	16,719 (3,079–30,359)[d]	−3386 to 5343
Probability of success with P/T	0.70 (0.5–0.9)[e]	−2809 to 4767
Cost of P/T 4.5 g, $	26.26 (13–39)	685 to 1262
Cost of hospitalization for success with P/T, $	7,610 (0–16,042)[f]	−4348 to 6882
Cost of hospitalization for failure with P/T, $	24,403 (3,876–44,930)[g]	−5179 to 7137

[a]Range based on standard deviation for costs and ±20% for probabilities.
[b]Threshold value of 0.57.
[c]Threshold value of $6212.
[d]Threshold value of $21,140.
[e]Threshold value of 0.75.
[f]Threshold value of $10,576.
[g]Threshold value of $19,778.
ABBREVIATIONS: I/C, imipenem/cilastatin; P/T, piperacillin/tazobactam.
SOURCE: From Marra et al. (51). Reproduced from Ann Pharmacother 33(2):161, with permission.

a. For all cost values of imipenem/cilastatin, it is the preferred agent.

b. When the cost of hospitalization for treatment failure with imipenem/cilastatin is at its minimum ($3079), piperacillin/tazobactam is the preferred agent.

c. When the probability of success with imipenem/cilastatin is 0.6, it is the preferred agent.

d. When the probability of success with piperacillin/tazobactam is 0.8, it is the preferred agent.

e. When the cost of hospitalization for success with piperacillin/tazobactam is $10,000, imipenem/cilastatin is the preferred agent.

References

1. Kassirer JP, Moskowitz AJ, Lau J, Pauker SG: Decision analysis: A progress report. Ann Intern Med 106:275–291, 1987.

2. Drummond M, Stoddard G, Torrance G: *Methods for the Economic Evaluation of Health Care Programmes.* Oxford, U.K., Oxford University Press, 1987.

3. Weinstein M, Fineberg H, Elstein A, et al: *Clinical Decision Analysis.* Philadelphia, WB Saunders, 1980.

4. Pauker SG, Kassirer JP: Decision analysis. N Engl J Med 316:250–258, 1987.

5. Sonnenberg FA, Roberts MS, Tsevat J, Wong JB, Barry M, Kent DL: Toward a peer review process for medical decision analysis models. Med Care 32:JS52–JS64, 1994.

6. Taylor WC, Aronson MD, Delbanco TL: Should young adults with a positive tuberculin test take isoniazid? Ann Intern Med 94:808–813, 1981.

7. Smith TJ, Hillner BE: The efficacy and cost-effectiveness of adjuvant therapy of early breast cancer in premenopausal women. J Clin Oncol 11:771–776, 1993.

8. O'Meara JJ, 3rd, McNutt RA, Evans AT, Moore SW, Downs SM: A decision analysis of streptokinase plus heparin as compared with heparin alone for deep-vein thrombosis. N Engl J Med 330:1864–1869, 1994.

9. Bloom BS, Hillman AL, Fendrick AM, Schwartz JS: A reappraisal of hepatitis B virus vaccination strategies using cost-effectiveness analysis. Ann Intern Med 118:298–306, 1993.

10. Oster G, Huse DM, Lacey MJ, Epstein AM: Cost-effectiveness of ticlopidine in preventing stroke in high-risk patients. Stroke 25:1149–1156, 1994.

11. Jorgenson G, Erramouspe J: Cost-effectiveness of selected management options for acute otitis media in ambulatory clinic patients. Consult Pharm 6:241–245, 1991.

12. Simon D: A cost-effectiveness analysis of cyclosporin in cadaveric kidney transplantation. Med Decis Making 6:199–207, 1986.

13. Paladino JA: Cost-effectiveness comparison of cefepime and ceftazidime using decision analysis. Pharmacoeconomics 5:505–512, 1994.

14. Drummond MF, Davies L: Economic analysis alongside clinical trials. Revisiting the methodological issues. Int J Technol Assess Health Care 7:561–573, 1991.

15. Evans RG, Robinson GC: Surgical day care: Measurements of the economic payoff. Can Med Assoc J 123:873–880, 1980.

16. Richardson WS, Detsky AS: Users' guides to the medical literature. VII. How to use a clinical decision analysis. B. What are the results and will they help me in caring for my patients? Evidence Based Medicine Working Group. JAMA 273:1610–1613, 1995.

17. Briggs A, Sculpher M, Buxton M: Uncertainty in the economic evaluation of health care technologies: The role of sensitivity analysis. Health Econ 3:95–104, 1994.

18. Welch WP, Miller ME, Welch HG, Fisher ES, Wennberg JE: Geographic variation in expenditures for physicians' services in the United States. N Engl J Med 328:621–627, 1993.

19. Messick CR, Mamdani M, McNicholl IR, et al: Pharmacoeconomic analysis of ampicillin-sulbactam versus cefoxitin in the treatment of intraabdominal infections. Pharmacotherapy 18:175–183, 1998.

20. Pauker SG, Kassirer JP: Therapeutic decision making: A cost-benefit analysis. N Engl J Med 293:229–234, 1975.

21. Pauker SG, Kassirer JP: The threshold approach to clinical decision making. N Engl J Med 302:1109–1117, 1980.

22. Ben-Menachem T, McCarthy BD, Fogel R, et al: Prophylaxis for stress-related gastrointestinal hemorrhage: A cost effectiveness analysis. Crit Care Med 24:338–345, 1996.

23. Heckerling PS, Verp MS: Amniocentesis or chorionic villus sampling for prenatal genetic testing: A decision analysis. J Clin Epidemiol 44:657–670, 1991.

24. Doubilet P, Begg CB, Weinstein MC, Braun P, McNeil BJ: Probabilistic sensitivity analysis using Monte Carlo simulation. A practical approach. Med Decis Making 5:157–177, 1985.

25. Decision Analysis by TreeAge (DATA), software package. Boston, TreeAge, 1999.

26. Kim WR, Poterucha JJ, Hermans JE, et al: Cost-effectiveness of 6 and 12 months of interferon-alpha therapy for chronic hepatitis C. Ann Intern Med 127:866–874, 1997.

27. Critchfield GC, Willard KE: Probabilistic analysis of decision trees using Monte Carlo simulation. Med Decis Making 6:85–92, 1986.

28. Critchfield GC, Willard KE, Connelly DP: Probabilistic sensitivity analysis methods for general decision models. Comput Biomed Res 19:254–265, 1986.

29. Hastings: *Statistical Distributions.* London, Butterworth, 1975.

30. Rothman KJ: Significance questing. Ann Intern Med 105:445–447, 1986.

31. Wakker P, Klaassen MP: Confidence intervals for cost/effectiveness. Health Econ 4:373–381, 1995.

32. Crystal Ball Pro. Denver, CO, Decisioneering, 1999.

33. Doyle JJ, Dezii CM, Sadana A: A pharmacoeconomic evaluation of cisplatin in combination with either etoposide or etoposide phosphate in small cell lung cancer. Semin Oncol 23:51–60, 1996.

34. Fleming C, Pauker S: An assessment of the performance of confidence measures obtained from probabilistic sensitivity analysis. Med Decis Making 7:281–289, 1987.

35. O'Brien BJ, Drummond MF, Labelle RJ, Willan A: In search of power and significance: Issues in the design and analysis of stochastic cost-effectiveness studies in health care. Med Care 32:150–163, 1994.

36. Gardiner J, Hogan A, Holmes-Rovner M, Rovner D, Griffith L, Kupersmith J: Confidence intervals for cost-effectiveness ratios. Med Decis Making 15:254–263, 1995.

37. Chaudhary MA, Stearns SC: Estimating confidence intervals for cost-effectiveness ratios: An example from a randomized trial. Stat Med 15:1447–1458, 1996.

38. McNamee P, Celona J: *Decision Analysis for the Professional with Supertree.* Redwood City, CA, Scientific Press, 1987.

39. Hollenberg J: SMLTREE: The all-purpose decision tree builder. Boston, Pratt Medical Group, 1985.

40. Pauker SG, Kassirer JP: Clinical decision analysis by personal computer. Arch Intern Med 141:1831–1837, 1981.

41. Franke D, Hall C: Arborist: Decision tree software. Dallas, Texas Instruments, 1984.

42. Morabia A, Steinig-Stamm M, Unger PF, et al: Applicability of decision analysis to everyday clinical practice: A controlled feasibility trial. J Gen Intern Med 9:496–502, 1994.

43. Clancy CM, Cebul RD, Williams SV: Guiding individual decisions: A randomized, controlled trial of decision analysis. Am J Med 84:283–288, 1988.

44. Silverstein MD, Albert DA, Hadler NM, Ropes MW: Prognosis in SLE: Comparison of Markov model to life table analysis. J Clin Epidemiol 41:623–633, 1988.

45. Albert DA, Silverstein MD, Paunicka K, Reddy G, Chang RW, Derus C: The diagnosis of polyarteritis nodosa. II. Empirical verification of a decision analysis model. Arthritis Rheum 31:1128–1134, 1988.

46. Carter BL, Butler CD, Rogers JC, Holloway RL: Evaluation of physician decision making with the use of prior probabilities and a decision-analysis model. Arch Fam Med 2:529–534, 1993.

47. Eddy D: *A Manual for Assessing Health Practices and Designing Practice Policies: The Explicit Approach.* Philadelphia, American College of Physicians, 1992.

48. Richardson WS, Detsky AS: Users' guides to the medical literature. VII. How to use a clinical decision analysis. A. Are the results of the study valid? Evidence-Based Medicine Working Group. JAMA 273:1292–1295, 1995.

49. Touchette DR, Rhoney DH: Cost-minimization analysis of phenytoin and fosphenytoin in the emergency department. Pharmacother 20:908–916, 2000.

50. Cagnoni PJ, Walsh TJ, Prendergast MM, Bodensteiner D, Hiemenz S, Greenberg RN, Arndt CA, Schuster M, Seibel N, Yeldandi V, Tong KB: Pharmacoeconomic analysis of liposomal amphotericin B versus conventional amphotericin B in the empirical treatment of persistently febrile neutropenic patients. J Clin Oncol 18(12):2476–2483, 2000.

51. Marra FO, Frighetto LO, Marra CA, Sleigh KM, Stiver HG, Bryce EA, Reynolds RP, Jewesson PJ: Cost-minimization analysis of piperacillin/tazobactam versus imipenem/cilastatin for the treatment of serious infections: A Canadian hospital perspective. Ann Pharmacother 33(2):156–162, 1999.

Ethical Concerns in Drug Research and Literature Evaluation

David J. Edwards

OUTLINE

Goals and Objectives

Introduction

*Ethical Issues in Conducting
   Biomedical Research*

  Respect for Persons

  Beneficence

  Justice

*Oversight of Research in the United
   States*

  Institutional Review Boards

  Informed Consent

Scientific Misconduct

Ethical Issues in Literature Evaluation

Study Questions

References

KEY WORDS

Beneficence
Justice
Institutional review board

Informed consent
Conflict of interest

Goals and Objectives

The objective of this chapter is to familiarize readers with the basic ethical principles that guide the conduct of modern biomedical research, as well as the role of institutional review boards (IRBs) and other agencies in ensuring that these guidelines are followed. Recent cases of scientific misconduct and the difficulties in detecting fraudulent data prior to publication are reviewed. In addition, current policies of several major medical journals for disclosure of conflicts of interest are discussed as a method for dealing with unethical behavior in the review and evaluation of drug literature. At the completion of this chapter, readers should:

1. Be familiar with the Declaration of Helsinki and the Belmont Report and the ethical principles of respect for persons, beneficence, and justice, as outlined in these documents.

2. Understand the role of the Food and Drug Administration (FDA) and the National Institutes of Health in overseeing research in the United States.

3. Understand the composition and role of IRBs in protecting human subjects from unacceptable risks.

4. Be able to examine a consent form to determine if the essential elements of informed consent are present.

5. Understand the role of the Office of Research Integrity in investigating cases of scientific misconduct in the United States.

6. Be aware of the ethical issues associated with the review and evaluation of drug literature, as well as journal policies, with respect to disclosure of conflicts of interest.

Introduction

In a utopian society, science would be concerned with the discovery of new information, scientific writing with the clear and accurate presentation of the data, and reviewers would objectively evaluate the quality and significance of the work. Unfortunately, biomedical scientists and health care practitioners are subject to the same pressures, conflicts of interest, and moral choices as the rest of society. Violation of ethical principles related to the conduct, publication, and interpretation of research occurs all too frequently and comes in many forms. It can involve any participant in the process, including investigators, sponsors, editors, and peer reviewers, as well as those using the primary literature to produce commentaries, editorials, and review articles. Clinicians who must evaluate the literature for the benefit of their patients need to be aware of potential unethical practices in the generation of primary and tertiary literature and must guard against external influences that may influence their own evaluation of the data.

Ethical Issues in Conducting Biomedical Research

The basic principles and guidelines under which modern biomedical research is conducted originated with the Nuremberg Code in 1947. Drafted as a set of standards for evaluating the conduct of physicians and scientists toward prisoners in concentration camps during World War II, its basic principles have since been incorporated into a number of other documents, including the Declaration of Helsinki (1964) and the Belmont Report (1979). Many journals have policies that require submitted manuscripts to contain a statement that the research described adheres to the principles outlined in these documents. The Belmont Report was issued by the National Commission for the Protection of Human Subjects of Biomedical and Behavioral Research under the authority of the Department of Health, Education, and Welfare in the United States and outlined three general ethical principles: (1) respect for persons, (2) beneficence, and (3) justice.

Respect for Persons

This principle implies that individuals are capable of making an informed decision as to whether to participate in biomedical research and that the choice of the individual must be respected. In addition, subjects with impaired or diminished capacity to make such a decision need to be protected. Examples include young children or adults whose mental capacity is diminished due to disease or illness. Investigators as well as parents or other caretakers must make difficult decisions in such situations and take special precautions to ensure that the rights of these subjects are respected. Although a level of protection is required, these subjects also deserve to receive the benefits that research can offer with respect to advances in health care. Few would argue that research into the effects of drugs in the pediatric population or diseases such as Alzheimer's disease is not needed. In addition, emergency research in critically ill patients under circumstances where obtaining an informed consent is not possible could ultimately save human life.[1]

The principle of *respect for persons* also suggests that individuals should not be coerced into participation. Although overt coercion may be rare, more subtle forms exist, which can interfere with the individual's free choice. Prisoners, health professional students, and the unemployed represent three categories of potential research subjects whose ability to freely choose to participate may be compromised by personal circumstances or a relationship with the investigators. This may also apply to patients who do not wish to offend their primary caregiver by refusing to participate in a study. The application of this principle is embodied in the consent form. Potential research subjects must read and sign this document as a way of certifying that they are truly providing informed consent to participate in a research study.

KEY CONCEPT

Respect for persons implies that subjects should be free to make an informed decision regarding participation in research. An appropriate consent form is essential if this principle is to be met.

Beneficence

The principle of *beneficence* refers to the obligation of the investigator to do his or her utmost to ensure that research subjects are not harmed. The risks of the research should be minimized and the potential benefits maximized. This principle is closely related to the fundamental tenet of the Hippocratic Oath to "do no harm" and can create conflicts for clinician-scientists. How does one weigh the potential benefits to individual subjects compared with the benefits that might accrue to society as a whole from the results? Certainly, it is the individual who accepts all of the risks associated with the research, and the investigator must base decisions on whether to enter patients into a study primarily on the needs of the patient not society.

Marquis[2] has pointed out the dilemma facing physicians who are considering enrolling patients in randomized clinical trials. If a physician believes that one treatment is superior to another, how can he or she permit the patient to enter the study knowing that the patient may receive the other treatment? The same concept applies to the inclusion of patients in studies involving placebo controls, although the issue is even more contentious since a physician cannot reasonably expect a true therapeutic response in subjects receiving a placebo. There has been considerable debate on this topic in the psychiatric community where some have taken the stand that the use of a placebo is akin to denying these patients treatment. These individuals view placebo-controlled research as unethical and immoral and believe that it could lead to behavior on the part of the research subject that is potentially dangerous to the individual and society. The position of the FDA is that placebo controls are required for drugs such as antihypertensives and those used for psychiatric disorders because the effectiveness of these agents is very difficult to demonstrate. In addition, a meta-analysis of the FDA database suggested that the incidence of suicide and attempted suicide was not different in depressed patients receiving a placebo compared with those receiving investigational new drugs or established therapeutic agents.[3]

For a physician, the decision to ask a patient to participate in a randomized study where he or she may receive a placebo or a treatment they view as inferior is a difficult one. However, the ethical dilemma can be resolved by recognizing that only a randomized clinical trial with a rigorous study design and statistical analysis can truly determine whether one treatment is superior to another or even a placebo. Nobody prefers to treat patients with drugs that are not superior to a placebo, and it is in the best interest of the patient population as a whole to know which treatment is best. Physicians and other health care professionals are obliged to do whatever they can do to alleviate human suffering. Personal views based primarily on anecdotal evidence concerning the efficacy or toxicity of a particular drug need to be set aside in the absence of quality data from a randomized trial.

Justice

The principle of *justice* relates to fairness or equitable distribution with respect to the risks and benefits associated with research. If justice is to be served, then those individuals who assume the risk should be the same people who benefit from the results. Extreme examples of injustice include experiments conducted on prisoners of war during World War II and the Tuskegee syphilis study conducted in the United States in the 1940s. In the latter study, rural black men were denied treatment for syphilis so that the natural course of the disease could be studied.[4] This research violated not only the principle of beneficence by denying these patients treatment but also the principle of justice since syphilis is clearly not a disease that is confined to the rural African-American male population. Presumably, cases of injustice such as these will not be repeated but more subtle examples may still occur today. Care must be taken to ensure that indigent patients or other economically disadvantaged groups are not the primary source of subjects for studies with drugs, medical devices, or surgical procedures that will ultimately only be affordable to affluent members of society or those with full health care coverage.

KEY CONCEPT

The principle of justice mandates that those individuals that assume the risks of research also be included among those able to reap the benefits.

The three ethical principles described in the Belmont Report are rather broad. More specific guidelines that encompass and expand upon these general principles are needed for the evaluation of modern clinical research. Emanuel et al.[5] have outlined seven ethical requirements that must be met in order for a clinical trial to be considered ethical: (1) value, (2) scientific validity, (3) fair subject selection, (4) favorable risk-benefit ratio, (5) independent review, (6) informed consent, and (7) respect for subjects. These requirements are listed and expanded upon in Table 14-1 and can serve as a useful model for those involved in the review and approval of biomedical research.

Oversight of Research in the United States

Research on human subjects in the United States is conducted under the authority and guidance of the FDA for products subject to FDA approval or the Office for Protection from Research Risks (OPRR) for research supported or regulated by the Department of Health and Human Services. The regulations of OPRR and the FDA, while distinct, were harmonized in 1991 and are similar in principle. Both agencies delegate direct responsibility for ensuring that the principles outlined in the Declaration of Helsinki and the Belmont Report are followed to an IRB as described by the Public Health Service Act, Part 46 ("Protection of Human Subjects"). Most universities and many hospitals have their own IRBs, while researchers at smaller institutions, private companies, or in private practice may establish a written agreement to use the services of an IRB of another institution. Oversight of IRB activity takes place by different mechanisms. The FDA conducts extensive on-site inspections of investigators, sponsors, and IRBs to evaluate compliance. The OPRR, on the other

TABLE 14-1.	Seven Requirements for Determining Whether a Research Trial Is Ethical*		
Requirement	**Explanation**	**Justifying Ethical Values**	**Expertise for Evaluation**
Social or scientific value	Evaluation of a treatment, intervention, or theory that will improve health and well-being or increase knowledge	Scarce resources and nonexploitation	Scientific knowledge; citizen's understanding of social priorities
Scientific validity	Use of accepted scientific principles and methods, including statistical techniques, to produce reliable and valid data	Scarce resources and nonexploitation	Scientific and statistical knowledge; knowledge of condition and population to assess feasibility
Fair subject selection	Selection of subjects so that stigmatized and vulnerable individuals are not targeted for risky research and the rich and socially powerful not favored for potentially beneficial research	Justice	Scientific knowledge; ethical and legal knowledge
Favorable risk-benefit ratio	Minimization of risks; enhancement of potential benefits; risks to the subject are proportionate to the benefits to the subject and society	Nonmaleficence, beneficence, and nonexploitation	Scientific knowledge; citizen's understanding of social values
Independent review	Review of the design of the research trial, its proposed subject population, and risk-benefit ratio by individuals unaffiliated with the research	Public accountability; minimizing influence of potential conflicts of interest	Intellectual, financial, and otherwise independent researchers; scientific and ethical knowledge
Informed consent	Provision of information to subjects about purpose of the research, its procedures, potential risks, benefits, and alternatives, so that the individual understands this information and can make a voluntary decision whether to enroll and continue to participate	Respect for subject autonomy	Scientific knowledge; ethical and legal knowledge
Respect for potential and enrolled subjects	Respect for subjects by (1) Permitting withdrawal from the research (2) Protecting privacy through confidentiality (3) Informing subjects of newly discovered risks or benefits (4) Informing subjects of results of clinical research (5) Maintaining welfare of subjects	Respect for subject autonomy and welfare	Scientific knowledge; ethical and legal knowledge; knowledge of particular subject population

*Ethical requirements are listed in chronological order from conception of research to its formulation and implementation.
SOURCE: From Emanuel et al. (5). Reprinted from JAMA 283:2701–2711, 2000.

hand, relies primarily on the assurance process by which institutions provide written assurance every 5 years that they are in compliance with the policies and procedures for protection of human subjects. On-site investigations of IRB compliance by the OPRR are uncommon, but the agency is increasingly active in conducting off-site reviews of documents. These reviews resulted in a suspension of federally funded research at seven universities between June 1998 and March 2000. In most cases, the root cause of compliance problems has been found to be a lack of institutional support for the IRB.[6] It is clear that the protection of human subjects is a moral obligation that requires significant institutional resources in today's environment to fulfill and document the functions of the IRB.

Institutional Review Boards

By law, an IRB must be composed of at least five members. The members should not consist entirely of one gender or one profession and should have at least one member who is not a scientist and one who is not otherwise affiliated with the institution. Lawyers, social workers, or members of the clergy often fill the latter positions. Individuals not employed by the institution sponsoring the IRB serve an important role since they do not have the inherent conflict of interest that exists for most of the other members. For example, denying approval for an investigator to conduct a project sponsored by a pharmaceutical company may represent a significant loss of revenue for a university. Most IRBs have considerably more than the minimum of five members and strive for diversity among the membership in order to obtain a wide range of views on the merits of individual projects.

The function of the IRB is to protect the rights of research subjects by reviewing and monitoring biomedical research. The IRB has the right to approve, request modifications, or deny the approval of protocols. Changes to a previously approved protocol must be resubmitted to the IRB prior to initiating the research. The study design is evaluated to ensure that the risks associated with the study are reasonable in view of potential benefits. An assessment of the scientific merits of the design is appropriate since a poorly designed study will not yield results of therapeutic value and will be exposing subjects to risk without the possibility of benefit. The criteria for inclusion and exclusion of subjects are reviewed to determine that subject selection is equitable. In addition, the methods for recruiting subjects must be examined. Advertisements that will be placed in newspapers, on television, or in any public place cannot mislead or attempt to induce subjects to participate by misstating the relative risks and benefits of the research.

KEY CONCEPT

The IRB has the ultimate responsibility for ensuring that the risks associated with biomedical research are appropriate given the potential value of the results.

Any adverse events that occur during the course of a study must be reported to the IRB even if the relationship between the adverse event and the drug under study is unclear or unlikely. In the case of multicenter studies, the sponsor must forward all reports of adverse events to each of the institutions involved in the study. The IRB must conduct a regular review of these reports to determine if the risk-benefit ratio has been altered to the point where approval of the study should be revoked. Despite these precautions and safeguards, unexpected and sometimes tragic events do occur. In September 1999, Jesse Gelsinger, a patient with a genetic deficiency in the enzyme ornithine transcarbamylase, which helps to regulate ammonia metabolism, died in a study testing an experimental gene therapy.[7] The death was thought to be related to a systemic inflammatory response to the administration of a massive dose of the gene vector, a modified adenovirus. Whether investigators or IRB reviewers should have been able to predict such a response is a matter that is currently under investigation, but it points to the fact that experimental treatments can be dangerous and IRB oversight does not eliminate risks associated with participation in research.

Informed Consent

Much of the effort of the IRB is directed toward reviewing the consent form to ensure that all of the basic elements are in place, that risks and benefits are appropriately stated, and that the document will be understandable to those who will be asked to participate. Consent forms must include a number of elements, including an explicit statement that the subject is consenting to participate in a research study. This is important in distinguishing between research and routine care in patients who may also be asked to provide consent for surgery or other procedures that are part of their medical treatment. The purpose of the study along with the foreseeable risks and potential benefits must be explained as well as any alternative treatments that the patient may have access to. Investigators must take care that the benefits are not overstated while the risks are trivialized. Phone numbers or some other convenient way of contacting the investigator must be provided. In addition, the subject must be told that their participation is voluntary and that they may withdraw at any time without compromising their standard medical treatment.

If compensation is to be offered either for participation in the study or for injuries incurred as a result of the study, this must also be stated. Compensation for participation in research is an ethical issue that goes to the heart of the issue of coercion. Suppose, for example, a Phase I study requires healthy human volunteers to take a new drug in order to study its pharmacokinetics and metabolism in humans. The sponsor is willing to pay $1000 to participants who will be required to undergo a prestudy physical exam and spend 2 days at the clinic taking the drug and providing several blood and urine samples. It is highly unlikely that many middle-aged adults with full-time, well-paying jobs will volunteer for this study. On the other hand, students or unemployed individuals may view this as an economic opportunity. It is clear that the level of compensation offered can interfere with the ability of potential research subjects to make an informed choice strictly based on the merits of the project. While compensation for the time and expenses of research participants is acceptable, it should not be in itself an inducement to participate. For example, a reasonable honorarium might cover parking, gas, and meals, as well as compensation for time at an hourly rate similar to the minimum wage. A study requiring a subject to spend 4 days at the clinic could reasonably provide more compensation than a project completed within a single day.

KEY CONCEPT

Compensation for participation in research should not be so great as to induce subjects to participate since this interferes with the ability of individuals to freely choose based solely on the risks and benefits of the study.

Research subjects come from a variety of backgrounds in terms of level of education, comprehension of the English language, and ability to understand medical terminology or jargon. An important feature of the consent form is that it should be written in a style that can be understood by individuals with limited education and little or no background in health care. Studies conducted in several countries or involving subjects speaking different languages pose a special problem since consent documents must be translated into the language of fluency in order to be useful.

Subjects must also be informed about provisions for maintaining confidentiality of their records. In general, the FDA has the right to view study records, but disclosure to other external parties is prohibited. In the case of publications, data are typically coded so that individuals cannot be identified. Case reports or other types of papers involving photographs of subjects to illustrate a point about a disease or treatment certainly have the potential to threaten patient confidentiality. It is the policy of some journals, for example the *British Medical Journal*, to require a separate written consent from the patient to allow publication of any material that might allow identification. Issues of confidentiality can become quite complex. Virginia Commonwealth University was ordered by the OPRR to halt all research for a short period in January 2000 after the father of a participant in a genetics study complained that the family history provided by his daughter violated the family's privacy.[8] Whether informed consent must be sought from the entire family in addition to the primary research subject in cases like this remains an issue for debate in the field of genetic research.

Additional elements of informed consent that may be present when appropriate include the consequences to the patient related to early withdrawal from the study and a statement that any significant new findings developed during the course of a study will be divulged to the patient. Studies with new drugs, for example, may identify an unexpected side effect that could affect the willingness of subjects to continue their participation. While the consent form is a written document, it is common practice for investigators to review the information verbally to ensure that the potential subject really understands the nature and extent of their obligation. Subjects must be given a copy of the consent form for their files, which will allow them to review the procedures, risks, and benefits at any time should they desire.

Scientific Misconduct

Scientific misconduct can be defined as fabrication, falsification, plagiarism, or deception in proposing, carrying out, or reporting results of research and deliberate, dangerous, or negligent deviations from accepted practice in carrying out research.[9] Although recent cases have been highly publicized by the media, it appears that such practices have been going on since humans started engaging in research and are certainly not confined to the biomedical field. As documented in the book *Betrayers of the Truth* by Broad and Wade (Simon and Schuster, New York, 1982),[10] the famed Egyptian astronomer Ptolemy catalogued the positions of over 1000 stars in his seminal work *Almagest*, published in the second century A.D. Unfortunately, a number of stars visible from Alexandria where Ptolemy was located are not listed. It has been suggested that this is because Ptolemy plagiarized the earlier work of the Greek astronomer Hipparchus of Rhodes. None of the neglected stars are visible from Rhodes, which has a latitude of 5° north of Alexandria. In 1912, Charles Dawson reported the discovery of a skull and jawbone with human and apelike characteristics in the Piltdown gravel pit near Sussex, Great Britain. The so-called Piltdown man was reported to be the elusive missing link proving that man evolved from apes. Ultimately, the skull was found to be that of a human and no more than 600 years of age while the jaw was that of a modern orangutan. Both had been altered to appear older than they really were.

The motivation for such activities is unclear. The pressure to publish may be one factor in today's highly competitive world of science. However, as pointed out by Drummond Rennie, former editor of *JAMA,* "laziness, desire for fame, greed and an inability to distinguish right from wrong are just as likely to be at the root of the problem."[11] The incidence of scientific misconduct is also unknown. Approximately 1 or 2 cases per million inhabitants are referred to Scandinavian authorities for further investigation each year.[12] In the United States, the Office of Research Integrity reviewed close to 1000 allegations between 1993 and 1997. Of these, 150 cases were formally investigated, and 76 resulted in findings of misconduct.[13] Estimating the true incidence is an impossible task, given difficulties in detection as well as differing interpretations among the scientific community as to what constitutes misconduct. While fabrication of data is clearly wrong, other practices are not so blatant. Scientists may exclude patients with extreme results in order to improve the quality of their data or to enhance the statistical validity of conclusions. The famed father of genetics, Gregor Mendel, has been accused of "trimming" experimental data to make the results fit the hypothesis. An analysis of Mendel's data by the statistician Ronald Fisher suggests that it is highly unlikely that the reported results (e.g., exactly 300 round peas and 100 wrinkled peas when theory predicts a 3:1 ratio) would occur in real-life experiments.[10]

Selective reporting is another questionable practice in which experiments that do not support the hypothesis proposed by the investigator or sponsor may not even be submitted for publication. Kahn and coworkers conducted a study in which they determined that there was no difference between HIV-1 Immunogen, a product designed to boost immune response, and placebo in the clinical progression of HIV.[14] The investigators were confronted with an ethical dilemma when they decided to publish the results of the study against the wishes of the sponsor, Immune Response Corp (IRC). The researchers decided that it would be unethical to allow other trials of this product to proceed without informing the scientific and medical communities of the negative results of their study. At the other extreme, supportive data may be published in more than one journal, a practice known as *duplicate,* or *redundant, publication.* It has been estimated that up to 13% of published papers may be redundant.[15]

Pharmaceutical companies may detect fraud and misconduct in clinical trials through the monitoring conducted by their clinical research associates. Misconduct in academic or hospital settings, however, is largely discovered either accidentally or due to whistle-blowing on the part of one or more coinvestigators. The *Journal of Bone and Joint Surgery* published a paper on allografted knee ligaments in animals, only to be informed by a reader that one of the electron micrographs had been taken from a previously published study on nerve endings in human ligaments.[16] Journals do not have access to original medical records or laboratory notebooks and must accept at face value that the data contained in a submitted manuscript is legitimate. Editors and reviewers may become suspicious particularly when data are too unique or too perfect, as evidenced by unrealistically small deviations in the data (e.g., Mendel's work). Excessive rates of publication can also be a tip-off. Janice Rymer[17] reported attending a conference at which a previously unknown investigator submitted 16 abstracts for publication, one of which received an award. Much of the data was subsequently found to be either plagiarized or fabricated. Between 1979 and 1981, John Darsee, a postdoctoral researcher in the laboratory of the esteemed cardiologist Eugene Braunwald, wrote close to 100 abstracts and papers, many of which had to be retracted when demonstrated to have been fabricated.[18] Modern biomedical research is increasingly a collaborative effort involving several investigators with expertise in highly specialized methods and techniques of analysis. This makes it more difficult for individual members of the research team to understand exactly how all of the data was generated. In most documented cases, the fraudulent activities of one investigator went unnoticed by most of the others. In the case of the plagiarized electron micrograph of knee ligaments mentioned earlier, there were three coauthors of the original paper in addition to the primary author, and all denied having any direct involvement in the original research. Although apparently not party to the fraudulent activities of the principal investigator, these individuals clearly violated ethical principles with respect to authorship of papers (see Chap. 3).

Many would agree that scientists who fabricate, misrepresent, or otherwise inappropriately manipulate the data from a research study are guilty of one of the most extreme violations of ethical and moral conduct. These cases have the potential to affect the well-being of patients everywhere since failure to detect scientific misconduct prior to publication may lead clinicians to base treatment decisions or public health practices on fabricated data. Robert Liburdy, a biologist at Lawrence Berkeley National Laboratory, published two papers in 1992 linking low-level electromagnetic fields to changes in cellular function. This supported the hypothesis that electromagnetic fields could cause cancer and led to a public scare regarding the health effects of living, working, or going to school in close proximity to power lines. Investigations at the university as well as the Office of Research Integrity found that Liburdy was guilty of publishing fraudulent information.[19] In 1998, the *British Medical Journal* retracted a paper[20] when one of the investigators, Cameron Bowie, was unable to document that his assistant had actually conducted the original research.[21] The project involved a home interview of severely disabled adults with a follow-up telephone interview 1 year later. The paper concluded that those individuals who had seen only a general practitioner or nurse had more unmet needs than those who were also seen by a social worker or who were associated with a patient organization. These results had significant implications for the community care of disabled individuals, but when Bowie attempted to contact some of these individuals 6 years later, none could recall the telephone interview and only one-third had any memory of a home visit.

In a more recent case, cancer researcher Werner Bezwoda was fired from his position at the University of the Witwatersrand in South Africa after an investigation revealed multiple violations of ethical conduct.[22] Dr. Bezwoda originally reported at the annual meeting of the American Society of Clinical Oncology that high-dose chemotherapy followed by bone marrow transplantation in patients with advanced breast cancer doubled the time of survival without relapse compared with patients receiving low-dose chemotherapy. This report was at odds with three other studies presented at the same meeting, which found no benefit to high-dose therapy and prompted the National Cancer Institute to send a team to South Africa to review the records of patients in Dr. Bezwoda's study. The results of the audit revealed several major problems.[23] Records on many of the patients who received high-dose treatment were missing, and several of those that were reviewed did not meet the stated inclusion criteria for the study. Perhaps more critical was the finding that no data could be found that any patients actually received the stated control regimen. Finally, no signed consent forms were available and the IRB had no record of approving the study.

The Bezwoda case represents an extreme and flagrant violation of the ethical principles of scientific conduct and one that could have had serious consequences had it gone undetected. Patients could have been exposed to a toxic high-dose chemotherapy regimen that did not in fact prolong their survival. It has been argued that the scientific process is inherently self-correcting since significant new results will only be viewed as valid if independently corroborated by other investigators. Indeed, it was the discrepancies between Bezwoda's results and those of other investigators that drew attention to this case. In most situations, however, independent confirmation of study results is not immediately forthcoming, and it may be months or years before results are either disputed or confirmed.

Since the scientific community is, for the most part, self-policing, the public must rely on the integrity of the investigators to ensure that unethical practices are not widespread. However, in view of the fact that the Public Health Service in the United States currently provides more than $11 billion annually toward extramural research, taxpayers have more than a passing interest in being assured that their money is being well spent. In 1989, the Department of Health and Human Services in the United States set up an agency, now known as the Office of Research Integrity, to develop policies and procedures related to preventing, monitoring, investigating, and imposing sanctions related to scientific misconduct (see http://ori.dhhs.gov/). Institutions receiving federal funds are required to have administrative procedures in place to deal with allegations of misconduct in a timely fashion. In addition, each institution must ensure that whistle-blowers, those who allege misconduct on the part of others, are protected from retaliation. Although this is never easy, it is much easier for a senior scientist such as Cameron Bowie, emeritus director of public health, to be forthright about misconduct on the part of a junior investigator as described in his essay, "Was the Paper I Wrote a Fraud?"[24] Researchers in training or at an early stage of their careers may be reluctant to bring allegations of fraud against established investigators who may be well respected within their field of study and influential with funding agencies and journals. Institutions are unlikely to welcome with open arms a junior researcher who may place millions of dollars of research funding in jeopardy by bringing charges of misconduct against a senior scientist. In the Liburdy case discussed previously, Lawrence Berkeley National Laboratory was asked to repay more than $800,000 in misspent funds. Naturally, the university feels that they have been penalized for having been forthright in exposing the misconduct of one of its employees.[19] The process of bringing forth and investigating scientific misconduct is one that raises ethical concerns and conflicts of interest for individuals and institutions. The service provided to the public in exposing fraudulent science mandates that whistle-blowers be rewarded not punished.

Ethical Issues in Literature Evaluation

It may come as a surprise to some that those who review and comment on the biomedical literature are also subject to breaches of ethical conduct. A glaring example was the review written by Jerry Berke of the book, *Living Downstream: An Ecologist Looks at Cancer and the Environment*, by Sandra Steingraber. Berke wrote a highly critical review of this book in the November 20, 1997, issue of the *New England Journal of Medicine*. Subsequent reports[25] have revealed that Berke was, at the time of the review, the medical director for W. R. Grace, a chemical company that has been the subject of more than one investigation into environmental pollution. Berke's affiliation with the chemical company was noticeably absent from the published review.

Unfortunately, a number of pieces of evidence point to the fact that unethical behavior and conflicts of interest are common in the review and publication of drug and other biomedical literature. Many of the problems associated with peer review of submitted manuscripts, including rejection of papers related to professional rivalry and outright theft of privileged information were detailed in Chap. 3. Stelfox et al.[26] searched the literature for papers discussing the controversy over the safety of calcium channel blocker usage in patients with cardiovascular disease. They concluded that there was a strong association between the authors' position on this issue and their financial relationship with a manufacturer of a calcium channel antagonist. Of those authors who were supportive of the use of these drugs, 96% had a financial relationship with a manufacturer. Sixty percent of those who were neutral on this issue had such a relationship, while only 37% of those who were critical of the use of these drugs in this situation were financially linked to a pharmaceutical company. Similar results have been reported in other investigations. Freidberg and coworkers found that pharmaceutical company-sponsored studies were approximately eight times less likely to report unfavorable qualitative conclusions with respect to the economic benefits of drugs such as hematopoietic colony-stimulating factors, antiemetics, and taxanes in oncology.[27] This is an important finding, given the importance of cost-effectiveness to the success of a new drug product in today's marketplace.

Clinical drug research in the United States and around the world is largely supported by the pharmaceutical industry, and it is to be expected that companies will act in their own economic best interest. It has been suggested that one explanation for the positive findings of studies sponsored by companies is related to the fact that intensive internal screening results in only products that are highly likely to have positive clinical and economic benefits reaching the final stages of drug testing. Indeed, while authors such as Freidberg have observed a tendency for company-sponsored studies in general to be more favorable to their drugs than other studies, overt bias can be difficult to detect in individual papers.

A much more insidious problem relates to commentaries, editorials, and review articles based on the primary literature. It can be argued that it is much easier for an author of a review or commentary to pick and choose specific papers or isolated results from papers that support his or her hypothesis while ignoring those that present an opposing view. An analysis of review articles into the health effects of passive smoking found that while only 37% of reviews concluded that passive smoking was not harmful, 74% of these papers were written by authors affiliated with the tobacco industry.[28] Indeed, the only factor in a multivariate analysis that was linked to whether a review concluded that passive smoking was not harmful was an affiliation with a tobacco company. For this reason, journals may have more stringent conflict-of-interest guidelines for authors of tertiary literature. For example, the conflict-of-interest guidelines for the *New England Journal of Medicine* state that authors of research articles should disclose any financial arrangements that they may have with a company whose product is a focal point of the investigation. However, "because the essence of reviews and editorials is selection and interpretation of the literature, the *Journal* expects that the authors of such articles will not have **any** financial interest in a company (or its competitor) that makes a product discussed in the article" ("Information for Authors," *New England Journal of Medicine*). Such a stringent policy can be difficult to enforce, given that most reviews are written by clinical scientists who are considered to be experts in the field, the same group of individuals who are likely to be approached by pharmaceutical companies to conduct research on their products. In fact, the editors of the *New England Journal of Medicine* recently published an apologetic letter related to this issue. They noted that almost half of the review articles published in the "Drug Therapy" section of the journal since 1997 were written by authors who had received major financial support or were consultants to companies at the time they were invited to prepare a review.[29]

KEY CONCEPT

The close ties between industry and the biomedical community makes conflicts of interest in drug research and evaluation inevitable. Full disclosure of potential conflicts is needed if readers are to conduct an informed evaluation of the merits of published research.

The *British Medical Journal* has taken a somewhat different approach to the issue of conflict of interest, a condition, which the editors acknowledge, is both widespread and to be expected in an area of science where much of the funding comes from the private sector.[30] The policy of the *BMJ* is that conflicts should be disclosed rather than prohibited. This may be a more feasible approach and allows the reader to draw his or her own conclusions regarding the possibility of external influences affecting the results of an investigation. Unfortunately, it appears that authors and reviewers often have a different view than editors as to what constitutes a conflict of interest and, therefore, fail to make any declaration. To combat this problem, the *BMJ* has replaced the term *conflict of interest* with *competing interests* in an effort to reduce the stigma that authors may attach to the former term. Authors and reviewers of papers are asked whether they have, in the past 5 years, been employed or received speaking fees, reimbursement for attending a symposium, research funds, or consulting fees from an organization that may gain or lose financially from the results of the study. They are also asked whether they hold stocks or have any other competing interests. Although questions are directed at financial interests, individuals are encouraged to report any personal, political, religious, or other interest that may be worthy of disclosure. George Lundberg was fired from his position as the editor of *JAMA* in 1999 after being accused of interjecting politics into the journal.[31] Lundberg reportedly fast-tracked the publication of a manuscript, entitled "Would You Say You 'Had Sex' if . . . ?"[32] at a time when the U.S. Congress was investigating the sexual conduct of President Clinton.

It is perhaps unreasonable to expect that those evaluating and reviewing the literature will apply a fresh and open mind to every paper. A lifetime of experience brings with it certain opinions and biases that cannot help but color one's approach. Papers that support a hypothesis diametrically opposed to one's own viewpoint provide a significant challenge to the reviewer. Nonetheless, science should be about facts not opinions. Scientists and reviewers should be able to present and evaluate the facts without allowing personal biases to distort the essential nature of the data. The general public has neither the access to primary literature nor the training required to appropriately evaluate the significance of research and places its trust in the biomedical community to perform this role. At a time when public trust in science and traditional health care practices appears to be low, unethical practices by researchers and reviewers have the potential to further undermine respect for the scientific process. Decreased public funding for research along with increased support of scientifically unproven therapies and health care practices could be the result.

Study Questions

1. What are the requirements for composition of an IRB?

2. Should the IRB evaluate the scientific merit of a protocol?

3. What are the basic elements of informed consent that must be provided to potential research subjects?

4. Why are conflicts of interest more of a concern with tertiary literature than primary literature?

References

1. Karlawish JH, Hall JB: The controversy over emergency research. A review of the issues and suggestions for a resolution. Am J Respir Crit Care Med 153:499–506, 1996.

2. Marquis D: How to resolve an ethical dilemma concerning randomized clinical trials. New Engl J Med 341:691–693, 1999.

3. Khan A, Warner HA, Brown WA: Symptom reduction and suicide risk in patients treated with placebo in antidepressant clinical trials: An analysis of the Food and Drug Administration database. Arch Gen Psychiatry 57:311–317, 2000.

4. White RM: Unraveling the Tuskegee Study of Untreated Syphilis. Arch Int Med 160:585–598, 2000.

5. Emanuel EJ, Wendler D, Grady C: What makes clinical research ethical? JAMA 283:2701–2711, 2000.

6. Ellis GB: Keeping research subjects out of harm's way. JAMA 282:1963–1964, 1999.

7. Marshall E: Gene therapy death prompts review of adenovirus vector. Science 286:2244, 2000.

8. Amber D: Case at VCU brings ethics to forefront. The Scientist, May 1, 2000, 1.

9. Evans I: Conduct unbecoming—the MRC's approach. BMJ 316:1726–1733, 1998.

10. Broad W, Wade N: *Betrayers of the Truth*. New York, Simon and Schuster, 1982.

11. Rennie D: An American perspective on research integrity. BMJ 316:1726–1733, 1998.

12. Riis P: Honest advice from Denmark. BMJ 316:1726–1733, 1998.

13. Pownall M: Falsifying data is main problem in US research fraud review. West J Med 170:377, 1999.

14. Kahn JO, Cherng DW, Mayer K, Murray H, Lagakos S: Evaluation of HIV-1 Immunogen, an immunologic modifier, administered to patients infected with HIV having 300 to 549×10^6/L CD4 cell counts. JAMA 284:2193–2202, 2000.

15. Waldron HA: Is duplicate publishing on the increase? BMJ 304:1029, 1992.

16. Fraud and Plagiarism, Committee on Publication Ethics Report, 1998; www.bmj.com/misc/cope/.

17. Rymer J: Fraud at conferences needs to be addressed. BMJ 317:1590, 1998.

18. Relman AS: Lessons from the Darsee affair. N Engl J Med 308:1415–1417, 1983.

19. Barinaga M, Kaiser J: Fraud finding triggers payback demand. Science 285:1189–1190, 1999.

20. Williams MH, Bowie C: Evidence of unmet need in the care of severely physically disabled adults. BMJ 306:95–98, 1993.

21. Retraction—Evidence of need in the care of physically disabled adults. BMJ 316:1700, 1998.

22. Hagmann M: Cancer researcher sacked for alleged fraud. Science 287:1901–1902, 2000.

23. Weiss RB, Rifkin RM, Stewart FM, Theriault RL, Williams WA, Herman AA, Beveridge RA: High-dose chemotherapy for high-risk primary breast cancer: An on-site review of the Bezwoda study. Lancet 355:999–1003, 2000.

24. Bowie C: Was the paper I wrote a fraud? BMJ 316:1755, 1998.

25. Josefson D: US journal embroiled in another conflict of interest scandal. BMJ 316:247, 1998.

26. Stelfox HT, Chua G, O'Rourke K, Detsky AS: Conflict of interest in the debate over calcium-channel antagonists. N Engl J Med 338:101–106, 1998.

27. Friedberg M, Saffran B, Stinson TJ, Nelson W, Bennett CL: Evaluation of conflict of interest in economic analyses of new drugs used in oncology. JAMA 282:1453–1457, 1999.

28. Barnes DE, Bero LA: Why review articles on the health effects of passive smoking reach different conclusions. JAMA 279:1566–1570, 1998.

29. Angell M, Utiger RD, Wood AJJ: Disclosure of authors' conflicts of interest: A follow-up. New Engl J Med 342:586–587, 2000.

30. Smith R: Beyond conflict of interest. BMJ 317:291–292, 1998.

31. Hopkins J: JAMA's editor fired over sex article. BMJ 318:213, 1999.

32. Sanders SA, Reinisch JM: Would you say you 'had sex' if? JAMA 281:275–277, 1999.

The Future of Drug Information and the Internet

Richard L. Slaughter

OUTLINE

Goals and Objectives

Introduction

The Internet as a Source of Drug Information

Reliability of Information on the Internet

The Internet and Biomedical Journals

Presentation of Information

Examples of Journals Online

E-Journals and E-Journal Servers

Summary

Study Questions

References

KEY WORDS

BioMed Central
Drug information
E-journal
E-journal server
HON

Internet
MedCERTAIN
NetPrint
Online
PubMed Central

Goals and Objectives

The goal of this chapter is to discuss issues concerning the use of the Internet for accessing drug information. After completing this chapter, readers should:

1. Appreciate the significance of the Internet as a source of health and drug information and understand issues centered around the delivery of information on the Internet.

2. Recognize organizations that address issues related to the reliability of information on the Internet.

3. Understand that the Internet is a medium for the delivery of traditional published biomedical information.

4. Understand how biomedical journals are approaching the Internet for dissemination of information.

5. Recognize e-journals and e-servers.

6. Understand the implications of prepublication servers and posting results of studies on the Internet prior to publication.

Introduction

The nature of how drug information is delivered to the end user is changing rapidly as the Internet becomes much more pervasive. It has been estimated that in 1998 there were 47 million Internet users in the United States.[1] By June 1999, this had grown to 63.4 million, and it had increased to 148.8 million users by July 2000.[2] Also, 14 million new U.S. households went online in 2000. This was double the number that went online in 1999. The average user spent over 7.5 h online a week in 1999, which was projected to increase to 8.2 h/week in 2000.[3]

Health-related sites have been among the most popular sites visited. For example, comparing activity from October to January 1999, www.Drkoop.com had the largest gain in visitors (726.4%) and www.Onhealth.com the sixth largest gain (298.7%).[4] It was estimated that $450 million would be spent purchasing drugs online in 2000. In one year (1997 to 1998) the number of adults who sought health related information almost doubled, from 12 to 22.3 million (see Fig. 15-1). Most people sought information about disease states (52%), while 33% surfed for information on pharmaceuticals (Fig. 15-2). It is projected that online health care businesses will dominate the Internet market in the coming years. It is estimated that business-to-business online health care will increase from a $6 billion market in 1999 to a huge $348 billion market in 2004. Further, by 2004, business-to-business online health care will make up one-sixth of the overall business trade in health care. The majority of this activity will be in processing claims. However, part of this growth will be in patient care–related activities such as electronic medical records, patient care documentation, and clinical applications such as online treatment guidelines. Clearly, the Internet is a major component of daily business, com-

> **KEY CONCEPT**
>
> The Internet is widely used to obtain health care information. By 2005, almost 90 million adults will be using the Internet for this purpose.

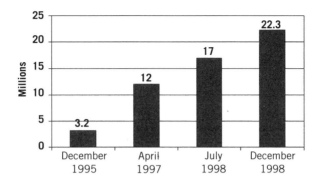

Figure 15-1. U.S. adults retrieving health or medical information online. *[Data adapted from Lake (3).]*

munication, and entertainment and an important source of information on health care and drugs.

It has been estimated that by 2005, 88.5 million adults will use the Internet to find health information, shop for health products, and communicate with affiliated payers and providers through online channels. Increased growth will be due to greater use of the Internet by people over 65 and because insurance companies will move customers to the Internet to purchase drugs, process claims, and obtain consumer education on health-related issues.

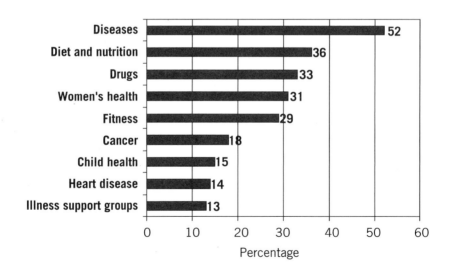

Figure 15-2. Health-related contents searched for on the Internet. *[Adapted from Lake (3).]*

The Internet as a Source of Drug Information

The Internet has become a means of rapidly accessing information about health care and prescription drugs. As mentioned in previous chapters, a wide range of sources of information can be accessed through the Internet. These sources include private individuals with an interest in a given health topic, health care organizations, health care agencies and foundations, and pharmaceutical companies. Some examples of novel uses of the Internet include video broadcasting of medical procedures and conferences. In 2000, the Detroit Medical Center launched an interactive Web site titled Morning Report Reviews, at www.mdmorningreport.com. This site is in the format of the morning report in which the most interesting cases that have been admitted to a hospital are reported. The histories of four to six patient cases that have been treated at Detroit Receiving Hospital will be presented each month. This site uses an interactive format targeted for physicians and medical students enabling them to learn more about evidence-based approaches to treatment through the case histories of actual patients. The use of the Internet for such activities will increase as technology allows the transference of greater amounts of data, particularly video and audio data, across communications networks. The use of the Internet as an important educational tool for the delivery and receipt of text, video, and audio information has increased substantially over the past few years and will continue to do so.

The Internet is a source of educational programs, including continuing education (CE) programs. These will continue to grow in the future as degree programs and individual courses are offered through the Internet. Currently, many colleges offer courses entirely through the Internet or use the Internet to enhance courses taught by conventional means. Examples of courses taught through a courseware program at Wayne State University can be found at www.wayne.edu:8000. Randy Trinkle recently published a review of the sources of accredited pharmacy CE programs, which is available on the Internet.[5] This is a good comprehensive source for Internet-related CE programs in pharmacy.

Some examples of routine Web sites include an industry site, www.merck.com and a professional organization site for the American Diabetes Association, www.diabetes.com. The Merck home page is divided into sections concerning general health, information about Merck products, and information about the company. For example, general information about the Merck product Fosamax, geared for either general consumers or health care professionals, can be found. Accessing the health information component provides what is best described as a traditional journal-type advertisement for Fosamax. There is access to the package insert, and there are links to the National Osteoporosis Foundation and the Bone Measurement Institute. This is an example of tertiary literature presented through a Web page.

The dissemination of information directly from manufacturers to consumers will continue. One current avenue is by tracking information at the point of access and requesting data from the user for the purpose of providing future product or disease state information. Technology is now available to identify the user's computer address and immediately send product information automatically. The ability to track this information is beginning to influence marketing strategies.

Another example of health information can be found at professional organization sites, such as that of the American Diabetes Association, www.diabetes.org. This site provides general information about diabetes, news about diabetes, information about the American Diabetes Association, and new information about the epidemiology and/or treatment of the disease. This site provides very high quality current, relevant, and unbiased information on the disease state.

The preceding examples provide some insight into the type of health-related information that is readily accessible from the Internet. This type of information is very user-friendly, consumer-oriented, and easy to obtain. These are reasons why the Internet is widely used to access health-related information.

KEY CONCEPT

Use of the Internet has grown because information can be easy to obtain, is user-friendly, and is consumer-oriented.

A frequently asked question concerns how Internet sources are to be referenced. Internet information is different from that in print media because of its dynamic nature. That is, information can readily be changed—it can be updated or removed at the discretion of the individual or organization that posted it. In contrast, printed media are constant. A reference source published in a journal will always have the same location, and the information will always be the same. A reference source posted on a Web site may or may not be present in the future. Further, the content of the posted information, if the source has not been removed, could very well have changed. That is the nature of the Internet. For this reason, some guidelines should be adhered to when referencing Internet sources. Here are examples from the *American Journal of Health-Systems Pharmacy*[6]:

11. National Cancer Institute Home Page [resource on World Wide Web]. URL: http://www.nci.nih.gov. Available from Internet. Accessed 1995 Apr 28.

12. Kulikowski S. Readability formula, in NL-KR (Digest vol. 5, no. 10) [electronic bulletin board]. Rochester, NY; 1988. Accessed 1998 Jan 31. Available from nl-kr@cs.rochester.edu; Internet.

Note that the information given includes the title, such as National Cancer Institute Home Page, the type of source (electronic bulletin board or World Wide Web), the URL address (e.g., www.nci.nih.gov) or e-mail address (nl-kr@cs.rochester.edu), and the date accessed. Note that this format has been used for the Internet references cited in this chapter.

Reliability of Information on the Internet

The Internet is one of the primary sources of information for consumers on health-related issues. Since there is high reliance on the Internet for information and there is no review process in place (as exists with printed media), there is justifiable concern about the quality of the information provided. Some authors have expressed concern about the public health consequences that could result from false or misleading drug information posted on the Internet.[7]

Kim et al.[8] have recently reviewed criteria that are used for the evaluation of health-related Web sites. These criteria should include an evaluation of the accuracy of the content, authority of the authors or sponsoring organization of the Web site, disclosure of the relationship of the Web site to its sponsoring agencies, appropriate referencing of the content, and provisions for feedback. These are summarized in Table 15-1.

Four Internet sites—MedicineNet, RxList, Drug InfoNet, and thriveonline—were evaluated by Hatfield et al.[9] against criteria very similar to those recommended by Kim et al. They sought information on 30 of the most commonly prescribed medications and found that the accuracy of information was >98% for all sites; however, only two of the sites had consumer information available. They concluded that most of the information provided was reliable. Note that this study

TABLE 15-1. **Important Factors in Evaluating Health-Related Web Sites**

Content	Is it accurate and reliable?
Web page design	Is the design appealing?
Disclosure statements	Is the nature of the organization and its relationship to sponsoring agencies (e.g., pharmaceutical companies) provided?
Currency of information	Are dated updates provided?
Authority of source	Is the source of information a known authority in the field?
Ease of use	Is the site easy to navigate?
Accessibility and availability	Is the site freely accessible or is there an access fee? Is it always available?
Links provided	Are links provided to other important sites?
Documentation	Is the information provided documented with references?
Feedback	Is there a means to provide feedback or ask questions?

SOURCE: Adapted from Kim et al. (8).

evaluated only four sites, which represents a small fraction of the sites on the Internet that can provide information on pharmaceuticals.

The Health on the Net Foundation (HON) has developed a code of conduct for medical and health sites. The sole purpose of this organization is to address the reliability and credibility of health-related information on the Internet. Figure 15-3 shows the symbol HON uses for site approval. A site's sponsors need to apply to HON for the use of its seal, and they must agree to adhere to the principles outlined by HON. As an example of a HON approved site, Achoo—Internet Health Directory (www.achoo.com), is designed to catalog, index, describe, and rate the health care information on the Internet. This site adheres to the HON code of conduct. Achoo.com serves as a gateway to free information from sites that display the HON code of conduct. Web users should look for sites that subscribe to the HON code. This will help to provide some degree of quality from Web sites. More information about HON has been published in the *American Journal of Health-Systems Pharmacy* [(July 1):57, 2000]. As stated in this article, display of HON certification by a Web site, while not a guarantee of the quality of the site, will help users to identify sites that are reliable and credible. See Table 15-2 for Web addresses of health-related organizations.

KEY CONCEPT

Reliability of information can be improved by looking for sites on the Internet that are approved by the Health on the Net Foundation (HON).

Another initiative by MedCERTAIN (MedPICS Certification and Rating of Trustworthy and Assessed Health Information on the Net; www.medpics.org/medcertain/, an international nonprofit project putting trust into health information on the net, has a goal of using filtering technologies to establish a third-party rating system that will allow consumers to filter harmful health information and to positively identify and select high-quality information. This effort uses panels of experts

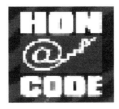

Figure 15-3. Health on the Net Foundation (HON) Code of Approval seal.

TABLE 15-2. **Web Addresses of Health-Related Organizations**

Organization	Web Address
Alzheimer's Association	www.alz.org
American Cancer Society	www.cancer.org
American Diabetes Association	www.diabetes.org
American Foundation for AIDS Research	www.amfar.org
American Heart Association	www.americanheart.org
American Liver Foundation	www.liverfoundation.org
American Lung Association	www.lungusa.org
Arthritis Foundation	http://arthritis.org
Cystic Fibrosis Foundation	www.cff.org
Epilepsy Foundation	http://efa.org
Fertility Foundation	www.fertilityfoundation.org
Hepatitis B Foundation	www.hepb.org
Multiple Sclerosis Foundation	www.msfacts.org
Muscular Dystrophy	www.mdausa.org
National Cancer Institute	www.nci.nih.gov/
National Center for Complementary and Alternative Medicine	http://nccam.nih.gov/
National Foundation for Depressive Illness	www.depression.org
National Headache Foundation	www.headaches.org
National Heart Lung and Blood Institute	www.nhlbi.nih.gov
National Institute of Arthritis and Musculoskeletal and Skin Diseases	www.nih.gov/niams/
National Institute of Diabetes and Digestive and Kidney Diseases	www.niddk.nih.gov/
National Institute of Mental Health	www.nimh.nih.gov
National Institute of Neurological Disorders and Stroke	www.ninds.nih.gov
National Institute on Aging	www.nih.gov/nia/
National Institute on Allergy and Infectious Diseases	www.niaid.nih.gov/
National Institute on Drug Abuse	www.nida.nih.gov
National Kidney Foundation	www.kidney.org
National Parkinson Foundation	www.parkinson.org
National Stroke Foundation	www.stroke.org
National Women's Health Information Center	www.4woman.org/

to screen sites and provide quality seals ranging from a "good standing" seal to a "gold" seal indicating that the site has undergone external peer review. This is a more proactive approach to assessing the quality of sites.

The Internet Healthcare Coalition (IHC) provided the framework for the e-Health ethics summit in Washington, D.C., January 31 to February 2, 2000. This code is published in the *Journal of Medical Internet Research* [2(1):e2, 2000; www. symposion.com/jmir/2000/1/e2]. This code of ethics provides guiding principles under five main headings: candor and trustworthiness; quality; informed consent, privacy, and confidentiality; best commercial practices; and best practices for provision of health care on the Internet by health care professionals. As can be seen, this effort by the IHC goes beyond issues related to content and enters into behavioral issues (e.g., confidentiality and privacy).

In summary, the quality of health information that is accessible on the Internet is a concern. Several approaches are being taken to try to ensure global access to high-quality, reliable, and accurate information. While these efforts will help to ensure that information provided is accurate, it should not replace scrutiny by the individual reader of this information.

The Internet and Biomedical Journals

In addition to consumer-related information, the Internet has begun to completely change the face of traditional journal publication. It has been projected that more than 90% of all published research will be available through electronic databases. The impact of the Internet on biomedical journals includes not only accessibility, but also how information is presented (e.g., printed and online formats; free and password-protected areas), the creation of new online-only journals, copyright issues, and cost issues. The remainder of this chapter focuses on these areas with the goal of identifying current trends that are likely to impact the future delivery of drug information to the end consumer.

Presentation of Information

The Internet provides a significant challenge for traditional biomedical journals—to interface a longstanding print media format that is very rigid in structure with an amorphous electronic format. While almost all journals now have their own Web sites, the amount of information provided, the accessibility of information, and the attitude of the journal toward the Internet varies drastically from journal to journal. This results in highly varied approaches to online publication of material among journals. Most journals provide tables of contents, abstracts, and possibly limited access to full-text versions of articles. Most will also provide topic searching through past journals and through affiliated journals.

Access to full-text versions of articles varies from journal to journal. Some journals provide access only through a username and password, which is provided free or for a fee. Others provide complete access to full-text articles. Once a full-text article is found, there are several ways of obtaining a printed copy. One is to print directly from a Web browser. This option typically provides text information, with tables and figures printed separately. The article as printed from the Web may differ somewhat from the published article. Another option is to convert the article to a PDF file and then print. Note that this version will provide a copy that is identical to the printed version. Copies of articles can also be delivered to an e-mail address for a fee. By limiting access to full-text articles, journals limit access and direct users to the format the journal prefers.

KEY CONCEPT

Journals vary widely in how they provide online access to information. Some journals provide free access, whereas others charge for access.

Examples of Journals Online

American Journal of Health-System Pharmacy (AJHP).   This is the official journal of the American Society of Health-System Pharmacists and is published every 2 weeks. The society provides an online version of the journal at http://ashp.org/public/pubs/ajhp/. This journal provides an exact copy of the printed version online. Full-text versions of articles are provided in PDF format, which are very easy to access. *AJHP* provides full-text articles back to August 1999 and access to *AJHP* news and article abstracts back to March 1997. The journal can be searched for information back to March 1997 using keyword searching only. Searching by citation or journal location is not possible. Other information available includes author information, advertising, career opportunities, reprints and permissions, supplements, and subscription.

New England Journal of Medicine (NEJM).   The *New England Journal of Medicine,* published by the Massachusetts Medical Society, is considered by many to be the most prestigious medical journal. It can be found online at www.nejm.org. The current issue is posted on the Web site at 5 P.M. on Wednesday of each week. This site provides limited access to information, with full-text versions available only to subscribers. For nonsubscribers, the online version provides access to abstracts of all scientific articles and to some other components of the journal. The site implies an interactive approach for the What's the Diagnosis? section, which links to the Case Records of the Massachusetts General Hospital section of the journal, and the Take the Images Quiz, which uses images from the Images in Clinical Medicine section of the journal. As mentioned, subscribers to *NEJM* are provided with full-text versions of published articles; these are easily accessed and used. The journal is available in full-text format from the first issue of 1993, and search capability back to 1990 is provided. The Search the Past Issues section provides for detailed and customized searches by title, topic, author, 1990 to present, article category, publication date, issue number, or page number. It is easy to perform general topic searches as well as to search for specific articles.

NEJM does place limitations on the use of electronic copies, as stated under Terms and Conditions, Section 2, Limitations on Use:

> The Service may be accessed, viewed or otherwise used only by a Registered Subscriber. As a Registered Subscriber, you are permitted to view, browse and/or download for temporary copying purposes only the contents of this website, provided these uses are for noncommercial, personal purposes, and further provided that you maintain all copyright and any other notices on all copies. However, except as provided by law or by this Agreement, the contents of this website may not be further stored, reproduced, distributed, transmitted, modified, adapted, performed, displayed (including adaptations/displays such as by "framing"), published or sold in whole or in part without the prior written permission from MMS.

Note that this is an adaptation of print media copyright policies to an electronic medium. The *NEJM* Web site is a limited-access site that provides information very close to that in the printed journal.

American Journal of Cardiology (AJC).   *The American Journal of Cardiology*, published by Elsevier Science, is a highly regarded specialty journal that focuses on the clinical diagnosis and treatment of cardiovascular disease. This journal boasts the shortest lag time from receipt of manuscript to publication of all scientific journals (<5 months). The online version, at www.cardiosource.com, is accessible only to paid subscribers. As pressure increases for greater accessibility of information, journals that limit accessibility are likely to be in the minority in the future. Levels of access will be an area of debate and contention between publishers of traditional journals and proponents of accessibility of information on the Internet.

The Lancet Interactive.   *The Lancet* provides an online version, *The Lancet Interactive*, at www.thelancet.com. This site expands the electronic journal beyond simply providing access to the traditional print version. Access is controlled through a username and password; however, a level of access is provided at no charge. Access to the traditional printed journal is provided; however, only abstract information is provided to nonsubscribers. Full-text articles are provided on only a limited basis. What is of interest on this site is the creation of discussion groups, including a Hot Papers section that serves as a point for initiating discussion. For example, on June 29, 2000, the paper "Regular Inhaled Salbutamol and Asthma Control: The TRUST Randomised Trial" (*Lancet* 355:1675–1679, 2000) was being discussed. Other discussion topics included pregnancy stretch marks, oral submucous fibrosis, holistic therapies, contact-lens-associated microbial keratitis, evidence-based illiteracy, and racism in health care. As is shown, a very wide range of topic areas is covered. In addition, users have the ability to begin their own discussion groups. This is an example of how a journal can use the Internet to expand services beyond what can be provided in print media.

Another area where *The Lancet Interactive* has taken initiative is in the creation of the Electronic Research Archive. As stated by *The Lancet,*[10] "The objective of this archive is to create a searchable electronic public library of research in international health. We are seeking content that covers all issues relevant to medicine in the developing world." This provides a forum for the posting and discussion of papers prior to acceptance for publication. Posting of papers electronically prior to acceptance by a journal for widespread review is quite controversial and is discussed in more detail in the section on e-journals.

British Medical Journal (BMJ).   The *British Medical Journal,* at www.bmj.com, represents one of the better attempts at moving a well-established printed journal into an electronic format. The *BMJ* site was started in 1995 and is fully accessible at no charge, with no registration required. Features offered at this site are in some ways unique and may represent how traditional journals will use the Internet in the future. Searching the *BMJ* is very easy; the search process allows for searches by author, keyword, or citation and allows for searches across multiple journals. It is very unusual for a journal to allow easy searching across nonaffiliated journals.

Full-text versions of accessed articles are provided, with several options available to the user. For example, the user can send a response to the article, go to other related articles in the *BMJ,* go to related articles in PubMed, or search Medline by the names of the authors of the article. At the end of each article, *BMJ* provides information on related articles published in the *BMJ* and on other articles that have cited the specific article. This is somewhat novel. The *BMJ* provides excellent connectivity from its published articles, and it offers easy and rapid comment on published articles through the Rapid Responses section. For example, seven letters were posted on June 28, 2000 (site accessed on June 29), on seven different topics published in the *BMJ,* including articles that had been published as recently as June 24. This provides for rapid and timely discussion of the printed version. The *BMJ* has sections on debates, theme issues and series, a bookstore, and access to Netprints, an electronic archive that posts prepublished articles (see following section). The *BMJ* also links to free books. This is a user-friendly, Internet-friendly site that represents very well how a printed journal can successfully interface with the Internet.

This section has reviewed how traditional journals have begun to use the Internet as a forum for the publication and presentation of biomedical information. The examples have shown how journals have taken different approaches to the Internet, ranging from an interactive, open-access policy (e.g., *BMJ*) to a very closed access (e.g., *AJC*). In the future, journals will continually have to deal with issues related to level of access and how they are reimbursed for information displayed on the Internet.

E-Journals and E-Journal Servers

The cost of biomedical journals, coupled with the accessibility of the Internet, has the potential of creating a revolution in the delivery of health-related research to end users. For example, the average subscription cost of a medical journal was

$663.21 in 2000; it had increased by 38.6% over the previous 3 years, whereas the Consumer Price Index increased by only 3.9% between 1997 and 1999 (154.5 to 160.5).[11] The increases in journal publication costs have greatly outstripped the ability of institutions to keep pace with them. In March 2000, the Association of American Universities, the Association of Research Libraries, and the Merrill Advanced Studies Center of the University of Kansas met solely to provide recommendations to academic communities concerning the crisis in journal pricing. It stated:

> The current system of scholarly publishing has become too costly for the academic community to sustain. The increasing volume and costs of scholarly publications, particularly in science, technology, and medicine (STM), are making it impossible for libraries and their institutions to support the collection needs of their current and future faculty and students.[11]

Further, it has been argued that these increases are particularly outrageous because most of the content of journals is already funded by public money (either through grants or subsidies provided by research universities), so the public is paying for the same information at least twice. Further, the bulk of the work on journals is provided free by academic faculty members. This includes serving as journal editors, performing the peer review process, and doing the copyediting.[12] Much of this activity is driven by the tenure process in universities that place high pressure on faculty members to publish and to become involved in the publication process. Over the next several years, the nature of the publishing media will change in direct response to the capabilities of the Internet.

KEY CONCEPT

The increasing cost of journals is placing increasing burdens on libraries, such that alternate sources of providing information are being evaluated.

One format that is emerging is *e-publishing*, or publishing the results of research in electronic format, in journals that publish only electronically. This is not necessarily a new concept to academia. In 1991, an automated archive was started at the Los Alamos National Laboratory that served as a means of electronic communication of research within the high-energy physics community. Articles could be submitted electronically directly to the archive and then accessed by anyone interested in the topic. This effort has been widely successful in the physics community. It has enhanced, not replaced, the peer review process and has in fact streamlined the process, as some journals will accept publication directly from this server. Further, feedback is broader than that provided by a selected number of peer reviewers, as articles are posted for anyone to comment on. The high usage of this site—2500 submissions per month serving 30,000 distinct hosts a week—indicates the success this site has had. This certainly can be used as a model for electronic publishing and review.[13]

Similar non-peer-reviewed archives have now been set up in other disciplines, and in some cases are replacing the traditional paper journals in these fields.[14] An example is an initiative by the Scholarly Publishing and Academic Resource Coalition (SPARC). This is a worldwide alliance of research institutions, libraries, and organizations that encourages competition in the scholarly communications market. Its purpose is to forge new solutions to current problems associated with scientific journal publishing. It states that "SPARC strives to return science to scientists." It has the following aims:

1. Increase competition in the scholarly communication marketplace.

2. Ensure fair use of electronic resources while strengthening the proprietary rights and privileges of authorship.

3. Use technology to reduce costs and improve scholarly communication.

Organic Letters was the first SPARC-sponsored journal. This collaborative effort of the American Chemical Society and SPARC delivers original articles reporting the latest developments in all areas of organic chemistry. A unique aspect of this journal is the use of electronic transmission for review and subsequent publication. The submission, review, and acceptance time for this journal can be as short as a few weeks.

PubMed Central.   These efforts have been initiated outside of health-related fields. However, in 1999 Harold Varmus, director of the National Institutes of Health, proposed to create a Web site titled E-biomed, where all biomedical research would be accessible. He proposed that this site would post peer-reviewed papers by traditional journals and that another would post almost any type of scholarly work, based on the recommendations of two reviewers. Examples of work that might be presented would include negative results from clinical trials, experimental techniques that are of interest to small subsets of the scientific community, or large data sets from biomedical studies.[15] These are examples of information that does not get into the printed media, and that can influence future research by its exclusion. That is, additional studies may be performed addressing research questions that have already been answered but have not been published because of the biases journals have against publishing studies with negative results. This proposal has been met with a high degree of controversy, particularly from traditional print media publishers. For example, the *New England Journal of Medicine* published an editorial by Arnold Relman titled "The NIH 'E-biomed' Proposal—A Potential Threat to the Evaluation and Orderly Dissemination of New Clinical Studies."[16] Relman concludes his editorial as follows:

> In clinical research, the best way to handle new data is to require rigorous peer review before their dissemination and, with few exceptions, to post the results

in electronic data bases only after they have been published in carefully edited, peer-reviewed journals. That is because prepublication evaluation of the reliability of clinical studies and impartial assessment of their implications for health care are usually more important than the speed with which the data are made available.

Despite the criticism, the E-biomed proposal led to the creation of PubMed Central, www.pubmedcentral.nih.gov, which began accepting articles in January 2000. This is a barrier-free repository that archives, organizes, and distributes peer-reviewed reports as well as reports that have been screened but not peer reviewed. The scope has expanded to include plant and agricultural research in the life sciences, in addition to biomedical research. Organizations supportive of PubMed Central include the Association of Academic Health Science Libraries, the Association of Research Libraries, and the Medical Library Association, among others. All material presented is indexed by one of the major abstracting and indexing services. Content and input on material that will appear in PubMed Central are controlled by the scientific publishers, professional societies, and groups other than the NIH. This control includes the screening of non-peer-reviewed reports. Copyright resides with the submitting group or author, not with PubMed Central. Journals that are available through PubMed Central (as of October 2000) and those that are to become available are shown in Table 15-3.

As an example, the journal *Critical Care* can be accessed through PubMed Central. *Critical Care* publishes commentaries, reviews, and original research. Only the original research articles are provided free of charge through PubMed Central. The full content of the journal is available on a subscription basis online and in print form. The subscription rates for this journal are as follows:

- Personal—online and print, $295; online only, $109
- Institutional—online and print, 1 to 20 employees, $590; 20 to 999 employees, $1474; 1000 to 2000 employees, $2950

This example illustrates the tiered pricing of journals and shows the impact of journal pricing at the institutional level. So while PubMed Central provides some free access and is moving toward an open environment, it is still heavily tied to the traditional journal format. It will be interesting to see how PubMed Central changes in the future and in particular how it will handle the publication of non-peer-reviewed research, which it had placed aside as of July 2000.[17]

BioMed Central. In May 2000, Vitek Tracz, head of the Current Science Group, started his own Internet publication services, BioMed Central, at www.biomedcentral.com. BioMed Central provides fast online publishing of peer-reviewed research in biomedicine with no barriers. It is run by a group of biomedical editors and a growing number of respected biological and medical researchers. As an example, the subject advisor list in cardiology includes the

TABLE 15-3. Journals Available Through PubMed Central

First Journals

Arthritis Research

BMC Biochemistry and Structural Biology

BMC Bioinformatics

BMC Family Practice

BMC Genetics

BMC Genomics

BMC Nephrology

Breast Cancer Research

Critical Care

Genome Biology

Molecular Biology of the Cell

Proceedings of the National Academy of Sciences of the United States of America

Forthcoming Journals

British Medical Journal

BioMed Central—many new journals

Canadian Medical Association Journal

Journal of Medical Entomology

Nucleic Acids Research

The Plant Cell

Plant Physiology

SOURCE: Adapted from http://pubmedcentral.nih.gov.

well-known scholars Julien Bogousslavsky, Eugene Braunwald, and Laurence Cohn. This high caliber of editorial staff adds substantially to the service's credibility. An interesting aspect of the papers BioMed publishes is that the original submitted article is provided as well as the peer review critique and the authors' response. This certainly opens up the peer review process for all readers to evaluate. For example, the article "Who Should Get the Pneumococcal Vaccine?" by R. Andrew Moore, published October 4, 2000, was submitted as "Are Pneumococcal Polysacharride Vaccines Effective? Meta-analysis of Prospective Trials" on July 26, 2000. The reviewer responded on September 9,

2000, and the author's response to the review was dated September 29, 2000. The manuscript was published less than 1 week after its acceptance. This is certainly a time line that would be difficult for any print journal to match. Articles published in BioMed Central journals are immediately posted on PubMed Central and indexed in PubMed. Also, in contrast to almost all printed journals, authors retain copyright for publication in BioMed Central. In addition, all research articles from the existing journals *GenomeBiology, Arthritis Research, Breast Cancer Research, Respiratory Research, Current Controlled Trials in Cardiovascular Medicine,* and *Critical Care* will be freely available through BioMed Central. As an example, *Current Controlled Trials in Cardiovascular Medicine* is an online and print media cardiovascular journal that provides access to current research in cardiovascular medicine. The aim of this journal is to stimulate debate; facilitate communication among investigators and users of trial results; provide tools, advice, and support for investigators and users of trial results; and bring readers the best available information relating to the application of clinical trials to cardiovascular practice. The journal aims to publish both positive and negative findings and to make data from clinical trials easily accessible.[18] A unique aspect of this journal is the depository for non-peer-reviewed articles. This is for authors who wish to disseminate information that may not be suitable for a conventional journal. Subjects of articles considered include the following:

- Improvements in techniques
- Detailed laboratory protocols
- Design of experiments
- Unexpected observations
- Preclinical work on drug development
- Design of clinical trials
- Genome data
- Microarrays
- DNA sequences

The efforts of PubMed Central, BioMed Central, and journals such as *Current Controlled Trials in Cardiovascular Medicine* are sure to affect the nature of biomedical publishing in the future. A more interactive approach as well as means of publishing a broader array of data such as peer reviewed reports from studies with negative results, and data that are not peer reviewed will increase in the future.

In a similar vein, the British Medical Society in collaboration with Stanford University Libraries and High Wire Press decided not to wait for the E-biomed proposal to develop, but instead created their own prepublication e-server, called Netprints. This is a repository of non-peer-reviewed original research. The user is warned prior to entering the site with the following caution statement:

Articles posted on this site have not yet been accepted for publication by a peer reviewed journal. They are presented here mainly for the benefit of fellow researchers. Casual readers should not act on their findings, and journalists should be wary of reporting them.

The purpose of this effort is to attempt to transform the peer review process from the current highly structured "black-box" approach that is mired with problems (see Chap. 3) to an entirely open process. These efforts are met with resistance in the traditional journal environment, as some journals, such as the *New England Journal of Medicine* and *JAMA,* will not accept publications that have been presented on prepublication servers such as Netprints.

Other prepublication archives include one sponsored by *The Lancet,* the Electronic Research Archive (ERA), which is designed for research into international health and for the posting of articles accepted by the journal for peer review. In addition, *The Lancet* provides an e-print server for the posting of articles for review prior to publication and as an alternative route to formal publication in *The Lancet.* The aim of this service is to widen the peer review process to strengthen the quality of the subsequent print version of articles. The primary goal of this server is to improve the peer review process with the goal of increasing the quality of published manuscripts. This is in comparison to servers that are designed to post non-peer-reviewed manuscripts.

KEY CONCEPT

Prepublication servers can allow for dissemination of information that might not otherwise be published (e.g., negative results) and can allow for broader review of studies prior to publication.

Summary

It will be of interest to both the scientific and lay communities how the relationships between traditional and electronic journals evolve over time. It is quite evident that the Internet will play an important role in the dissemination and accessibility of information. However, it will also play a very important role in the type of research that is presented, the type of data and results that are presented, and how the public reviews that information for use. There are very significant differences of opinion and approach. Some feel that the posting of non-peer-reviewed information will harm society because of the potential use of information that has not undergone rigorous scientific review. Others are of the opinion that the posting of information on the Internet will enhance and streamline the peer review process and ultimately provide higher quality literature to the end user. This chapter attempts to highlight some of the issues that are likely to influence how drug information is presented and obtained in the future. Hopefully, this has provided some insight into just some of the forces that will influence how drug information, and particularly biomedical journal formats, will be presented and accessed in the future.

Study Questions

1. Describe the HON Code of Conduct.

2. List five factors that are important in evaluating the reliability of a Web site.

3. Compare the online accessibility of the *American Journal of Cardiology* to that of the *British Medical Journal.*

4. What are the advantages and disadvantages of publishing research results on a prepublication server such as Netprints?

5. Describe PubMed Central and BioMed Central.

References

1. About the Internet Home Page. http://internet.about.com, August 1, 1999. Accessed June 23, 2000.

2. Nielson/Netratings Home Page. www.nielsennetratings.com. Accessed October 5, 2000.

3. Lake D: Forecasts for the year 2000: From Internet business to online gaming, researchers predict a big year for the Net in 2000. http://internet.about.com/industry/internet, January 17, 2000. Accessed June 23, 2000.

4. Thompson MJ: Web spotlight: The hot sites of 1999. http://internet.about.com/industry/internet, December 20, 1999. Accessed June 23, 2000.

5. Trinkle R: Pharmacy continuing education available on the Internet. Pharmacotherapy 19:909–921, 1999.

6. American Society of Health System Pharmacists Home Page. www.ashp.org/public/pubs/ajhp/vol56/num01/procforsub.html. Accessed October 5, 2000.

7. Kassirer JP, Angell M: The Internet and the *Journal.* N Engl J Med 332:1709–1710, 1995.

8. Kim P, Eng TR, Deering MJ, Maxfield A: Published criteria for evaluating health related web sites (review). BMJ 318:647–649, 1999.

9. Hatfield CL, May SK, Markoff JS: Quality of consumer drug information provided by four web sites. ASHP 56:2308, 1999.

10. Lancet electronic research archive in international health and eprint server. Lancet 354:2–3, 1999.

11. Albee B, Dingley B: U.S. periodical prices—2000. www.ala.org/alonline. Accessed June 23, 2000.

12. Principles for emerging systems of scholarly publishing. www.arl.org/scomm/tempe.html. Accessed June 23, 2000.

13. Delamothe T, Smith R: Moving beyond journals: The future arrives with a crash. BMJ 318:1637–1639, 1999.

14. Delamothe, T: The paper mindset. Lancet 351 (suppl I):5–6, 1998.

15. The Blue Sheet. September 1, 1999, p. 10.

16. Relman AS: The NIH 'E-biomed' proposal—A potential threat to the evaluation and orderly dissemination of new clinical studies. N Engl J Med 340 (23), 1999.

17. Marshall E: Publish and perish in the internet world, Science 289:223–225, 2000.

18. Furberg C, Pitt B: Current controlled trials in cardiovascular medicine: A new journal for a new age. http://cvm.controlled-trials.com. Curr Control Trials Cardiovasc Med 1:1–2, 2000.

Answer Key

Chapter 1

1. The paper describes the results of a research study, so it would be appropriately characterized as a primary literature source.

2. This paper is a review paper compiled from primary sources, so it would be appropriately characterized as a tertiary reference.

3. This is a report of three case reports, which would characterize this reference as a primary literature source.

4. Embase is an abstracting service that provides access to international journals, so it is best characterized as a secondary reference.

5. Advantages of obtaining information from the Internet include readily accessible information and ease of use. Disadvantages include the lack of formalized review of material posted, resulting in potential misinformation. Users of Internet information need to be more critical of interpreting information that has been found.

Chapter 2

1. Medline would be the most appropriate database to use. The two NLM services that can be used to access Medline at no cost are the IGM and PubMed.

2. This search was performed on October 19, 2000, and there were 288 references on *St. John's wort* and 317 for *hypericum*. Using the MeSH browser indicates that *hypericum* is an indexed term and *St. John's wort* is a free-text term. A more comprehensive search is conducted using indexed terms, which is why more references were found using *hypericum* as opposed to *St. John's wort*.

3. The search terms used can be *hypericum* (or *St. John's wort*, although *hypericum* will screen more references), *drug interactions*, and *lancet*. Individually, the following shows the number of references for each term used alone:

Hypericum:	317 references
Drug interactions:	83,969 references
Lancet (limited by journal name):	87,407 references

The search can be constructed as follows:

Hypericum AND Drug Interactions AND Lancet

This should identify those articles that relate to hypericum and drug interactions that are published in the *Lancet*. Seven articles were found. The printout of the search performed on October 19, 2000, is shown in Fig. 2-9.

4. Note this search was performed on October 19, 2000.

    a. Five references were cited under the name Fugh-Berman A.

    b. Twelve hits occurred for this article between January and October 2000.

    c. LC Tsen, S Segal, M Pothier, et al: Alternative medicine use in presurgical patients. Anesthesiology 93(1):148, July 2000.

    d. This is a tertiary reference that provides a good overview of important drug interactions with herbal products, including St. John's wort. It would be appropriate to answer this question using this as a reference source.

5. Searches can be limited by publication type such as clinical trial, editorial, letter, meta-analysis, practice guideline, randomized clinical trial, and review. Limiting the search by clinical trial, meta-analysis, or randomized clinical trial would ensure that a primary reference source would be obtained.

Chapter 3

1. *Bias against the null hypothesis* refers to the observation that papers describing negative results (i.e., where the drug under study did not show an effect) are more likely to be rejected for publication. This tends to produce a body of literature that is skewed in favor of the statistically significant outcomes and can create difficulties if only published data is used for a subsequent review of the literature (e.g., meta-analysis).

2. The *impact factor* is dependent on the number of times papers published in a journal are cited in future papers. Although there are a number of limitations with the impact factor, it is based on the assumption that more important papers will be cited more frequently than less important research. The circulation of a journal may be influenced to some extent by the impact factor, in that there will likely be more subscribers to a journal that publishes a larger number of important papers. However, many biomedical journals serve as the official publication of an organization or society, and circulation will be primarily dependent on the number of members of the organization.

3. "Uniform Requirements for Manuscripts Submitted to Biomedical Journals" contains instructions to authors on how to prepare manuscripts that are accepted by over 500 journals. The document also provides guidelines regarding duplicate publication, authorship, style, content, and citations.

4. The demographic characteristics of the study population can only be described after the study has been completed and should be placed in the "Results" section

of the manuscript. This should not be confused with the inclusion and exclusion criteria for selection of patients, which should be in the "Methods."

Chapter 4

1. A cohort study has some characteristics in common with a clinical trial. Both involve a comparison between a group of patients receiving a drug and a control group. In addition, both designs follow the patients prospectively to determine the effect on a specified outcome measure. The primary difference between these types of studies is that the cohort study is observational; patients are placed in the study group because they have a clinical indication for the drug, not specifically because they are part of a study. The consequence of this is that there is no randomization in a cohort design making it critical that careful attention be paid to the selection and characteristics of the control group.

2. Retrospective studies tend to be less expensive to conduct and can usually be completed more quickly because new data does not have to be generated. This is particularly true if the drug effect of interest takes months or years to occur. The primary disadvantage of the retrospective study is that the investigator usually has no control over the quality of the data and important information may be missing or inaccurate.

3. Since relative risk was used to assess the outcome of interest, this must have been a cohort study. A cohort of subjects was identified in 1986 and consumption of coffee and other caffeinated beverages determined. They were then followed through 1996 for the development of symptomatic gallstones. Because the relative risk in coffee drinkers was less than 1, consumption of coffee showed a protective effect and appears to prevent gallstones in some patients.

4. Recall bias (also known as selective recall) is a problem that can confound the assessment of exposure to the drug of interest in a case-control study. Subjects who have experienced an adverse event (case group) may be more likely to remember or report use of a drug under investigation than those in the control group.

Chapter 5

1. No. Even if an adequate number of representative subjects are studied, the results will be meaningless if confounding factors are not accounted for. Internal validity can be thought of as a prerequisite for external validity. Studies that lack internal validity do not produce reliable conclusions regarding the effects of the test drug. There would be no value in extrapolating confounded results from the sample studied to the population at large.

2. Most papers describing clinical trials provide a table in which the variables known or likely to affect the outcome measures are compared between the treatment groups. These may include demographic characteristics as well as indicators

of the severity or duration of disease. If there are no statistically significant differences between groups, it is assumed that randomization has been successful. It is important to remember that randomization should also result in even distribution of unknown factors that have yet to be identified as having an influence on the effect of the drug.

3. The purpose of blinding is to lessen the effects of expectations on the outcome being studied. Therefore, blinding is most important for studies where the measure of drug effect is subjective, that is, dependent on human ratings or evaluations. Blinding the subjects is less critical in studies where the outcome is highly objective. However, in this case, it is considered good scientific practice to blind those individuals involved in the measurement (e.g., lab technicians) of the identity of the samples.

4. In an extreme example, suppose that 100 patients are treated with a new drug and that 70% respond well and complete the study. The other 30% drop out and cannot be examined at the time of the final assessment. If only patients completing the study are analyzed, the response rate will be 100%. Using an intention-to-treat analysis, the response rate is only 70%. Certainly patients who are responding to an active treatment are less likely to drop out of a study than those who are not responding. However, the true response rate is likely greater than 70% since some of the dropouts may have been responders who failed to complete the study for any number of other reasons (lack of motivation, adverse events, moved to another part of the country, etc.). By assuming that all of those who do not finish the study are nonresponders, the intention-to-treat analysis will tend to underestimate the treatment effect.

Chapter 6

1. The sensitivity of the test is $958/985 = 97.3\%$. The specificity of the test is $738/746 = 98.9\%$.

2. The estimated population of the United States in 2000 is 276,000,000. The incidence of breast cancer per million is $(182,000/276,000,000) \times 1,000,000$. The result is 659 new cases of breast cancer for each million citizens. It should be noted that this is not a particularly informative figure since breast cancer is a disease that primarily occurs in adult women. It would be more useful to estimate incidence using the population of adult women in the United States rather than total population.

3.

	EBT	Ratio of DM/3MM
Mean	2.21	28.07
Median	2.185	13
Standard deviation	0.63	32.58
Coefficient of variation (%)	28.5	116.1

For the EBT, the mean and median are similar, suggesting that the data is not highly skewed. Variability is reasonable with a coefficient of variation of 28.5%. The ratio of DM/3MM was clearly much more variable, with a coefficient of variation of 116.1%. The data is highly skewed, with a mean that is more than double the median. Inspection of the data indicates an extreme value (109) that is almost 10 times higher than the median. For the ratio of DM/3MM, the mean is not a good measure of central tendency.

Chapter 7

1. a. The z-score for an albumin concentration of 3.5 g/dL is 2.0. In other words, a concentration of 3.5 g/dL would be 2 standard deviations below the mean. According to App. A, 95.45% of observations lie within 2 standard deviations of the mean, 2.28% are more than 2 standard deviations above the mean, and 2.28% are more than 2 standard deviations below the mean. Therefore, the chance of obtaining an albumin concentration of 3.5 g/dL or less in an individual randomly selected from the population is 2.28%.

   b. No. With a sample of 20 subjects, the standard error of the mean is 0.11. The calculated value for t with a sample mean of 3.5 g/dL is 1.0/0.11 = 9.1. In other words, the mean in the hospitalized patients is approximately 9.1 standard errors of the mean below the population value. For a sample with 19 degrees of freedom, 95% of sample means in which subjects are randomly selected from the population should lie within ±2.093 (see App. B). Since the mean in the sample is far below this range, it must be concluded that these patients are not representative of the general population.

2. a. The appropriate t-value for a 95% confidence interval and 10 subjects ($v = 9$) is 2.26. The 95% confidence interval is equal to 22.0 ± 6.9, or from 15.1 to 28.9.

   b. Because it can be stated with 95% confidence that the mean peak simvastatin concentration with grapefruit juice is between 15.1 and 28.9 ng/mL, which is substantially above the mean of 9.3 ng/mL with water, it is highly likely that grapefruit juice increases peak concentrations of simvastatin.

3. Treatment with bupropion alone as well as the combination of bupropion and a nicotine patch result in a statistically significant improvement in the abstinence rate compared to both placebo and nicotine patch treatments. The nicotine patch was not significantly different from the placebo, and bupropion alone was not significantly different from the bupropion-nicotine patch treatment. A Type II error is possible whenever the null hypothesis is accepted (p-values > 0.05).

Chapter 8

1. A paired t-test is the most appropriate test because the data are parametric, follow a normal distribution, and are from a crossover design so that each subject serves as its own control.

2. The differences are as follows:

Subject Number	Difference
1	8.7
2	9.9
3	1.8
4	14
5	4.1
6	−5.3
7	0.7
8	2.6
9	9.8
10	4.3
11	14.8
12	8.4
13	3.2

There is consistency in that almost all of the subjects demonstrate an increase in urinary 6-β-hydroxycortisol/cortisol ratio. There is some variation in the amount of change, however, within each subject (−5.3 to 14.8). The magnitude of change is large—over an 80% increase in this ratio.

3.

	Increases the Chance of Statistical Significance	Decreases the Chance of Statistical Significance
Degree of change in consistency of change in urinary 6-β-hydroxycortisol/cortisol ratio D_m	A large change increases the chance	
Consistency of change in urinary 6-β-hydroxycortisol/cortisol ratio SEM_d	A consistent change since almost every subject increased	
Subject number		Small subject number

4. A p-value of 0.003 indicates that there is a 0.3% chance that the null hypothesis statement is true, or a 99.7% chance that it is false. Since this value is well under 5%, the null hypothesis would be rejected. This is an expected result since the degree of change D_m is large and there is a reasonable, consistent change among the subjects. So, even though the subject number is small, a statistically significant change would be expected.

5. St. John's wort did increase the 6-β-hydroxycortisol/cortisol ratio.

6. The data are parametric in nature and normally distributed; since there are two groups compared and they are independent from one another, an unpaired t-test should be used.

7. The CV for men is 36% and for women 31%, so the variances are very similar.

8. a. The mean values appear to be different, with the value in the women's group almost 80% higher than that in the men's.

b. The CV values are 36% for men and 31% for women, showing similar variances that are not that large.

c. The subject number is small, particularly in the women's group ($n = 5$).

9. There is less than a 5% chance that labetalol clearance is the same in women as in men, so the null hypothesis is rejected. This result is what would be expected, with caution because of the small number of subjects in the women's group.

10. The data is parametric and most likely normally distributed. However, note the CV of >100% for renal clearance in the carbon monoxide group. Subjects are being evaluated after three phases using a crossover design, so changes in nicotine disposition will be evaluated within each subject. A repeated measures ANOVA would be appropriate to use.

11. Variances are not similar. Note the following CVs:

Cigarette smoking	62%
Carbon monoxide	106%
Air	55%

12.

	Clearance	Renal Clearance
SS_{bet}	Mean values are modestly different (11–12%)	Mean values are substantially higher in CM and A group (45–47%)
SS_{wit}	CVs are low in each group (19–20%)	CVs are high in each group (55–106%)
Subject number	Subject number is small	Subject number is small

13. A Tukey posttest is a post hoc test that is used when an ANOVA is statistically significant.

14. Despite the fact that the mean values for renal clearance appear to be different, the subject number ($n = 12$) was too small to detect a difference given the high variances (CVs ranging from 55 to 106%). That is why this result was not significant. The mean values for clearance are modestly different; however, the variances are small. Even though the individual data is not shown, it can be assumed that there

was a consistent change between groups such that a statistical difference was reached with an n of 12.

15. A multifactorial ANOVA allows for simultaneous analysis of more than one independent variable on a dependent variable, such as gender and age on drug clearance.

Chapter 9

1. The data presented is nominal in nature, and the two groups compared are independent from one another, so a chi-square test would be appropriate to use.

2. Differences in adverse events: the imipramine group had a substantially higher rate of side effects ranging from twofold higher for headache (6 vs. 2) to twelvefold higher for nausea (12 vs. 1).

3. Number of observations: a total of 314 patients were studied, so that there is a reasonable number of subjects overall. Some of the adverse events reported for St. John's wort were low, so this study may not be able to determine the incidence of these events, but it can determine if the incidence is different from imipramine.

4. By looking in the chi-square table in App. C, it should be seen that the χ^2 value of 51.12 is greater than the last value in the table (20.52) when v is equal to 5 [no. rows − 1 (5) ∗ no. columns − 1 (1)]. The p-value is therefore <0.001, so there is less than a 0.1% chance that the null hypothesis statement is true or a greater than 99.9% chance that it is false. It is concluded that there is a difference in adverse events comparing hypericum to imipramine.

5. The data can be formatted into a 2 × 2 table as shown:

	Patients with an Adverse Event	Patients Without an Adverse Event
Hypericum, $n = 157$	62	95
Imipramine, $n = 157$	105	52

There is 1 v, so that it would be appropriate to use the chi-square with the Yates correction factor.

6. The p-value from the χ^2 table in App. C for 1 v is <0.001 (χ^2 of 22.56 is greater than the value of 10.83 in the table). The null hypothesis would be rejected. In this case, since such a large difference was seen, it would not be expected that the Yates correction factor would make a difference. The χ^2 value calculated without the Yates correction factor is 23.65.

7. The number of observations in the hypericum group is small (3 or 4%), so it would be appropriate to use the Fisher's exact test to compare these results.

8. The data presented in this table is from a prospective randomized controlled study, the data is nominal in format, and each data set can be formatted into a 2 × 2 table, so it would be appropriate to use the risk ratio to analyze this data.

9. Using Eq. (8-4), the risk ratio is calculated to be 3.71 and 3.76.

10. The 95% CI is wider in the ulcers within 30 days group. The range in this group is 9.99 (11.3 − 1.31) as compared to 6.6 (8.28 − 1.68). The reason for this is the difference in subject numbers between these two comparisons ($n = 118$ for ulcers with 30 days group; $56 + 62 = 118$) and 240 in the recurrent bleeding by day 7 group ($120 + 120 = 240$). Note that the range or width of the 95% CI is indirectly proportional to subject number.

11. The data is ordinal in nature and the study design is randomized parallel, so a Mann-Whitney U test could be used to analyze these results.

Chapter 10

1. a. The dependent variable is SBP in Fig. 10-15a and DBP in Fig. 10-15b. These are the dependent variables because blood pressure could be affected or influenced by concentrations of tamsulosin. That is, SBP and DBP could be dependent on tamsulosin concentration.

> b. The independent variable is tamsulosin concentration. This is because factors that influence tamsulosin concentration, such as hepatic and renal function, are completely independent from SBP and DBP.

> c. These are examples of negative correlations since the changes in blood pressure (SBP or DBP) appear to move in an inverse manner to tamsulosin concentration. The r-values in both graphs are below 0.5, so this is an example of a weak correlation.

> d. The r^2-values are for SBP 0.18 $[(-0.42^2)]$ and for DBP 0.13 $[(-0.36^2)]$, so 18% of the variability in change in SBP is related to tamsulosin concentration and 13% of the variability in the change in DBP is related to tamsulosin concentration.

2. a. The statistical conclusion is that the null hypothesis in both cases is accepted—there is no correlation between the change in blood pressure (SBP and DBP) and plasma concentration of tamsulosin.

> b. The factors that influence the statistical result of a correlation analysis are the number of observations and the r-value.

> c. Even though the numbers are not large, there appears to be a reasonable number of data points ($n = 18$) and the correlation has been evaluated as weak, so while both of these parameters affect the statistical result, the low r-values would have the primary influence in the statistical result.

3. This statement is technically accurate; however, it gives the impression that there is a negative correlation between change in blood pressure and tamsulosin concentration. The authors want the reader to believe a relationship exists. Given the low r- and r^2-values and the fact that the relationship is not statistically significant, a conclusion should be reached that there is no correlation between these variables. This is not how the data is presented by the authors.

4. a. The dependent variables are the response measurements (ACT and aPTT), which are influenced or dependent on the concentration of argatroban. The independent variable is argatroban concentration, because it is not influenced or dependent on ACT or aPTT. It is influenced by factors that influence drug clearance, such as renal and hepatic function.

b. This is an example of a linear regression analysis.

c. The correlation coefficient (r-value) for ACT is 0.85 and for aPTT 0.87, so this is a very good correlation that may be predictive.

d. Response can be predicted with some degree of reliability. Certainly, response is lower at an argatroban concentration of 200 ng/mL, as compared to 600 or 1000 ng/mL. However, at a given concentration there still is a very wide range in response (twofold or higher at any given concentration). At an argatroban concentration of 600 ng/mL, aPTT could range from 30 to 70 s or ACT from 90 to 220 s. This may limit the degree to which this regression analysis can be applied in predicting response of patients to argatroban concentration.

5. a. A Spearman rank correlation is a nonparametric correlation analysis. Since the data presented is parametric, the data was not normally distributed in the opinion of the authors, so a nonparametric analysis was used.

b. This graph shows two very distinct outliers in the upper right section. Visually removing these will alter the correlation such that almost no correlation is apparent. When results can be altered by removing one or two data points, interpretation of the results must be done with caution.

6. a. A survival analysis should be used to compare the outcome (remission rate) in patients with Crohn's disease who receive methotrexate as compared to those who receive placebo.

b. Similar numbers of patients started the study (methotrexate, $n = 40$; placebo, $n = 36$); however at 40 weeks the numbers were different, with 19 methotrexate patients evaluated at 40 weeks (47% of those that started the study) as compared to 12 placebo patients (36% of those that started). In this case, the difference is due to the effect of methotrexate on increasing the remission rate, as opposed to other reasons for a difference in numbers, such as dropout rates because of adverse effects.

Chapter 11

1.

Feature	Narrative Review	Systematic Review
Clinical question	Broad in scope	Focused clinical question
Search strategy/ source(s) for literature	Rarely specified, potentially biased	Comprehensive sources/ explicit search strategy

Feature	Narrative Review	Systematic Review
Selection of studies	Rarely specified, potentially biased	A priori inclusion criteria rigorously applied
Appraisal of studies	Variable	Rigorous critical appraisal
Synthesis of studies	Usually a qualitative summary	Quantitative synthesis (meta-analysis includes statistical synthesis)
Confidence in using results for patient care	Sometimes evidence-based	Usually evidence-based

2. Does warfarin improve outcomes in elderly patients with chronic atrial fibrillation compared with no treatment. Need to consider the following:

a. Type of exposure (e.g., could also include unfractionated heparin, low-molecular-weight heparin, ASA)

b. Type of outcome (e.g., stroke, myocardial infraction, death)

c. Type of person (e.g., age, acute versus chronic atrial fibrillation)

d. Type of control (e.g., placebo, another therapy)

e. Type of study (e.g., randomized controlled trials only?)

3. The fail-safe N method is a tool to detect the impact of publication bias, should it be present, on the overall results of the meta-analysis. Assuming that studies not showing significant results are unpublished or not identified, it calculates the number of additional studies that would need to be added to the meta-analysis to alter its results. It is highly unlikely that 26 studies have been performed and not published that, on average, showed no difference between β-adrenergic blockers and placebo.

4. CDD does not have a significant effect on the CD4 + T cell count in asymptomatic HIV patients, but it has a dramatic effect on CD4 + T cell counts in patients with AIDS. Note that the 95% CI crosses 1 for the asymptomatic HIV meta-analysis and, therefore, is not statistically significant.

Chapter 12

1. Statement c is false. Cost-effectiveness analyses measure costs in monetary terms and outcomes using a clinical measure.

2. Answer b. Cost of lost patient productivity would not normally be considered from a managed care perspective, as this cost does not impact the managed care organization.

3. Answer b. The expected value of Antibiotic A is $122. It is calculated as follows: $(0.8 \times 0.9 \times \$100) + (0.8 \times 0.1 \times \$200) + (0.2 \times 0.8 \times \$150) + (0.2 \times 0.2 \times \$250)$

4. Statement b is false. Hotel costs are generally considered as variable costs, not fixed costs.

Chapter 13

1. a. Fosphenytoin is preferred.

   b. Approximately $80.

   c. No. The cost difference distribution favors phenytoin and does not include zero.

2. a. Conventional amphotericin B is preferred.

   b. The approximate total treatment cost of conventional amphotericin B is $43,000. The total treatment cost of conventional amphotericin B does not change as the cost of liposomal amphotericin B is varied.

3. a. False

   b. False

   c. True

   d. True

   e. True

Chapter 14

1. An institutional review board must have at least 5 members. The members must have enough expertise and diversity to provide a competent review of the submitted protocols. The committee should not be composed entirely of individuals from the same profession or gender. At least one of the members should be a nonscientist and there should be at least one member who is not employed by or otherwise affiliated with the institution (the same person could fulfill both of these criteria).

2. Yes. Protocols that lack scientific merit will ultimately provide no benefit to either the study participants or society in general. An assessment of scientific merit is required in order to accurately evaluate the risk/benefit ratio of a study.

3. All consent forms must include the purpose, a statement that the study involves research, duration of involvement, description of procedures, reasonably foreseeable risks, possible benefits to subjects or others, alternative treatments, procedures for maintaining confidentiality, availability of compensation for injury, contact person for information on the study as well as the rights of research subjects, and an assurance that participation is voluntary and may be discontinued without penalty at any time.

4. The authors of a paper reporting the results of a clinical study (primary literature) may have a vested interest in the outcome of the study (e.g., research conducted or sponsored by the pharmaceutical industry). However, the reader should be able to determine whether the results are valid on the basis of the description provided of the study design, patient population and methods of data analysis. In the case of tertiary literature (review articles, textbook chapters, etc.), the task of

selecting and evaluating the primary literature has already been completed by the author. Readers rely on the author to perform a complete and objective evaluation since the conclusions cannot be verified without direct access to the primary literature.

Chapter 15

1. This is a code of conduct established by the Health on the Net Foundation (HON) medical and health sites. A site must apply for the use of this seal of approval and adhere to principles outlined by HON.

2. Any one of the following:

- Web page design
- Disclosure statements
- Currency of information
- Authority of source
- Ease of use
- Accessibility and availability
- Links provided
- Documentation provided
- Feedback

3. The accessibility of these two journals is widely different. Access to the *American Journal of Cardiology* is restricted to paid subscribers, while the *British Medical Journal* is accessible to everyone.

4. Advantages of publishing on a prepublication server are that data that might not be applicable for print media (e.g., results from negative studies, results from clinical trials, experimental techniques) can be published and made accessible. A broader peer review process can occur through critique provided by a wide audience. The disadvantage is that the reliability of information that has not been peer reviewed in the traditional sense is less certain.

5. PubMed Central is an effort by the National Institutes of Health to create a Web site that would make all biomedical research accessible. Peer-reviewed papers from traditional journals would be posted as well as non-peer-reviewed work such as results from clinical trials or data sets from biomedical studies. As of October 2000, PubMed Central had focused on providing access to peer-reviewed research manuscripts from traditional journals. BioMed Central provides for rapid, efficient online publication of peer-reviewed research. Authors retain copyright for articles published. An experienced, well-respected editorial board runs BioMed Central.

Appendix A

z-Score for a Normal Distribution

z	Percent of Normal Curve Whose Distance from the Mean Is:			
	Within z SD	>z SD	<z SD	Outside z SD
0.00	0.00%	50.00%	50.00%	100.00%
0.10	7.97	46.02	46.02	92.03
0.20	15.88	42.97	42.07	84.15
0.30	23.58	38.21	38.21	76.42
0.40	31.08	34.46	34.46	68.92
0.50	38.29	30.85	30.85	61.71
0.60	45.15	27.43	27.43	54.85
0.70	51.61	24.20	24.20	48.39
0.80	57.63	21.19	21.19	42.37
0.90	63.19	18.41	18.41	36.81
1.00	68.27	15.87	15.87	31.73
1.10	72.87	13.57	13.57	27.13
1.20	76.99	11.51	11.51	23.01
1.30	80.64	9.68	9.68	19.36
1.40	83.85	8.08	8.08	16.15
1.50	86.64	6.68	6.68	13.36
1.60	89.04	5.48	5.48	10.96
1.70	91.09	4.46	4.46	8.91
1.80	92.81	3.59	3.59	7.19
1.90	94.26	2.87	2.87	5.74
2.00	95.45	2.28	2.28	4.55

Continued

Percent of Normal Curve Whose Distance from the Mean Is:

z	Within z SD	>z SD	<z SD	Outside z SD
2.10%	96.43%	1.79%	1.79%	3.57%
2.20	97.22	1.39	1.39	2.88
2.30	97.86	1.07	1.07	2.14
2.40	98.36	0.82	0.82	1.64
2.50	98.76	0.62	0.62	1.24
2.60	99.07	0.47	0.47	0.93
2.70	99.31	0.35	0.35	0.69
2.80	99.49	0.26	0.26	0.51
2.90	99.63	0.19	0.19	0.37
3.00	**99.73**	**0.13**	**0.13**	**0.27**
3.10	99.81	0.10	0.10	0.19
3.20	99.86	0.07	0.07	0.14
3.30	99.90	0.05	0.05	0.10
3.40	99.93	0.03	0.03	0.07
3.50	99.95	0.02	0.02	0.05

The *t* Distribution

2 p	0.5	0.4	0.2	0.1	0.05	0.01
p	0.25	0.2	0.1	0.05	0.025	0.005
ν						
1	1.00	1.38	3.08	6.31	12.71	63.66
2	0.72	1.06	1.89	2.92	4.30	9.92
3	0.76	0.98	1.64	2.35	3.18	5.84
4	0.74	0.94	1.53	2.13	2.78	4.60
5	0.73	0.92	1.48	2.02	2.57	4.03
6	0.71	0.91	1.44	1.94	2.45	3.71
7	0.71	0.90	1.42	1.89	2.36	3.50
8	0.70	0.89	1.40	1.86	2.31	3.36
9	0.70	0.88	1.38	1.83	2.26	3.25
10	0.70	0.88	1.37	1.81	2.23	3.17
11	0.70	0.88	1.36	1.80	2.20	3.11
12	0.70	0.87	1.36	1.78	2.18	3.05
13	0.70	0.87	1.35	1.77	2.16	3.01
14	0.69	0.87	1.35	1.76	2.14	2.98
15	0.69	0.87	1.34	1.75	2.13	2.95
16	0.69	0.86	1.34	1.75	2.12	2.92
17	0.69	0.86	1.33	1.74	2.11	2.90
18	0.69	0.86	1.33	1.73	2.10	2.88
19	0.69	0.86	1.33	1.73	2.09	2.86
20	0.69	0.86	1.33	1.72	2.09	2.85

Continued

30	0.68	0.85	1.31	1.70	2.04	2.75
40	0.68	0.85	1.30	1.68	2.02	2.70
50	0.68	0.85	1.30	1.68	2.01	2.68
100	0.68	0.84	1.29	1.66	1.98	2.62
∞	0.68	0.84	1.28	1.65	1.96	2.58

The χ^2 Distribution

p	0.25	0.2	0.1	0.05	0.025	0.001
ν						
1	0.45	0.71	1.07	3.84	5.02	10.83
2	1.386	1.83	2.41	5.99	7.38	13.82
3	2.366	2.95	3.67	7.82	9.35	16.27
4	3.357	4.04	4.88	9.49	11.14	18.47
5	4.351	5.13	6.06	11.07	12.83	20.52
10	9.342	10.47	11.78	18.31	20.48	29.59
20	19.34	20.95	22.78	31.41	34.17	45.32
40	39.34	31.32	33.53	55.76	59.32	66.77
50	49.34	51.89	54.72	67.51	71.42	79.49
100	99.34	102.95	106.91	124.34	129.56	140.17

F-Table for $p < 0.05$ (Lightface) and $p < 0.01$ (Boldface)

ν_n

ν_d	1	2	3	4	5	6	7	8	9	10	20	50	100
1	161	200	216	225	230	234	237	239	241	242	250	252	253
	4052	**4899**	**5403**	**5625**	**5764**	**5859**	**5928**	**5981**	**6022**	**6056**	**6208**	**6302**	**6334**
2	18.51	19.00	19.16	19.25	19.30	19.33	19.36	19.37	19.38	19.39	19.44	19.47	19.49
	98.49	**99.00**	**99.17**	**99.25**	**99.30**	**99.33**	**99.37**	**99.37**	**99.39**	**99.40**	**99.45**	**99.48**	**99.49**
3	10.13	9.55	9.28	9.12	9.01	8.94	8.88	8.84	8.81	8.78	8.64	8.58	8.56
	34.12	**30.82**	**29.46**	**28.71**	**28.24**	**27.91**	**27.67**	**27.48**	**27.34**	**27.13**	**26.60**	**26.35**	**26.23**
4	7.71	6.94	6.59	6.39	6.26	6.16	6.09	6.04	6.00	5.96	5.80	5.70	5.66
	21.20	**18.00**	**16.69**	**15.98**	**15.52**	**15.21**	**14.98**	**14.80**	**14.66**	**14.54**	**14.02**	**13.69**	**13.52**
5	6.61	5.79	5.41	5.19	5.05	4.95	4.86	4.82	4.78	4.74	4.56	4.44	4.40
	16.26	**13.27**	**12.06**	**11.39**	**10.97**	**10.67**	**10.45**	**10.29**	**10.15**	**10.05**	**9.55**	**9.24**	**9.13**
6	5.99	5.14	4.76	4.53	4.39	4.28	4.21	4.15	4.10	4.06	3.87	3.75	3.71
	13.74	**10.92**	**9.78**	**9.15**	**8.75**	**8.47**	**8.26**	**8.10**	**7.98**	**7.87**	**7.39**	**7.09**	**6.99**
7	5.59	4.74	4.35	4.12	3.97	3.87	3.79	3.73	3.68	3.63	3.44	3.32	3.28
	12.25	**8.55**	**8.45**	**7.86**	**7.46**	**7.19**	**7.00**	**6.84**	**6.71**	**6.62**	**6.15**	**5.85**	**5.75**

v_d													
8	5.32	4.46	4.07	3.84	3.89	3.58	3.50	3.44	3.39	3.34	3.15	3.03	2.98
	11.26	**8.65**	**7.59**	**7.01**	**6.63**	**6.37**	**6.19**	**6.03**	**5.91**	**5.82**	**5.36**	**5.06**	**4.96**
9	5.12	4.26	3.86	3.63	3.48	3.37	3.29	3.23	3.18	3.10	2.98	2.80	2.76
	10.56	**8.02**	**6.99**	**6.42**	**6.06**	**5.80**	**5.62**	**5.47**	**5.35**	**5.18**	**4.32**	**4.51**	**4.41**
10	4.96	4.10	3.71	3.48	3.33	3.22	3.14	3.07	3.02	2.97	2.77	2.64	2.59
	10.04	**7.96**	**6.55**	**5.99**	**5.64**	**5.39**	**5.21**	**5.06**	**4.95**	**4.85**	**4.41**	**4.12**	**4.01**
15	4.54	3.68	3.29	3.06	2.90	2.78	2.70	2.64	2.55	2.55	2.39	2.18	2.12
	8.68	**6.36**	**5.42**	**4.89**	**4.56**	**4.32**	**4.14**	**4.00**	**3.89**	**3.80**	**3.36**	**3.07**	**2.97**
20	4.35	3.49	3.10	2.87	2.71	2.60	2.52	2.45	2.40	2.35	2.12	1.96	1.90
	8.10	**5.85**	**4.34**	**4.43**	**4.10**	**3.87**	**3.71**	**3.56**	**3.45**	**3.37**	**2.94**	**2.56**	**2.53**
50	4.03	3.18	2.79	2.56	2.40	2.29	2.20	2.13	2.07	1.99	1.78	1.60	1.52
	7.17	**5.06**	**4.20**	**3.72**	**3.41**	**3.18**	**3.02**	**2.88**	**2.78**	**2.62**	**2.28**	**1.94**	**1.82**
100	3.94	3.08	2.70	2.48	2.30	2.19	2.10	2.02	1.97	1.92	1.68	1.48	1.39
	6.90	**4.82**	**3.98**	**3.51**	**3.20**	**2.99**	**2.82**	**2.69**	**2.59**	**2.51**	**2.06**	**1.73**	**1.59**

NOTE: v_n = degrees of freedom for the numerator; v_d = degrees of freedom for the denominator. When v_n and v_d = infinity, $F = 1.0$

Health Care–Related Web Sites

E-Servers

BioMed Central	www.biomedcentral.com
NetPrints	www.clinmed.netprints.org
PubMed Central	www.pubmedcentral.nih.gov

Health Care Organizations

Alzheimer's Association	www.alz.org
American Cancer Society	www.cancer.org
American Diabetes Association	www.diabetes.org
American Foundation for AIDS Research	www.amfar.org
American Heart Association	www.americanheart.org
American Liver Foundation	www.liverfoundation.org
American Lung Association	www.lungusa.org
Arthritis Foundation	www.arthritis.org
Cystic Fibrosis Foundation	www.cff.org
Epilepsy Foundation	www.efa.org
Fertility Foundation	www.fertilityfoundation.org
Hepatitis B Foundation	www.hepb.org
Muscular Dystrophy	www.mdausa.org
National Cancer Institute	www.nci.nih.gov
National Center for Complementary and Alternative Medicine	www.nccam.nih.gov
National Foundation for Depressive Illness	www.depression.org
National Headache Foundation	www.headaches.org
National Heart Lung and Blood Institute	www.nhlbi.nih.gov
National Institute on Aging	www.nih.gov/nia
National Institute on Allergy and Infectious Diseases	www.niaid.nih.gov

National Institute of Arthritis and Musculoskeletal and Skin Diseases	www.nih.gov/niams
National Institute of Diabetes and Digestive and Kidney Diseases	www.niddk.nih.gov
National Institute on Drug Abuse	www.nida.nih.gov
National Institute of Mental Health	www.nimh.nih.gov
National Institute of Neurological Disorders and Stroke	www.ninds.nih.gov
National Kidney Foundation	www.kidney.org
National Parkinson Foundation	www.parkinson.org
National Stroke Foundation	www.stroke.org
National Women's Health Information Center	www.4woman.org
Multiple Sclerosis Foundation	www.msfacts.org

General Health and Drug Information

Dr. Koop.com	www.dr.koop.com
Rxlist	www.rxlist.com
Mosby's GenRx	www.mosby.com/mosby/PhyGenRx
HealthWeb	www.healthweb.com

National Organizations

Food and Drug Administration	www.fda.gov
National Agricultural Library	www.nalusda.gov
National Cancer Institute	www.nci.nih.gov
National Library of Medicine	www.nlm.nih.gov
Center for Disease Control	www.cdc.gov
National Institutes of Health	www.nih.gov

Other

Cochrane Collaboration	www.hiru.mcmaster.ca/cochrane
MedCertain	www.medcertain.org
Achoo—Internet Health Directory	www.achoo.com

Pharmaceutical Companies

Listing of companies	www.pharminfo.com/phrmlink.html#drugs_RandD
Abbott	www.abbott.com
Astra Zeneca	www.astrazeneca.com
Aventis	www.aventis.com
Bristol Myers Squibb	www.bms.com
Eli Lilly	www.lilly.com
Glaxo-Wellcome	www.glaxowellcome.co.uk
Merck	www.merck.com

Novartis	www.novartis.com
Pfizer	www.pfizer.com
Pharmacia	www.pnu.com
SmithKline Beecham	www.sb.com

Professional Organizations

American Society of Health-System Pharmacists	www.ashp.org
American Pharmaceutical Association	www.aphanet.org
American College of Clinical Pharmacy	www.accp.com
American Association of Colleges of Pharmacy	www.aacp.org
American Heart Association	www.amhrt.org
American Diabetes Association	www.diabetes.org
American Cancer Society	www.cancer.org
American Council on Pharmaceutical Education	www.acpe-accredit.org

Searchable Databases

Gateway to All NLM databases	www.gateway.nlm.nih.gov
PubMed	www.nlm.nih.gov/PubMed/
Current Contents	www.isinet.com/
Science Citation Index	www.isinet.com/
Biosis	www.biosis.org
Cancerlit	www.cancernet.nci.gov
Center Watch	www.centerwatch.com
Internet Grateful Med	www.igm.nlm.nih.gov
Medscape	www.medscape.com
Toxnet	www.toxnet.nlm.nih.gov
Web of Science	www.webofscience.com

Journals

American Journal of Health-System Pharmacy	www.ajhp.org/public/pubs/ajhp
Annals of Internal Medicine	www.acponline.org/journals/annals/annaltoc.htm
The Lancet	www.thelancet.com/newlancet
New England Journal of Medicine	www.nejm.com
Archives of Internal Medicine	www.ama-ssn.org/public/journals/inte/intehome.htm
Journal of the American Medical Association	www.ama-assn.org/public/journals/jama/jamahome.htm
British Medical Journal	www.bmj.com

Glossary

abstract   A short (1550 to 2000 word) summary of a paper.

analysis of variance (ANOVA)   A statistical test that compares parametric data obtained from three or more groups.

bias   An effect that causes results to deviate in a systematic manner from their actual value.

boolean   A combinatorial system devised by George Boole that combines propositions with the logical operators AND, OR, IF, THEN, EXCEPT, and NOT; commonly used in creating drug literature searches.

case-control study   A retrospective study in which subjects are identified because they have experienced an adverse effect or have a disease being studied (the case group). Patients are compared to a defined control group.

case report   Report of interesting observations from a single patient or a small number of patients.

censored data   A description in survival analysis for patients or data that have been included at the start but not at the end of the analysis.

chi-square   A nonparametric statistical test that compares nominal data.

citation   A reference source such as a published article that has been quoted.

Cochrane Collaboration   An Internet-based worldwide initiative to prepare, maintain, and disseminate systemic reviews of the effects of health care.

coefficient of determination (r^2-value)   A statistical parameter used in correlation analysis that determines how much variance in the dependent variable is explained by the independent variable.

cohort study   Typically, a prospective study that follows patients who are exposed to a given drug or treatment.

correlation   A statistical test that determines whether two variables are related to one another.

correlation coefficient (r-value)   The statistical parameter that indicates the degree to which two variables are related to one another.

crossover design   An experimental design where the subjects serve as their own control (i.e., each subject receives two or more treatments).

cross-sectional study   A study that provides insight into the state of affairs at the time the study was performed.

database   An organized collection of information, such as references, that are arranged for ease and speed of search and retrieval.

dependent variable   A variable that is reliant or dependent on another variable (e.g., renal drug clearance is dependent on creatinine clearance).

descriptive study   Study that collects data that may suggest associations that lead to the formation of a hypothesis.

editorial board   A group of well-respected individuals in a given clinical or scientific field who advise the editor of a specific journal.

evidence-based medicine   Incorporating timely, pertinent evidence from the primary medical literature when caring for patients.

experimental study   Study that involves the formulation of a hypothesis and testing of that hypothesis through a specific study design.

Fisher's exact test   A nonparametric test that compares nominal data formatted into a 2×2 table when the number of observations is small.

free-text term   A word or term that is used for searching a database for information but is not indexed by the database. Also called *keyword*.

heterogeneity   Refers to methodological differences between studies (e.g., patients, drug exposure or treatment, outcome, etc.) that may compromise the ability to combine results in a meta-analysis.

hypothesis testing   A research test or study that is designed to determine the probability that a specific research question is true or false.

impact factor   The average number of times recent articles (previous 2 years) in a journal have been cited in a given year.

independent variable   A variable that is not dependent or reliant on another variable.

indexed term   A term or word that has been indexed by a database.

Internet   A global network connecting millions of computers.

interventional study   A prospective study in which the subject receives an intervention, such as a drug.

Kruskal-Wallis test   A nonparametric test that compares ordinal data obtained from three or more experimental groups.

Mann-Whitney U test   A nonparametric statistical test that compares ordinal data obtained from two independent groups in a parallel-design study.

McNemar's chi-square test   A nonparametric statistical test that compares nominal data obtained from the same subject in a crossover-design study.

Medline   The world's foremost database for searching biomedical literature.

meta-analysis   A quantitative synthesis, using statistical techniques, of two or more studies of the same outcome.

multifactorial ANOVA   An ANOVA procedure that allows for the simultaneous testing of several independent factors on one dependent variable.

nonparametric   Tests performed on data that are categorical in nature, such as nominal or ordinal data.

null hypothesis   A statement that says there is no difference in the measured outcome among all of the groups tested.

observational study   Study in which the investigator is a passive observer and recorder of data.

online   Turned on and connected. Users are considered to be online when they are connected to a computer service through a modem.

paired *t*-test   A statistical test that compares parametric data obtained from the same subject in a crossover design comparing two treatments.

parallel design   A study design in which the effects of a drug or treatment are compared in two or more separate groups during the same period of time.

parametric   Describes data that follows a pattern of normal distribution and can be expressed as a mean and standard deviation.

Pearson product-moment correlation   A correlation analysis performed on parametric data.

peer review   Prepublication critique of a manuscript by experts in the field.

pharmacoeconomic study   Study that evaluates the cost impact of drug therapy.

primary literature   The published results of research studies.

prospective study   A study in which all elements of the design are established prior to the generation and collection of data.

PubMed   An electronic service provided by the National Library of Medicine which allows users to search Medline with a Web browser.

randomization   A method in which subjects are assigned by chance to different experimental groups or treatments.

reference   A note in a publication that refers back to another published work.

regression analysis   A statistical test that correlates data to a specific equation, such as that for a straight line.

repeated measures ANOVA   A statistical test that compares parametric data obtained in the same subject from a crossover-design study using three or more treatments.

research study   Study that involves answering a question or hypothesis through specific study methodology.

retrospective study   Study that examines past events and previously collected data.

secondary literature   Literature sources that are used to find primary and tertiary sources of information.

Spearman rank correlation   A correlation analysis performed on nonparametric data.

survival analysis   A statistical analysis that evaluates how an outcome variable, such as survival, changes over time.

tertiary literature   Literature compiled from primary literature references.

unpaired *t*-test   A statistical test on parametric data obtained from a parallel-design study in two independent groups of subjects.

World Wide Web   A system of Internet servers that supports specially formatted documents.

INDEX

A

Abbott, Web address, 13, 355
Absolute risk reduction (ARR), 242
Abstracts, 53–54, 357
Accuracy, 56–57, 108
Accuracy, brevity, and clarity (ABCs), 56–58
Achoo—Internet Health Directory, 355
Active placebo, 98
Adverse drug reactions (ADRs), 7, 10–11
Adverse events (AEs), 88, 255
AHFS Drug Information, 3, 18
AIDSline database, 21, 23
American Association of Colleges of Pharmacy, 8, 13, 356
American Cancer Society, 13, 356
American Chemical Society, 326
American College of Clinical Pharmacy, 8, 13, 356
American Council on Pharmaceutical Education, 356
American Diabetes Association, 13, 316, 317, 356
American Heart Association, 13, 356
American Heart Journal, 7
American Journal of Cardiology, 323
American Journal of Health-System Pharmacy (AJHP):
  guidelines for referencing Internet sources, 317
  impact factor, 49
  online version, 322
  peer-reviewed articles, 8, 46
  Web address, 356
American Journal of Pharmaceutical Education, 8

American Pharmaceutical Association, 8, 13, 356
American Pharmacy, 8
American Review of Respiratory Diseases, 7
American Society of Consultant Pharmacists, 8
American Society of Health-System Pharmacists, 3, 8, 12, 13, 356
Analysis of extremes, 279, 280
Analysis of variance (ANOVA), 155, 164–174, 357
Analytical research design, 65
Annals of Emergency Medicine, 43–44
Annals of Internal Medicine:
  impact factor, 49
  peer review process, 43, 46–47
  primary drug literature, 7
  rejected papers, 47
  searching through OVID, 24
  structure of papers, 53
  Web address, 13, 356
Annals of Pharmacotherapy, 8, 49
Annual Review of Pharmacology and Toxicology, 50
Archives of Internal Medicine, 7, 13, 356
Area under the curve (AUC), of drug clearance, serum concentration vs. time, 8
Astra Zeneca, Web address, 355
Attrition of research subjects, 79, 101–102
Authorship, 51–53, 237
Aventis, Web address, 355

B

Bell curve, 129
Belmont Report, 297, 299

Beneficence, in biomedical research, 298
Bias (*see* Publication bias)
BIDS Embase, 6
Bioequivalence, 135
Bioethicsline database, 21, 23
BioMed Central, 327–330, 354
Biomedical research:
  ethical issues in, 296–299
  the Internet and, 321–330
  scientific misconduct in, 304–307
Biosis, 6, 356
Blinding control groups, 96–98
Boolean operators, 28, 357
Bootstrap analysis, 281–282
Boston Collaborative Drug Surveillance
  Program, 74
Brevity, 56–57
Bristol Myers Squibb, Web address, 13,
  355
British Journal of Clinical Pharmacology,
  49
British Medical Journal (BMJ):
  conflict-of-interest guidelines, 309
  online version, 324
  searching through OVID, 24
  Web address, 13, 356
British Medical Society, 329

C
Cancer, 7
Cancerlit, 356
Case-control designs, 69, 357
Case-control studies, 73–76
Case reports, 6–7, 11–12, 71–73, 357
Censored data, 357
Center for Disease Control, Web address,
  13
Center Watch, 6, 356
Central limit theorem, 131–133
Central tendency, 118–122
Chemical Carcinogenesis Research
  Information System (CCRIS), 25
ChemID database, 21, 22
Chi-square analysis, 180–188, 357
Chi-square distribution, 351
Citation analysis, 49, 357
Citation databases, 26, 32–35
  (*See also* ISI)
Clarity, 57–58

Clinical outcomes in cost-effectiveness
  analyses, 255
Clinical Pharmacokinetics, 49
Clinical Pharmacology and Therapeutics, 7,
  48–50
Clinical questions, 233–234, 237
Clinical significance, 140
Clinical trials:
  attrition of subjects in, 79, 101–102
  effectiveness studies of, 254–255
  in primary drug literature, 7–9
  validity of, 85–87
  volunteer subjects in, 100
Cochrane Collaboration, 235, 355, 357
Code of ethics, 321
Coefficient of determination of r^2-value,
  207–208, 357
Coefficient of variation, 122–124
Cohort study designs, 68, 76–79, 357
Colleges of pharmacy, Web addresses, 13
Commercial vendors, 22–25
Compendia, examples of, 4, 18
Competing interests, 309
Confidence intervals, 133–138
Confidentiality, 303
Conflicts of interest, 308–310
Consultant Pharmacist, 8
Continuing education (CE) programs, 316
Continuous data, 114, 117–118
Convenience sampling, 99–100
Correlation analysis, 203–212, 357
Correlation coefficient (*see* r-value)
Cost-benefit analysis, 9, 251–253
Cost-effectiveness analysis, 9, 10, 251, 255
Cost-minimization analysis, 9–10, 251
Cost-utility analysis, 9, 10, 251
Critical variable, 274
Crossover design, 155, 157, 169, 358
Crossover studies, 93–95
Cross-sectional studies, 68–70, 358
Current Contents, 5, 6, 356

D
Data (*see* Measurement; Statistics;
    Validity)
  (*See also* Parametric tests)
Database, 358
Decision analysis:
  advantages of, 286–287

Decision analysis (*Cont.*):
  for pharmacoeconomics, 257–258
  uncertainty and, 270–271
  (*See also* Sensitivity analysis)
Decision threshold values, 273
Decision trees, 258–261
Declaration of Helsinki, 297, 299–301
Degrees of freedom, 124
Department of Health, Education, and
    Welfare, 297
Dependent variable, 212, 358
DerSimonian-and-Laird method, 239
Descriptive studies, 66–67, 358
Developmental and Reproductive
    Toxicology and Environmental
    Teratology Information Center
    (DART/ETIC), 25
Dirline database, 23
Discounting, 257
Discrete data, 114
Discussion section, 55–56
Distribution of data, 129–131
  (*See also* Confidence intervals;
    Hypothesis testing)
Distribution of sample means, 131–133
Double-blind studies, 97
Drug Facts and Comparisons, 18
Drug Information Full Text database, 27
Drug literature:
  ethical issues, 307–310
  general health and drug information, 355
  primary drug literature, 6–12, 359
  secondary drug literature, 5–6, 360
  systematic reviews, 231, 232, 246
  tertiary drug literature, 3–4, 360
  therapeutic reviews, 230–231
  (*See also* Evaluation process; Internet;
    Journals; Observational research
    designs; Pharmacoeconomics;
    Research studies; Search strategies;
    Validity)
Drug Metabolism and Disposition, 49
Drug Topics, 7

E
Editorial board, 358
Effect size, 242–243
Effectiveness studies, 254–255
Efficacy, 254–255

E-journals, 324–330
Electronic Research Archive (ERA), 330
Eli Lilly, Web address, 13, 355
Embase Drugs database, 27
Empirical distribution, 129
Environmental Protection Agency (EPA),
    25
E-publishing, 325
E-servers, 324–330, 354
Ethical issues, 307–310
Evaluation process criteria:
  authorship, 51–53
  considerations, 47–48
  reliability of information, 12, 14, 40–42,
    318–321
  selecting appropriate journals, 48–51
  structure of papers, 53–56
  style guidelines, 56–59
  (*See also* Validity)
Evidence-based medicine, 231–233, 358
  (*See also* Pharmacoeconomics)
Evidence-Based Medicine database, 27
Experimental research design, 65, 67,
    84–85, 358
  (*See also* Clinical trials; Validity)
Explanatory research design, 65
Exploratory research design, 66
External validity, 86, 99

F
F-table, 362–363
Facts and Comparisons, 4
Fail-safe *N* method, 235–236, 237
False negative results, 110
Fisher's exact test, 180, 185–186, 358
Fixed costs, 256
Fixed-effects model, for combining
    studies, 240
Follow-up studies, 76–79
Food and Drug Administration (FDA),
    11, 13, 299
Framingham Heart Study, 76
Free text, 27, 358
Funnel plots, 235–236, 237

G
Gateway to all Databases, 17, 356
Gaussian curve, 129
Glaxo-Wellcome, Web address, 13, 355

Global assessment measures, 111
Goodman & Gilman's Pharmacological Basis of Therapeutics, 18

H
Hawthorne effect, 96
Hazardous Substances Data Bank (HSDB), 22, 25
Health care costs, 250–251
Health care organizations, Web addresses, 354–355
Health on the Net Foundation (HON), 319
HealthStar database, 21, 23
Heterogeneity, 239, 240–241, 242, 243, 358
High Wire Press, 329
HSRProj database, 23
Hypothesis, 84–85
Hypothesis testing, 138–143
   (*See also* Statistics)

I
IGM (Internet Grateful Med):
   databases, 21, 23
   delivery of Medline, 20
   home page, 22
   Web address, 17, 356
Impact factor, 49, 50, 358
Incremental cost-effectiveness analysis, 242–253
Independent variable, 212, 358
Index Medicus, 5, 20
Indexed term, 358
   (*See also* Search strategies)
Informed consent, 302–304
Infoseek search engine, 12
Institutional review board (IRB), 295–296, 299–304
Instrumental analysis, 109
Intention-to-treat analysis, 101–102
Internal validity, 85–87
International Committee of Medical Journal Editors, 51, 53
International Congress on Biomedical Peer Review and Global Communication, 45–46
International Pharmaceutical Abstracts (*IPA*), 5, 27

International Pharmaceutical Abstracts database, 27
Internet:
   biomedical journals, 321–330
   definition, 358
   health-related sites, 314–315, 320
   role in growth of drug literature, 2–3
   search engines, 12
   as a source of drug information, 316–317
   (*See also* Online drug literature; Web)
Internet Healthcare Coalition (IHC), 321
Interobserver reproducibility, 109
Interval measurement, 112–113, 115–118
Interventional studies, 70, 358
Introduction section, 54–55
Iowa Drug Information Service database, 27
Iowa Drug Information System, 5
Institute for Scientific Information (ISI):
   accessing databases, 19, 25, 26
   citation databases, 26
   Journal of Citation Reports, 50
   search strategies, 32–35
   Web address, 17
Integrated Risk Information System (IRIS), 25
Internet service provider (ISP), 18

J
Journal of Allergy and Clinical Immunology, 7
Journal of Citation Reports, 50
Journal of Clinical Pharmacology, 7
Journal of Infectious Diseases, 7
Journal of Managed Care Pharmacy, 8
Journal of Pharmaceutical Sciences, 49
Journal of Pharmacology and Experimental Therapeutics, 49, 50
Journal of Pharmacy Teaching, 8
Journal of the American Medical Association (*JAMA*):
   impact factor, 49, 50
   peer review process, 46, 330
   primary drug literature, 7
   Web address, 13, 356
Journals:
   biomedical, 321–330
   electronic, 22–25
   Medline indexes, 19–20

Journals (*Cont.*):
  peer-reviewed articles, 6–7, 8, 42–47
  Web addresses, 13, 356
  (*See also* Evaluation process criteria;
      Meta-analyses; PubMed; Validity)
Justice, in biomedical research, 298–299

K
Kaplan-Meier method, 218
Keywords, 27–28
Kruskal-Wallis test, 180, 358

L
Lag time, 51
The Lancet:
  Contributors section, 52–53
  impact factor, 49
  online version, 323
  prepublication archives, 330
  Web address, 13, 356
Learning effect, 109
Life years saved (LYS), 255
Linear regression analysis, 204, 205, 213
Loansome Doc, 20

M
Mann-Whitney U test, 180, 358
Mantel-Haenszel test, 239
Markov models, 261
Matched controls, 93
McNemar's chi-square, 186, 358
Mean:
  central limit theorem, 131, 132
  confidence interval of, 135
  Greek symbol for, 128
  measuring central tendency, 118–122
  sample size and, 147–148
  standard error of (SEM), 131–132, 135,
      156
  z-distribution of, 131–132
Measurement:
  assessing outcome in rheumatoid
      arthritis, 113–114
  of central tendency, 118–122
  definition, 106
  degrees of freedom, 124
  discrete compared to continuous data,
      114
  effectiveness of consequences, 254–256

Measurement (*Cont.*):
  of interval data, 115–118
  of ordinal data, 114–115
  of ratio data, 115–118
  of relevant costs, 256–258
  scales for, 111–114
  subjective compared to objective
      measures, 106–107
  surrogate measures, 107–108
  validating, 108–111
  of variability, 122–124
  (*See also* Nonparametric tests;
      Parametric tests; Statistics; Validity)
MedCERTAIN, 319–320, 355
Median, measuring central tendency,
      118–122
Medical Journal of Australia, 47
Medical subject headings (MeSH), 20, 23,
      29–31, 235–236
Medline:
  definition, 359
  indexes of journals, 19–20
  locating meta-analyses, 230, 235–236
  preliminary search, 26, 27
  searching through IGM, 23
  searching through ISI, 25
  secondary drug literature, 5
Medscape, 6, 356
Merck, Web address, 13, 316, 355
Meta-analyses:
  applying results of, 243–246
  appraising validity of studies, 236–238
  combining studies, 239–242
  defining clinical questions, 233–234
  definition, 359
  identifying heterogeneity, 239
  identifying relevant studies, 235
  interpreting results, 242–243
  Medline searches for, 230
  role in evidence-based medicine,
      231–233
  selecting articles for inclusion, 234–235
Methods section, 55
Mode, measuring central tendency,
      118–122
Monte Carlo simulation, 281–282, 283, 284
Mosby's GenRx, Web site, 4
Multiple factorial ANOVA, 171–173, 359
Multiway sensitivity analysis, 275–279

N

National Agriculture Library, 19
National Cancer Institute, 19, 317
National Commission for the Protection of Human Subjects of Biomedical and Behavioral Research, 297
National Heart, Lung, and Blood Institute, 100
National Institutes of Health (NIH), 12, 13
National Library of Medicine (NLM), 13, 17, 18–22
National organizations, Web addresses, 13, 355
Nature, 44, 49
NetPrints, 329, 330, 354
New England Journal of Medicine:
  clinical studies, 8–9
  conflict-of-interest guidelines, 308–309
  impact factor, 49, 50
  letters to the editor, 40–41
  peer-reviewed articles, 7, 330
  searching through OVID, 24
  Web address, 13, 322–323, 356
Nominal measurement, 111–112, 114–115, 180
Nonexperimental research design, 66
Nonlinear regression analysis, 213, 216–217
Nonparametric data, 195
Nonparametric tests:
  chi-square analysis, 180–188
  definition, 359
  odds ratio (OR), 180, 191–193
  of ordinal data, 193–196
  risk ratio (RR), 180, 188–191
  (*See also* Parametric tests; Statistics)
Normal curve, 129
Normal distribution, 129–131, 347–348
Novartis, Web address, 13, 355
Null hypothesis, 138–142, 203, 359
  (*See also* Type I errors; Type II errors)
Number necessary to treat (NNT), 242
Nuremberg Code, 296

O

Objective measures, 106–107
Observational studies:
  case-control studies, 73–76
  case reports, 71–73
  chi-square analysis and, 186–188

Observational studies (*Cont.*):
  cohort (follow-up) studies, 76–79
  considerations, 70–71
  definition, 359
Obstetrics and Gynecology, 44
Odds ratio (OR), 74–75, 180, 191–193
Office for Protection from Research Risks (OPRR), 299–301
Oldmedline database, 20
One-tailed hypothesis testing, 141
One-way ANOVA, 164–166
One-way repeated measures ANOVA, 172
One-way sensitivity analysis, 273–275, 284–285
Online drug literature:
  accessing databases, 19
  definition, 359
  reliability, 12, 14, 40–42, 318–321
  resources, 13
  (*See also* Internet; Journals; Web)
Ordinal measurement, 112, 114–115, 180, 193–196
Organic Letters, 326
Outlying data points, in correlation analysis, 211
OVID Technologies, 17, 19, 22–25

P

p-values, 138–139, 362–363
Paired *t*-test, 155–160, 359
Parallel design, 359
Parametric data, 154–155
Parametric tests, 359:
  analysis of variance (ANOVA), 155, 164–174
  definition, 156
  paired *t*-test, 155–160
  unpaired *t*-test, 160–163
  (*See also* Nonparametric tests; Statistics)
Payoffs, 259
Pearson product-moment correlation, 208–209, 359
Peer-reviewed journals, 6–7, 8, 42–47, 359
Period effect, 94–95
Pfizer, Web address, 355
Pharmaceutical companies, 12, 13, 355–356
Pharmaceutical Information Network, 12
Pharmacia, Web address, 356

Pharmacists, evaluating drug literature, 2–3
Pharmacoeconomics:
  definition, 359
  historical perspective, 250–251
  literature, 9, 253–261, 262–266
  types of analyses, 251–253
  validity of conclusions, 261–266
Pharmacological Basis of Therapeutics, 3–4
Pharmacotherapy, 7, 8, 43, 48, 49
*Pharmacotherapy: A Pathophysiologic
  Approach*, 3
Physician's Desk Reference (PDR), 4, 18
Placebo control, 89
Post hoc tests, 166
Power of research studies, 142–150
Practice effect, 109
Precision, 108–109
Prepublication servers, 324–330
Principles of Pharmacoeconomics, 9
Probabilistic sensitivity analysis, 281–283
Probability sampling, 99
Probability theory, 139
  (*See also* Parametric tests)
Professional organizations, Web addresses,
  13, 356
Proportion, 136–138, 148–150
Prospective studies, 68, 359
Public Health Service Act, 299–301
Publication bias, 235–237, 357
PubMed:
  accessing databases, 29
  definition, 359
  delivery of PubMed, 20
  search strategies, 29–32
  Web address, 6, 17, 356
PubMed Central, 326–327, 328, 354

Q

Qualitative systematic reviews, 232
Quality-adjusted life year (QALY), 255,
  280
Quality of research studies, 236–237
Quantitative measures, 111
Quasi-experimental designs, 67

R

r-value, 207–208, 357
Random-effects model, for combining
  studies, 239–241

Randomization, 67, 89–93, 239–240, 359
Range, role in variability, 122–124
Ratio measurement, 112–113, 115–118
Recall bias, 76
Recursive decision trees, 258–259, 261
Red man syndrome, 101
Redundant publication, 305
References section, 56, 359
Regression analysis, 202, 212–217, 359
Relative risk, 76–78
Relative risk reduction (RRR), 242
Repeated measures ANOVA, 169–170, 359
Reproducibility, 108–109
Research studies:
  biomedical, 296–299
  classification of study design, 64–70
  complex, 52
  definition, 359
  effectiveness of consequences, 254–256
  power of, 143–150
  in primary drug literature, 6–7
  quality of, 236–237
  reliability of information, 40–42
  scientific misconduct, 304–307
  (*See also* Measurement; Meta-analyses;
    Statistics; Subjects; Validity)
Respect for persons, in biomedical
  research, 297
Results section, 55
Retrospective studies, 68, 360
Review articles, 4, 5
Rheumatoid arthritis, measurement scales
  to assess outcome, 113–114
Risk ratio (RR), 180, 188–191
Rolling back the trees, 260
Rosenthal effect, 96, 97

S

Sampling, 98–100, 145–150
Scenario analysis, 279–281
Scholarly Publishing and Academic
  Resource Coalition (SPARC), 326
Science, 49
Science Citation Index:
  impact factor, 50
  search strategies, 32–35
  searching through ISI, 25
  secondary drug literature, 5, 6
  Web address, 356

Scientific misconduct, 304–307
Search strategies:
  boolean operators, 28
  case examples, 29–35
  database considerations, 26–28
  meta-analyses and, 235–236
  tips, 35–36
Semifixed costs, 256
Sensitivity analysis:
  calculations, 284–287
  conducting, 283–284
  heterogeneity and, 243
  identifying bias, 237
  meta-analyses and, 241, 246
  probabilistic, 281–283
  specificity and, 109–111
  validating considerations, 271–273
  validation with scenario analysis,
    279–281
  validation test methods, 273–379
  variables and, 260
Signal-to-noise ratio, 109
Significance, in hypothesis testing,
    140–144
Simple decision trees, 258–259
Single-blind studies, 97
SmithKline Beecham, Web address, 13,
    356
Spearman rank correlation, 208–209,
    360
Specificity tests, 109–111
Standard deviation:
  Greek symbol for, 128
  role in variability, 122–124
  z-distribution, 130–131
  (*See also* Confidence intervals)
Standard error of the mean (SEM),
    131–132, 135, 156
Standard normal deviate, 131
Stanford University Libraries, 329
Statistics:
  appropriate usage, 41
  central limit theorem, 131–133
  confidence intervals, 133–138
  correlation analysis, 203–212
  normal distribution, 129–131
  regression analysis, 212–217
  survival analysis, 218–221

Statistics (*Cont.*):
  (*See also* Hypothesis testing;
    Measurement; Meta-analyses;
    Nonparametric tests; Parametric
    tests; Validity)
Subject attrition, 79
Subjective measures, 106–107
Subjects:
  attrition of, 101–102
  biomedical, 296–299
  informed consent by, 302–304
  t-distribution and, 135
  in the United States, 299–304
Surrogate measures, 107–108
Survival analysis, 218–221, 360
Systematic reviews, 231, 232, 246

T
t-distribution, 132–133, 349–350
Terminal nodes, 259
Text words, 27
Textbooks, examples of tertiary
    literature, 4
Therapeutic Drug Monitoring, 49
Therapeutic reviews, 230–231
Three-way sensitivity analysis, 275–279
Threshold analysis, 275
Time orientation of research, 67
Time series analysis, 218
Toxics Release Inventory (TRI), 25
Toxline database, 21, 23
Toxnet, 17, 21–22, 25, 26, 356
Traditional model, for combining studies,
    239, 241
True values, 217
t-tests, 155
Two-tailed hypothesis testing, 141
Two-way ANOVA, 172–173
Two-way sensitivity analysis, 275–279,
    285–286
Type I errors, 141–143
Type II errors, 143–144

U
Uniform Requirements for Manuscripts
    Submitted to Medical Journals, 48,
    51
Unpaired t-test, 160–163, 360

U.S. National Library of Medicine (*see* National Library of Medicine)
US Pharmacist, 7

V
Validity:
  enhancing with control groups, 87–93, 95–100
    blinding, 96–98
    historical controls, 95–96
    importance of, 87–89
    matched controls, 93
    randomly assigned, 89–93
    sampling, 98–100
  meta-analyses and, 236–238
  of pharmacoeconomic conclusions, 261–266
  types of, 85–87, 99
  (*See also* Measurement)
Variability, 122–124
Variable costs, 256
Variables, 106, 259–260

Variance, 122–124
Virtual Library of Pharmacy, 12

W
Washout period, 94
Web, 18–19, 354–356, 360
Web of Science, 25, 32–35, 356
Weighted average, 260
Wilcoxan rank sum test, 180, 193–194
World Wide Web (*see* Web)

X
x-axis, in correlation analysis, 203

Y
y-axis, in correlation analysis, 203
Yates correction factor, 184–185

Z
z-distribution, 130–131
Zero point, 113
z-score, 130, 131, 133, 347–348